American Public Health Association
VITAL AND HEALTH STATISTICS MONOGRAPHS

TUBERCULOSIS

Tuberculosis

I. Tuberculosis Morbidity and Mortality and Its Control

Anthony M. Lowell

II. Tuberculous Infection

Lydia B. Edwards and Carroll E. Palmer

1969 / HARVARD UNIVERSITY PRESS

Cambridge, Massachusetts

Contents

Tables / I

Tables/II

Appendix B

Appendix C

Figures / I

Figures / II

Foreword

Rapid advances in medical and allied sciences, changing patterns in medical care and public health programs, an increasingly health-conscious public, and the rising concern of voluntary agencies and government at all levels in meeting the health needs of the people necessitate constant evaluation of the country's health status. Such an evaluation, which is required not only for an appraisal of the current situation, but also to refine present goals and to gauge our progress toward them, depends largely upon a study of vital and health statistics records.

Opportunity to study mortality in depth emerges when a national census furnishes the requisite population data for the computation of death rates in demographic and geographic detail. Prior to the 1960 census of population there had been no comprehensive analysis of this kind. It seemed appropriate, therefore, to develop for intensive study a substantial body of death statistics for a three-year period centered around that census year.

A detailed examination of the country's health status must go beyond an examination of mortality statistics. Many conditions such as arthritis, rheumatism, and mental diseases are much more important as causes of morbidity than of mortality. Also, an examination of health status should not be based solely upon current findings, but should take into account trends and whatever pertinent evidence has been assembled through local surveys and from clinical experience.

The proposal for such an evaluation, to consist of a series of monographs, was made to the Statistics Section of the American Public Health Association in October 1958, and a Committee on Vital and Health Statistics Monographs was authorized. The members of this Committee and of the Editorial Advisory Subcommittee created later are:

Committee on Vital and Health Statistics Monographs

Mortimer Spiegelman, Chairman
Paul M. Densen, D. Sc.
Robert D. Grove, Ph.D.
Clyde V. Kiser, Ph.D.
Felix Moore
George Rosen, M.D., Ph.D.

William H. Stewart, M.D. (withdrew June 1964)
Conrad Taeuber, Ph.D.
Paul Webbink
Donald Young, Ph.D.

Editorial Advisory Subcommittee

The early history of this undertaking is described in a paper that was presented at the 1962 Annual Conference of the Milbank Memorial Fund.* The Committee on Vital and Health Statistics Monographs selected the topics to be included in the series and also suggested candidates for authorship. The frame of reference was extended by the Committee to include other topics in vital and health statistics than mortality and morbidity, namely fertility, marriage, and divorce. Conferences were held with authors to establish general guidelines for the preparation of the manuscripts.

Support for this undertaking in its preliminary stages was received from the Rockefeller Foundation, the Milbank Memorial Fund, and the Health Information Foundation. Major support for the required tabulations, for writing and editorial work, and for the related research of the monograph authors was provided by the United States Public Health Service (Research Grant CH 00075, formerly GM 08262). Acknowledgment should also be made to the Metropolitan Life Insurance Company for the facilities and time that were made available to Mr. Spiegelman, now retired from its service, who proposed and administered the undertaking and served as general editor. The National Center for Health Statistics, under the supervision of Dr. Grove and Miss Alice M. Hetzel, undertook the sizable tasks of planning and carrying out the extensive mortality tabulations for the period 1959–1961. Dr. Taeuber arranged for the cooperation of the Bureau of the Census at all stages of the project in many ways, principally by furnishing the required population data used in computing death rates and by undertaking a large number of varied special tabulations. As the sponsor of the project, the American Public Health Association furnished

* Mortimer Spiegelman, "The Organization of the Vital and Health Statistics Monograph Program," *Emerging Techniques in Population Research (Proceedings of the 1962 Annual Conference of the Milbank Memorial Fund;* New York: Milbank Memorial Fund, 1963), p. 230. See also Mortimer Spiegelman, "The Demographic Viewpoint in the Vital and Health Statistics Monographs Project of the American Public Health Association," *Demography,* Vol. 3, No. 2 (1966), p. 574.

assistance through Dr. Thomas R. Hood, its Deputy Executive Director.

Because of the great variety of topics selected for monograph treatment, authors were given an essentially free hand to develop their manuscripts as they desired. Accordingly, the authors of the individual monographs bear full responsibility for their manuscripts, and their opinions and statements do not necessarily represent the viewpoints of the American Public Health Association or of the agencies with which they are affiliated.

Berwyn F. Mattison, M.D.
Executive Director
American Public Health Association

Preface

Tuberculosis, once the chief cause of death in our population, and more recently the principal fatal infectious disease in the middle years of life, has dropped in the last two decades to low levels of morbidity and mortality. It has by no means gone from our midst, however, and a penetrating assessment of its recent and current significance as a public health problem is needed to place it in proper perspective. Such an assessment we now have in this two-part volume, which is one of a series of monographs on vital and health statistics brought out under the sponsorship of the Statistics Section of the American Public Health Association. This volume presents a picture, statistically oriented, of tuberculous infection, morbidity, and mortality. Each of these aspects of the total problem must be considered for a comprehensive evaluation of the progress being made in controlling this still prevalent malady.

Tuberculosis was a disease of the utmost gravity in colonial times and early years of the United States republic. In those years, in both the cities and most populated rural areas, it accounted for at least a fifth of all deaths each year. As many as 500 per 100,000 of the population died from it annually in the cities of the eastern seaboard. Rates were similar in comparable regions in other parts of the world.

It is noteworthy, though, that throughout the years of industrial development and improving standards of living a slow but steady decline in the prevalence of the disease took place. This was at first without the benefit of an effective specific therapy, but a time came when such therapy was available, and with its use the decline accelerated.

In the accelerated decline in tuberculosis mortality the results of organized effort in its control are clearly evident. Much of the work in the early years of the twentieth century was by voluntary bodies of dedicated citizens without medical training, as well as by public-health minded physicians. Goals were first measured in terms of declining mortality, and when the death rate dropped, in the mid-1920's, below 100 per 100,000, it was a time for celebration for these devoted workers. Their efforts were heavily reinforced in later years by increased state, local, and federal participation in tuberculosis programs, and the deaths from tuberculosis have now reached the astonishingly low average rate of 4 per 100,000 per year.

As the mortality rate dropped, attention was focused more sharply on the case rates, as determined by representative mass studies of significant segments of the population. New goals were established, and voluntary and official forces alike attacked the tuberculosis problem with this more refined measure of accomplishment. Case rates were found to be dropping too, although generally not so rapidly as the mortality rates. More difficulties attended this type of evaluation, because of deficiencies in reporting and lack of general agreement on what constituted a case.

The next step logically was determination, as precisely as possible, of the prevalence of tuberculous infection in the population, as revealed by the tuberculin test. This index, too, has its pitfalls, but by and large it furnishes the best measure we have of the total hazard, present and future, from tuberculosis.

These three elements in evaluation of the course of progress in the decline of tuberculosis in the United States, that is, mortality, case rates, and the frequency of old and new infections as established by the tuberculin test, form the subject matter of the monograph here made available for students of the epidemiology of tuberculosis.

In Part I Anthony M. Lowell has presented an extraordinarily detailed summary of the past history of tuberculosis and medical and administrative measures that have been applied in its control. The account includes sections on improvements in treatment and facilities for care, methods for prevention, procedures in case finding and registration of cases, and a wealth of material on changes in the extent and character of tuberculosis in the last decade, in relation to age, sex, race, place of residence, economic state, environment, and other factors. An abundance of documentation of statements and conclusions is set forth in numerous figures and tables. Little that one would wish to know, in the respects named, cannot be found in this huge assemblage. The account is largely confined to objective facts, but occasionally the author ventures into some consideration of the future in the light of past experience, in such statements as this: "Today there is ample evidence that tuberculosis can become a rare, if not extinct, disease in the United States by the end of the twentieth century."

Certain epoch-making events are conspicuous in the story, such as the requirements of case reporting (1897ff), the founding of the National Tuberculosis Association (1904), the establishment of a Tuberculosis Control Division in the U.S. Public Health Service (1944), and the recent (1963) completion of a task force report containing recommendations for a ten-year plan raising the level of tuberculosis control through federal project grants to states. In all these events there was a remarkable alignment of the forces of the voluntary and official agencies in tuberculosis control. Lowell's account includes a relatively brief but broadly representative bibliography, marked by special attention to original sources.

Part II, by Lydia B. Edwards and Carroll E. Palmer, deals with tuberculosis infection rates as determined by the tuberculin test. It approaches the general problem on a somewhat different basis, that is, the authors' own research on the acquisition of tuberculosis infection and on its manifestations and their significance. Their report represents the culmination of a long and a highly detailed examination of some 600,-000 adolescents and young adults from all parts of the country. The study, in the authors' words, had as its objective "a nationwide picture of tuberculous infection."

The largest group of persons covered in the study was a half a million Navy recruits who were tuberculin tested as part of a cooperative program between the medical service of the U.S. Navy and the Tuberculosis Program of the U.S. Public Health Service. The most striking finding after a decade of study, as the authors note, is the low rate, about 4 percent, of tuberculin reactors in the group as a whole. This country's texts on tuberculosis, most of which antedate today's circumstances, generally place the tuberculin reaction rate at a much higher figure. Indeed the situation is improving so rapidly that, in the authors' opinion, the rate of new infections with tubercle bacilli in the group studied might now (that is, 1968) be substantially less than one per thousand per year. Such a low rate would have been inconceivable in even the most optimistic forecasts in the first half of the century.

The Edwards–Palmer account, in addition to its yield of noteworthy averages, such as those cited, reveals significant differences in rates of infection as affected by varying circumstances, including age within the rather narrow range studied, race and sex, place of residence (that is, metropolitan and nonmetropolitan), and known contact with tuberculosis patients. As an overall summary, the authors were in a position to state that the Navy recruit population, which was believed to be representative of the same age group in the general population, could be separated into two categories: a relatively low-rate group, composed of native-born white recruits without a history of contact with tuberculosis, and a relatively high-rate group composed of nonwhites, tuberculosis contacts, and recruits born and raised abroad.

As in the case of Part I, the report of findings in Part II is documented by a wealth of tabular material and charts. Standardized materials and procedures were used throughout the long, meticulous study. The nature of these is set forth in several detailed appendices.

These two parts of the monograph supplement each other admirably, bringing together in a single volume a comprehensive picture of the epidemiology of tuberculosis in the United States today, as disclosed, on the one hand, by a statistical study of its general mortality and number of living patients, and, on the other, by a highly detailed study, by the best of modern methods, of that subtle infection that might or might not, under certain circumstances, lead to overt tuberculous disease.

Esmond R. Long
Henry Phipps Institute
University of Pennsylvania
Philadelphia, Pennsylvania

Notes on Tables and Figures

1. Regarding 1959–1961 mortality data:
   a. Deaths relate to those occurring in the United States (including Alaska and Hawaii);
   b. Deaths are classified by place of residence (if pertinent);
   c. Fetal deaths are excluded;
   d. Deaths of unknown age, marital status, nativity, or other characteristics have not been distributed into the known categories, but are included in their totals;
   e. Deaths were classified by cause according to the *Seventh Revision of the International Statistical Classification of Diseases, Injuries, and Causes of Death* (Geneva: World Health Organization, 1957);
   f. All death rates are average annual rates per 100,000 population in the category specified, as recorded in the United States census of April 1,1960;
   g. Age-adjusted rates were computed by the direct method using the age distribution of the total United States population in the census of April 1, 1940 as a standard.[1]
2. Symbols used in tables of data:
   --- Data not available;
   ... Category not applicable;
   - Quantity zero;
   0.0 Quantity more than zero but less than 0.05;
   * Figure does not meet the standard of reliability or precision:
      a) Rate or ratio based on less than 20 deaths;
      b) Percentage or median based on less than 100 deaths;
      c) Age-adjusted rate computed from age-specific rates where more than half of the rates were based on frequencies of less than 20 deaths.
3. Case rates and death rates are annual rates per 100,000 mid-year population in the categories specified.
4. Geographic classification: [2]
   a. Standard Metropolitan Statistical Areas (SMSA's): except in the New England States, "an SMSA is a county or a group of contiguous counties which contains at least one city of 50,000 inhabitants or more or 'twin cities' with a combined population of at least 50,000 in the 1960 census. In addition, contiguous counties are included in an SMSA if, according to specified criteria, they are (a) essentially metropolitan in character and (b) socially and economically integrated with the central city or cities." In New England, the Division of Vital Statistics of the National Center for Health Statistics uses, instead of the definition just

[1] Mortimer Spiegelman and H. H. Marks, "Empirical Testing of Standards for the Age Adjustment of Death Rates by the Direct Method," *Human Biology,* 38:280 (September 1966).

[2] *Vital Statistics of the United States, 1960* (Washington, D.C.: National Center for Health Statistics, 1963), Vol 2 (*Morality*), Part A, Section 7, p. 8.

cited, Metropolitan State Economic Areas (MSEA's) established by the Bureau of the Census, which are made up of county units.

b. Metropolitan and nonmetropolitan: "Counties which are included in SMSA's or, in New England, MSEA's are called metropolitan counties; all other counties are classified as nonmetropolitan."

c. Metropolitan counties may be separated into those containing at least one central city of 50,000 inhabitants or more or twin cities as specified previously, and into metropolitan counties without a central city.

Part I / Tuberculosis Morbidity and Mortality and Its Control

Anthony M. Lowell

Author's Preface

By the historical method alone can many problems in medicine be approached profitably. For example the student who dates his knowledge of tuberculosis from Koch may have a very correct, but he has a very incomplete appreciation of the subject.
Sir William Osler (1849–1919)

The history of tuberculosis as a cause of illness and death in the United States during this century is in many respects easier to document than is the case for other diseases. State and city archives are replete with accumulated statistical information, much of it untapped and unevaluated. However, availability of these rich reservoirs of data exacts penalties when it becomes necessary to choose without bias and with objectivity those few facts which are of significance in research on tuberculosis.

In Part I the status of tuberculosis as an important morbid condition in the United States is reviewed by going beyond a mere examination of current vital and health statistics. Taken into account are trends of the disease, significant concepts of modern treatment and epidemiology, facilities available for the care of tuberculous patients, how the reporting and registration of tuberculosis deaths and cases developed, and a brief recapitulation of the more important milestones in the history of the disease in this country.

Statistics that contribute to a better understanding of tuberculosis as it exists today are given special emphasis, but it is true that a serious student of the problem will want to investigate original sources.

References at the end of the book were selected to document the major statements included in the text and to suggest sources of information but were not intended to be bibliographic in scope.

The author acknowledges the invaluable assistance given by Helen Anglin, Elizabeth Hughes, and Carole Long of the Tuberculosis Program with the compilation of statistical data.

January 1969   Anthony M. Lowell

1 / Tuberculosis in the United States and Programs for Control

NOTES ON THE HISTORY OF TUBERCULOSIS

Commentaries on tuberculosis in America during the colonial period and the nineteenth century reflected an acceptance of it as an ubiquitous scourge of humanity which was a common inheritance of the poor and rich alike.[1] Today, there is ample evidence that tuberculosis can become a rare, if not extinct, disease in the United States by the end of the twentieth century.

Tuberculosis is an ancient disease with a lineage that can be traced to the earliest history of mankind.[2] That it was extant in remote antiquity is affirmed by findings among Egyptian and Nubian remains of bone deformities characteristic of tuberculous disease. Percival Pott (1714–1788),[3] a distinguished British surgeon, described this form of tuberculosis in 1779 and it was subsequently named after him. The writings of Hippocrates (c. 460–377 B.C.), the "father of medicine," gave an excellent clinical account of the disease.[4] Tuberculosis was well known in the ancient Mediterranean world, where it was diagnosed and treated by Greek medical men, among others the imperial physician Galen (130–200 A.D.), who practiced in Rome and whose great authority profoundly influenced medical thought of the Middle Ages and remained unchallenged for twelve centuries.[5] Historians note that in India the medical luminary Suśruta (c. 500 A.D.) mentioned the "royal disease" in his writings. In the period of the Renaissance, Girolamo Fracastoro (1483–1553), regarded by some as the first epidemiologist, recognized the contagious nature of tuberculosis. In the last millennium tuberculosis has been universally distributed among all branches of the human race.[6]

Understanding of tuberculosis in modern terms began in the seventeenth century with the revival of the study of anatomy. The Dutch physician, Franciscus Sylvius (1614–72) deduced from autopsies that "phthisis," a wasting disease, was due to the formation of small, round masses or nodules, which he named "tubercles" and which he believed to be diseased lymph nodes. Somewhat later, Richard Morton (1637–98), an English physician, first associated autopsy findings with specific traits of the disease. In 1761 Leopold Auenbrugger (1722–1809) of Austria introduced percussion into diagnosis of chest disease, but it was not until René Laënnec (1781–1826), a French physician, invented the stethoscope in 1816 that modern physical diagnosis began.[7] Laënnec and other investigators learned much about tuberculosis, but why this disease process occurred was not demonstrated. Many theories were advanced, among them that tuberculosis was inherited or that the tubercle was a cancer-like destructive growth of certain tissues. Jean-Antoine Villemin (1827–92), a French army surgeon, drawing upon his experience with soldiers, deduced that tuberculosis might be contagious. After some experiments he reported to the French Academy of Medicine in 1865 that tuberculosis was transmissible.[8]

Robert Koch (1843–1910) of Germany isolated the bacillus *Mycobacterium tuberculosis* and proved that it was the sole cause of tuberculosis.[9] He reported upon his findings on March 24, 1882, before the Berlin Phthisiological Society. This event finally brought about an organized attack against tuberculosis, and it illustrates Sir William Osler's (1849–1919) [10] aphorism that "In science the credit goes to the man who convinces the world, not to the man to whom the idea first occurs."

In the colonial period and very early history of this country the acute and devastating epidemics of cholera, smallpox, yellow fever, and many other diseases which accounted for so much sickness and death, overshadowed the slow epidemic caused by tuberculosis. Its progress in time and space was difficult to evaluate, and its infectious nature although suspected by some was questioned or denied by others. The specificity of tuberculosis was not generally accepted until 1882, when Koch discovered the tubercle bacillus.

"Consumption, phthisis, scrofula" or the "white plague" was by no means ignored in the contemporary literature of the last century. Much earlier, in fact three hundred years ago, John Bunyan (1628–88) referred to tuberculosis somewhat euphemistically as the captain of the men of death, an invidious distinction it retained until the twentieth century. "The captain of all these men of death that came against him to take him away, was the Consumption, for it was that that brought him down to the grave." (The Life and Death of Mr. Badman)

Early in the eighteen hundreds thoughtful men began to study the epidemiology of "phthisis" and recognized that this disease too had an epidemic cycle although its specific characteristics were not well understood. But it was not until elementary record-keeping systems for reporting causes of death and, years later, the official registration of communicable diseases were created that the true extent of tuberculosis was dramatized.

Remedies to cope with so widespread a disease phenomenon were unavailable and workable solutions seemed to be beyond the understanding and capacities of sanitarians and health authorities. This lack of knowledge as to what caused tuberculosis or certainty as to how it was transmitted frustrated attempts at its eradication. The approach to this complex problem was pragmatic at best. At first, progress in containing the profound ravages of tuberculosis was measured by the reduction in the death rate but it was soon realized that this statistical index alone was not entirely satisfactory. It was, therefore, eventually supplemented by the recording of known cases of tuberculosis and the reporting of newly found disease. In 1900, case registration of tuberculosis was carried out in only a few large cities but gradually the practice of reporting communicable diseases expanded to include the whole United States during the fourth decade of this century.

Because nationwide vital statistics records were not gathered until comparatively recent times, some idea as to the extent of tuberculosis as a public health problem, in the early part of the nineteenth century, can be deduced from mortality data for a few communities that systematically collected such information. These cities and states were almost entirely in the northeastern part of the country. It appears from published documents that about one fourth of all deaths were due to "phthisis" or "consumption," the old terms for pulmonary tuberculosis. Usually the statistics did not include such forms of nonpulmonary tuberculosis as scrofula, tabes mesenterica, cold abscess, white swelling, lupus, and Pott's disease. The general practice was to mention the latter forms of tuberculosis as separate entities.

In Salem, Massachusetts, during the five-year period from 1768 to 1773 "consumption" (pulmonary tuberculosis) accounted for 117 or 18.2 percent of 642 deaths from all causes, and for the period 1799 to 1808 the proportion rose to 25 percent. The "consumption" death rate is estimated to have been around 440 per 100,000 population.[11] Boston, from 1810 to 1820, recorded 1,891 deaths from "consumption," a pulmonary tuberculosis rate of 489 per 100,000 population. Other cities had somewhat similar high rates: New York City (1804–08), 550; Philadelphia (1811–20), 618; Baltimore (1821–30), 392; Providence (1841–45), 501; and Charleston (1822–30), 450. During this era, in large cities, the proportion of deaths ascribed to tuberculosis ranged from 14 to 30 percent.

A century ago, tuberculosis was the leading cause of death in most of the large cities in the United States as illustrated by data for New York City (see Table 1.1). For the period 1804 to 1808 the consumption

Table 1.1   Leading causes of death, Old New York (Manhattan and Bronx)

Five-year period 1804-1808			Five-year period 1849-1853		
Cause of death	Annual average		Cause of death	Annual average	
	Deaths	Rate		Deaths	Rate
All causes	2,204	2,767	All causes	21,416	3,972
Consumption	438	550	Consumption	2,322	431
Convulsions	188	236	Convulsions	1,576	292
Cholera infantum	129	162	Cholera	1,107	205
Marasmus, atrophia	124	156	Inflammation, chest, lungs	1,077	200
Inflammation, chest, lungs	101	127	Marasmus, atrophia	1,029	191
Croup	88	110	Dysentery	956	177
Dropsy	86	108	Cholera infantum	839	156
Casualties, violence	79	99	Dropsy in head	801	149
Smallpox	74	93	Diarrhea	651	121
Typhus, typhoid	73	92	Apoplexy	552	102
Yellow fever	54	68	Croup	476	88
Dysentery	43	54	Inflammation, bowels, stomach	470	87
Worms	42	53	Smallpox	454	84
Whooping cough	36	45	Scarlet fever	454	84
Teething	36	45	Debility	432	80
Inflammation, bowels	34	43	Inflammation, brain	405	75
Sprue	26	33	Dropsy	321	60
Dropsy in head	23	29	Heart disease	258	48
Apoplexy	21	26	Measles	230	43
Palsy	19	24	Congestion, lungs	219	41
Other causes	490	614	Other causes	6,787	1,258

Population 1806 = 79,653   Population 1851 = 539,107

Source: Downing, T. K., Table of Semicentennial Mortality of the City of New York, compiled from The Records of the City Inspector's Department, comprising the full period from January 1, 1804, to December 31, 1853, New York Public Library.

(pulmonary tuberculosis) death rate was 550 per 100,000 population. Twenty percent of deaths due to all causes were attributed to tuberculosis. A half century later (1849–53), the death rates were around 400 per 100,000 population and about 11 percent of the reported deaths from all causes were due to tuberculosis.

In 1849, Lemuel Shattuck (1793–1859) made what appears to be, in the light of subsequent events, a classic understatement. In the *Report of the Sanitary Commission of Massachusetts,* 1850, he commented, *"Consumption,* that great destroyer of human health and human life, takes the first rank as an agent of death; and as such, we deem it proper to analyze more particularly the circumstances under which it operates. Any facts regarding a disease that destroys *one-seventh* to *one-fourth* of all that die, cannot but be interesting." [12] Indeed his other observations in this remarkably prophetic document bear repeating: "The *causes of this disease,* and the means of removal, are the great objects of investigation; and they can be accurately ascertained only by an extensive series of systematic, uniform and exact observations of the external circumstances,—atmospheric, local and personal,—occurring in each case. And we cannot too strongly impress upon local Boards of Health, upon the members of the medical profession, and upon all others interested, the importance of making a united and energetic effort to obtain such observations concerning every case which occurs in every part of the Commonwealth. Near 3,000 cases, in this State, annually terminate in death; and if they were properly observed, for a series of five, ten, or more years, it is impossible to anticipate the good results which might follow. Possibly,—and even *probably,*—discoveries might be made which would reduce the annual number of cases, certainly by hundreds, and perhaps by thousands. We shall hereafter suggest a form of a Register of Cases adapted to this object; and the great importance of the disease, and the confident hope that some discovery can be made which will materially abate its melancholy ravages, should arouse us all to action."

Although tuberculosis death rates of 400 per 100,000 population were common a century ago, under unusual circumstances even in comparatively recent times very high death rates have been prevalent for short periods of time. In Puerto Rico the tuberculosis death rate was 333 in 1933 when 16 percent of all deaths were attributed to tuberculosis; in the Philippines a rate of 306 prevailed in 1930; in Athens the rate was 409 in 1935; and the astounding high rates of 575 in Vienna in 1919, and 642 in Budapest in 1919 were reported during World War I years. Until 1941, in the New York City Central Harlem health center district, a densely crowded area with over 200,000 residents, tuberculosis death rates were well over 200 per 100,000 population. The tuberculosis death rate was 274 as recently as 1935, or nearly eighty times the rate for the United States in 1968.

A Task Force on Tuberculosis Control in the United States,[13] appointed in 1963 by the surgeon general of the U.S. Public Health Service, to consider the unsatisfactory situation in tuberculosis control and to recommend steps that might be taken to remedy it, prepared a report that in essence and spirit reiterated Mr. Shattuck's concern. It emphasized that tuberculosis is still a stubborn and tenacious adversary—a continuing burden to society.

DEVELOPMENT OF ADMINISTRATIVE CONTROL: THE PIONEERS
Two men, Dr. Hermann M. Biggs (1859–1923) in New York [14] and Sir Robert W. Philip (1857–1939) in Edinburgh,[15] were prime movers in establishing organized systems for the control of tuberculosis. The first tuberculosis dispensary in the world was opened by Sir Robert in Edinburgh in 1887, which was the nucleus of the "Edinburgh Anti-Tuberculosis Scheme." The dispensary initiated what today is a

vast system of administrative medicine. Two years later in 1889 Dr. Biggs, who in 1914 became the New York State Commissioner of Health, in association with his colleagues T. M. Prudden (1849–1924) and H. P. Loomis (1859–1907), took steps in creating a plan for the administrative control of tuberculosis in New York City. At the behest of the Commissioner of Health, Dr. Joseph D. Bryant (1845–1914), Biggs formulated a statement regarding the contagiousness of tuberculosis, pointing out that it was preventable, not directly inherited and that it was acquired by transmission of tubercle bacilli from the sick to the healthy. The report proposed measures for the prevention of tuberculosis, by protecting the public through a system of official inspection of cattle, disseminating information to the public that a tuberculous person with active tuberculous disease could be a source of danger to his associates, and by the careful disinfection of rooms and hospital wards which had been occupied by "phthisical" patients.[16]

Although prominent physicians received with disfavor the recommendations that the Board of Health take action in the sanitary surveillance of tuberculosis, Commissioner Bryant issued a circular prepared by Biggs for physicians and laymen entitled "Contagious Consumption-Rules to be Observed for the Prevention of the Spread of Consumption," dated July 9, 1889. It was the first step in the subsequent nationwide educational campaign against tuberculosis in the United States. In November 1893 the major features of Biggs' report became part of the public health code of the City of New York, and the program adopted by the Health Department on December 13, 1893, formed the nucleus of a complete scheme for the control of tuberculosis. In 1897, in spite of some opposition, the compulsory notification of tuberculosis, both pulmonary and other forms, by all physicians, householders, and others coming in contact with the disease was adopted. These were the first definite actions taken by an agency of local government in attempting to control tuberculosis.

Reporting and registration of tuberculosis cases and deaths was soon recognized to be a very important public health function in the control of tuberculosis. Subsequently tuberculosis became a legally reportable communicable disease in all of the states. Because of many technical and administrative difficulties information on the number of newly reported cases for the entire United States did not become available until 1930 (see Chapter 3).

In the early part of the nineteenth century the peripatetic Frenchman, Alexis de Tocqueville (1805–59),[17] noted that one of the interesting features of American democracy was a willingness and an ability on the part of its citizens as individuals to initiate social movements for the welfare of the community. He observed that "Americans of all ages, all conditions, and all dispositions, constantly form associations. They have not only commercial and manufacturing companies, in which all take part, but associations of a thousand other kinds,—religious, moral, serious, futile, general or restricted, enormous or diminutive. The Americans make associations to give entertainments, to found seminaries, to build inns, to construct churches, to diffuse books, to send missionaries to the antipodes; they found in this manner hospitals, prisons, and schools. If it is proposed to inculcate some truth, or to foster some feeling, by the encouragement of a great example, they form a society. Wherever, at the head of some new undertaking, you see the government in France, or a man of rank in England, in the United States you will be sure to find an association . . .

"As soon as several of the inhabitants of the United States have taken up an opinion or a feeling which they wish to promote in the world, they look out for mutual assistance; and as soon as they have found each other out, they combine. From that moment they are no longer isolated men, but a power seen from afar, whose actions serve for an example and whose language is listened to."

Tocqueville's observation has been borne out by the establishment in the United States of numerous nonofficial health agencies for the control of tuberculosis and other diseases.[18] Dr. Lawrence F. Flick (1856–1938) [19] organized in April 1892 the first American voluntary antituberculosis organization, The Pennsylvania Society for Prevention of Tuberculosis. In 1895 he helped to organize in Philadelphia the Free Hospital for Poor Consumptives, and in 1903 established the Henry Phipps Institute, the first institute for tuberculosis research in the United States.[20] Dr. Edward Livingston Trudeau (1848–1915) has been called "the father of the anti-tuberculosis campaign in the United States." Although his interests were largely in the field of research and sanatorium care of tuberculosis, his personal influence was national in scope as was the work of the Trudeau Sanatorium, the Trudeau Laboratory, and the Trudeau School of Tuberculosis located in the Saranac Lake region of upstate New York. Hundreds of physicians who "cured" or studied at "Trudeau" were responsible for spreading throughout the nation the philosophy of good sanatorium care.[21]

Dr. S. Adolphus Knopf (1857–1940) of New York [22] was one of the men responsible for the movement that in 1902 launched the Committee on the Prevention of Tuberculosis of the Charity Organization Society of New York City. He focused attention in 1903 and 1904 on the need of a national tuberculosis association. Edward T. Devine (1867–1948),[23] pioneer in the profession of social work, also of New York, at the beginning of the twentieth century introduced into organized associations a strong lay influence as a complement to that of physicians. Homer Folks (1867–1963), a sociologist and one time Commissioner of Charities for New York City, 1902–03, contributed to the technique of tuberculosis organization and the application of basic principles laid down by Biggs and others. In 1907 through the cooperation of the Russell Sage Foundation he helped organize, under the State Charities Aid Association of New York, the first comprehensive statewide campaign against tuberculosis, a model that was followed by other states.

DEVELOPMENT OF ADMINISTRATIVE CONTROL: VOLUNTARY AND GOVERNMENTAL ACTIVITY

In the United States, the first private sanatorium was erected in Asheville, North Carolina. Dr. Trudeau established the first sanatorium for the poor in 1884—the Adirondack Cottage Sanitarium. The first municipal sanatorium was erected in 1897 at Cincinnati, and the first state sanatorium was opened on October 1, 1898, at Rutland, Massachusetts. A tuberculosis dispensary was established at Philadelphia in 1891 by Rush Hospital for Consumption and Allied Diseases, and under municipal auspices in 1903 at Gouverneur Hospital in New York City. In May 1913, a Division of Tuberculosis was established under the Ohio State Board of Health. However, it took several decades before each state and most large cities had organized tuberculosis control programs under official auspices.[24]

The National Tuberculosis Association,[25] a nonofficial voluntary health agency, was organized in 1904 (National Association for the Study and Prevention of Tuberculosis) to create public understanding and stimulate programs for the control of tuberculosis. This agency is financed by the sale of Christmas seals, a method originated in Denmark in 1904 by Einor Holbøll, a Danish postal clerk, and introduced in this country in 1907 by Miss Emily P. Bissell (1861–1948) of Wilmington. Since then, efforts of the NTA (from 1968, the National Tuberculosis and Respiratory Disease Association) have been highly successful in promoting and maintaining public interest in tuberculosis through hundreds of local and state affiliates.

The Sixth International Congress on Tuberculosis [26] held in Washington in 1908, focused on tuberculosis as a worldwide problem and helped promote the idea of an overall national program in the United States. One of the derived benefits of this conclave was the stimulus given to state and local governments to seek legislation for tuberculosis control activities and the building of hospitals and sanatoria. In time a greater proportion of public funds was assigned for tuberculosis. With the increased interest, as governments began to shoulder the institutional burden, the monies involved grew in proportion. The total public appropriations by 1910 had reached more than $9,000,000 annually, of which over $4,000,000 came from the states, almost an equal amount from municipalities, and about $1,000,000 from the national government for federal hospitals. By way of contrast, in 1963 it was estimated by the Task Force on Tuberculosis Control that the annual hospital cost for tuberculosis was $335,800,000. Annual expenditures available in 1962 for various activities that could be used for tuberculosis programs were: state and local governments $32,500,000; tuberculosis associations $8,000,000; federal grants to the states $4,500,-000. Approximately $20,800,000 in additional funds were needed annually to implement an increased effort that would bring about more rapid progress against tuberculosis. The overall cost of tuberculosis to the nation's economy is estimated to be one billion dollars each year. The direct cost is around $600 million, for research, hospital care, control activities by federal, state, and local health agencies, compensation, and private physicians services; the indirect cost (due to loss of income from death and disease caused by tuberculosis) is estimated at over $400 million.

However, the early history of effort toward administrative control on a federal level was not encouraging. In 1917 the Kent Bill, which was amended to provide for a division of tuberculosis in the U.S. Public Health Service, failed to pass, as did similar bills introduced in the next session of Congress.[27] There were no significant developments until soon after Pearl Harbor when the surgeon general, Dr. Thomas Parran (1892–1968), established a small tuberculosis control section in the States Relation Division of the Bureau of State Services. In 1944 the Public Health Service Act (Public Law 78-410) authorized establishment of a tuberculosis control program. It placed upon the Public Health Service the responsibility of administering grants-in-aid to state health departments and of conducting demonstrations and research in tuberculosis. On July 6, 1944, the surgeon general established a Tuberculosis Control Division in the Bureau of State Services of the Public Health Service and it was approved on the same day by Paul V. McNutt (1891–1955), the Federal Security Administrator. Senior Surgeon Herman E. Hilleboe (1906–1974), who had been in charge of the Public Health Service emergency tuberculosis program since 1942, was appointed chief of the new division with rank of medical director, in which capacity he served until 1946. Beginning in 1944 casefinding was one of the principal activities of the Public Health Service in tuberculosis control (see Chapter 2).

The role of the Tuberculosis Program of the U.S. Public Health Service, since 1960 a branch of the National Communicable Disease Center in Atlanta, has been to exercise leadership in improving tuberculosis control efforts throughout the nation, conduct long-term research investigations, provide professional assistance and promote educational programs, stimulate other organizations and groups to participate in various anti-tuberculosis programs, and give the American public a comprehensive view of the tuberculosis problem as it relates to the nation's health.[28]

The Public Health Service provides supplemental fiscal support to state and local health departments for tuberculosis control activities through formula and special project grants-in-aid. Assistance is also given by Tuberculosis Program consultants with the development of tuberculosis programs when such help is requested. The tuberculosis control grant was first authorized by Section 314(b) of the Public Health Service Act, as approved July 1, 1944, to assist states in establishing and maintaining adequate measures for the prevention, treatment, and control of tuberculosis. In order to focus greater attention on the need for casefinding, Congress in the 1955 Appropriation Act (Public Law 83-472), directed that federal formula grants and state and local matching funds could only be used for prevention and casefinding activities. Public Law 87-290, approved September 22, 1961, provided for project grants for tuberculosis control. Furthermore, it specified that these project grants were to be used exclusively for improving services to known tuberculosis patients outside hospitals. Casefinding activities under this authority were to be limited to examination of contacts and diagnosis of suspects known to health departments. The Comprehensive Health Planning and Public Health Service Amendments of 1966 amended the Public Health Service Act to authorize Health Services Development Project Grants for the purpose of

(1) providing services to meet health needs of limited geographic scope or of specialized regional or national significance and (2) developing and supporting for an initial period new programs of health services. Tuberculosis project grants are awarded under the provision of (1) above.*

In December 1963, the surgeon general's task force completed its report, which contained recommendations for a ten-year plan to raise the level of nationwide tuberculosis control services through greater federal participation by means of increased formula and project grants to the states. The activities recommended were for services to unhospitalized active cases, inactive cases, and contacts to new active cases; identification of persons at risk through tuberculin testing of school-children and hospital admission X-ray programs; and continuing periodic examination as well as prophylactic treatment of persons at risk of developing tuberculosis. In 1967 there were 82 special tuberculosis projects in operation. The federal appropriations for tuberculosis control had reached $3,000,000 for formula grants and $14,950,000 for tuberculosis project grants.

The influence of these activities by the federal government is difficult to assess with precision, but there is ample evidence that control of tuberculosis is being improved, and that there is a resurgence of interest in this disease. One criterion is the number of professional and ancillary personnel added to already established health department tuberculosis programs and supported directly through project grants. On July 1, 1968, there were 2,316 approved positions available to these projects, for 139 physicians, 37 Public Health Service medical officers and 82 Public Health advisors, 689 nurses, 680 clerical personnel, and other persons in a variety of positions augmenting the regular staff assigned to tuberculosis control work in health departments.

TUBERCULOSIS IN THE UNITED STATES SINCE 1900:
AN OVERALL VIEW

It is significant that even before the development of public health programs for the control of tuberculosis, the fragmentary evidence available points to a decline in mortality from the disease during the nineteenth century.[29] According to data recited previously for New York

* Section 314(e) of the Public Health Service Act, as amended by the Comprehensive Health Planning and Public Health Services Amendments of 1966, Public Law 89-749, and the Partnership for Health Amendments of 1967, Public Law 90-174.

City (although of uncertain quality), during the first half of that century the death rate fell by about 25 percent; during its second half the rate was cut almost in two but still remained at an inordinately high level.[30] In Massachusetts the death rate for tuberculosis of the respiratory system fell from 365 per 100,000 in 1861 to 190 in 1900. It would appear that the improving socioeconomic milieu of the previous century included, among its benefits, a decline in tuberculosis mortality. Socioeconomic factors may have played an even more significant role in the present century, but this would be very difficult to evaluate if, indeed, it is at all possible to do so. Because both these factors and the public health movement were gradual in their development it is not surprising that the trend of tuberculosis mortality up to the late forties of this century was steady—dramatic in slope and not by abrupt drops (see Fig. 1.1).[31]

In the early years public health practice was in transition, undergoing a metamorphosis from the concepts of the sanitary era to those of contemporary epidemiological thinking. Gradually, the state of knowledge and general attitude of both the medical profession and the public began to change and tuberculosis was finally acknowledged to be curable and preventable. Discoveries of new methods and techniques raised the hope that tuberculosis could be controlled and possibly eradicated. Perhaps this early optimism was premature but at least it served as an incentive to spur the social conscience toward a broad and intensive approach to the problem.

Sanatorium care, with long periods of "rest cure," was augmented in the nineteen thirties and forties with collapse therapy of the lung by means of surgical procedures. With discovery and introduction of chemotherapeutic drugs into the medical treatment of tuberculosis, during the late nineteen forties and early fifties, the incidence and mortality from tuberculosis began to decline rapidly (see Fig. 1.1). These new antituberculosis drugs brought about changes in therapeutic procedures, which no longer required prolonged stays in sanatoria or special hospitals, where most tuberculosis specialists were to be found. By 1960 there were very few specialists who limited their medical practice exclusively to tuberculosis.

By 1967, treatment of tuberculosis with a variety of new drugs had become a complex matter calling for a high degree of medical sophistication. Problems posed by drug resistant organisms require more laboratory support as well as greater use of hospital facilities in the early treatment of the disease. Discovery of the so-called atypical mi-

17

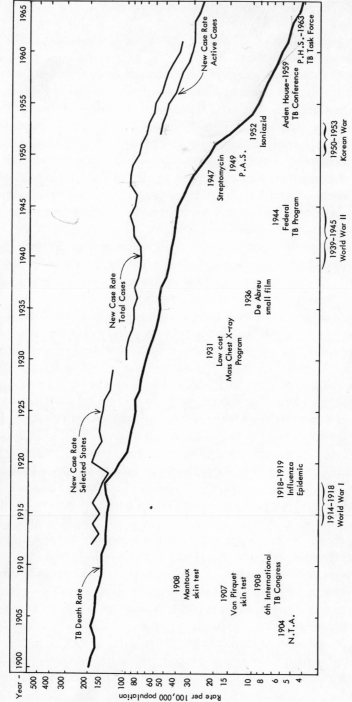

Figure 1.1. Tuberculosis, new case rates and death rates, United States, since 1900.

croorganisms, which simulate tuberculosis, have added to the difficulties of differential diagnosis.

During the early years of the twentieth century in most large cities almost all adults reacted to the tuberculin test, giving evidence that they had been infected with the tubercle bacillus. As late as 1946 this was still true in some sections of the country, but there was growing evidence that a steady decline in the rate of new infection was becoming the common trend. Generally, infection with the tubercle bacillus occurs more frequently in congested parts of the cities and large industrial centers where tuberculosis is more prevalent than in scattered agricultural communities. However, on rare occasions outbreaks of small epidemics are still reported in rural areas.[32]

By the 1940's it appeared as if Wade Hampton Frost's (1880–1938) concept of biological attrition, that the balance of nature was in favor of man against the tubercle bacillus, was being borne out in fact.[33] Recent developments in treatment of tuberculosis, with the important adjuvant of new drugs, have reduced tuberculosis mortality. On the other hand, the number of new active cases reported each year continues to decline rather slowly. Several studies show that approximately 75 to 80 percent of these newly reported cases arise from the large pool of persons who were exposed to and infected with tubercle bacilli years ago. The remaining 20 to 25 percent of the new cases reported during a year are the product of very recent infection. It is estimated that out of the total population of about 200 million people in this country, around 25 million would show a positive reaction to a tuberculin test, most of them having been infected prior to the current year. The proportion of the population found to be already infected is small in the younger ages but increases for those persons in the older ages who were exposed to tuberculosis years ago when the probability of becoming infected was much greater. (Figure 1.2 approximates very roughly the situation in this regard about 1960.)

As the surgeon general's 1963 task force on tuberculosis pointed out, society cannot permit or tolerate a status quo, when there are at hand the tools that can accelerate eradication of the ancient "white plague." Furthermore, it noted that "Tuberculosis is still a problem of considerable magnitude, that measures for its control are complex, that increased reduction in the incidence of tuberculosis disease and infection is achievable but will require augmented public health efforts, wisely directed."

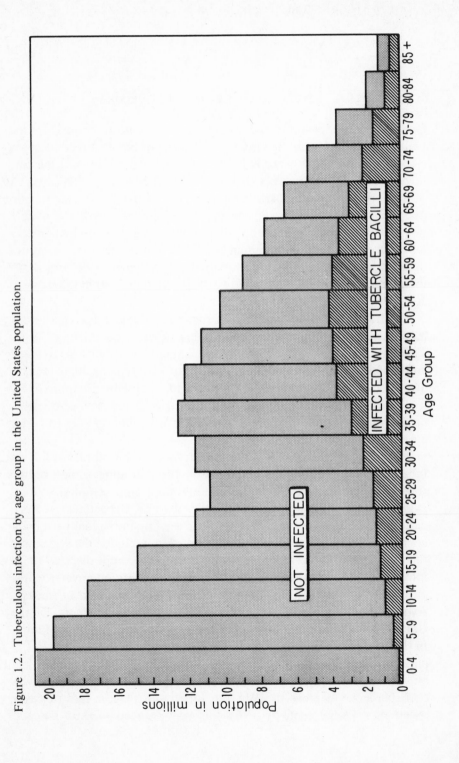

Figure 1.2. Tuberculous infection by age group in the United States population.

STATE-FEDERAL TUBERCULOSIS ERADICATION PROGRAM IN CATTLE

One of the important achievements in tuberculosis control in the United States has been the virtual elimination of bovine tuberculosis as a serious public health problem. It has been well established that the bovine tubercle bacillus is pathogenic for man and that it can cause all of the forms of tuberculosis the human type of bacillus is able to produce. In the past, mainly during the era when pasteurization of milk was not universally practiced, tuberculous cattle provided an important source of infection in human beings. A half century ago it was not unusual for children to become fatally ill or permanently deformed due to bovine tuberculosis contracted from drinking milk from tuberculous cows.[34]

The bovine tubercle bacillus as an etiological agent was clearly differentiated from other types of acid-fast tubercle bacilli in 1898 by Theobald Smith (1859–1934).[35] Most animals, whether fish, fowl, or amphibians, may develop tuberculosis, but of a type peculiar to their own species. Wild animals when brought into captivity are more likely to develop the disease than the domestic variety. However, only cattle, swine, and fowl, among domestic animals, are common prey to tuberculosis.

The economic loss to the cattle industry and serious threat of bovine tuberculosis to the health of the country brought about action on the state and federal level. In 1917 a national program to eliminate tuberculosis among cattle was instituted under the U.S. Department of Agriculture, although the tuberculin test was used by individual herd owners before the national program. This program included the systematic tuberculin testing of cattle and herds of cattle, prompt disposal of all infected cattle, adequate disinfection, and regulations governing the movement of cattle. It has become a universally accepted procedure. Avoidance of tuberculosis infection from dairy products in the United States has been reinsured by the general pasteurization of milk. In the program when infection in an area was reduced to less than 0.5 percent, that area became accredited. The entire United States became an accredited area in 1940 when the overall rate of infection was 0.46 percent. Whereas in 1918 the tuberculin reactor rate of cattle tested was 4.9 percent, by 1965 this was reduced to 0.08 percent.

However, systematic testing of cattle continues in order to prevent possible spreading of the disease (see Table 1.2).

Sporadic confined epidemics in cattle in recent years underscore the need for continued supervision. Cattle are usually infected by the bovine type of bacilli, and infrequently by the avian type, but there have been reports to suggest that human type bacilli were transmitted to cattle and other mammals.

Table 1.2   Bovine tuberculin testing: United States, 1917-65

Fiscal year	Cattle tested for tuberculosis	Reactors to tuberculin test		Fiscal year	Cattle tested for tuberculosis	Reactors to tuberculin test	
		Number	Percent			Number	Percent
Total	457,103,149	4,158,724	0.9	1940	12,222,318	56,343	0.46
				1941	12,229,499	40,702	0.3
1917	20,101	645	3.2	1942	10,983,086	28,008	0.26
1918	134,143	6,544	4.9	1943	9,308,936	17,167	0.18
1919	329,878	13,528	4.1	1944	8,894,466	18,338	0.2
1920	700,670	28,709	4.1	1945	8,105,480	19,534	0.24
1921	1,366,358	53,768	3.9	1946	8,454,463	19,464	0.23
1922	2,384,236	82,569	3.5	1947	8,312,919	16,666	0.2
1923	3,460,849	113,844	3.3	1948	8,294,423	15,943	0.19
1924	5,312,364	171,559	3.2	1949	8,737,501	17,007	0.19
1925	7,000,028	214,491	3.1	1950	9,439,811	17,733	0.19
1926	8,650,780	323,084	3.7	1951	8,847,228	12,353	0.14
1927	9,700,176	285,361	2.9	1952	9,164,265	10,351	0.11
1928	11,281,490	262,113	2.3	1953	9,675,245	10,811	0.11
1929	11,683,720	206,764	1.8	1954	10,234,665	10,886	0.11
1930	12,845,871	216,932	1.7	1955	9,210,810	11,133	0.12
1931	13,782,273	203,778	1.5	1956	9,220,244	14,363	0.15
1932	13,443,557	254,785	1.9	1957	8,976,409	13,974	0.156
1933	13,073,894	255,096	2.0	1958	8,883,813	15,361	0.17
1934	15,119,763	232,368	1.5	1959	8,187,161	18,914	0.23
1935	25,237,532	376,623	1.5	1960	9,439,706	14,149	0.15
1936	22,918,038	165,496	0.7	1961	9,788,386	14,579	0.15
1937	13,750,308	94,104	0.7	1962	9,219,298	10,940	0.12
1938	14,108,871	89,359	0.6	1963	8,394,790	8,314	0.10
1939	11,186,805	60,338	0.5	1964	8,252,855	8,255	0.10
				1965	7,123,667	5,608	0.08

Source: Animal Disease Eradication Division, Agricultural Research Service, U. S. Department of Agriculture, Cooperative State-Federal Tuberculosis Eradication Program, Statistical Tables, Fiscal Year 1966 (April 1967).

CLASSIFICATION OF TUBERCULOSIS

Although tuberculosis is a communicable disease, it is relatively difficult for tubercle bacilli to invade the body and establish active disease. Most tuberculosis is passed on by airborne transmission of the tubercle bacilli.[1] Primary infection may occur in children or adults; it may remain latent, progress, activate later, or repeatedly relapse. With the onset of primary tuberculosis the tuberculin test becomes positive from three to ten weeks after infection. Childhood is still the most typical age for primary infection, but incidence of infection in children is decreasing. First infection is occurring relatively more frequently in young adults when contact with the adult world becomes much more common than when their normal environment was comparatively limited. Most childhood infections show a benign course and the lesions heal without treatment. With a few exceptions the pattern of development of primary infection is the same in adults as in children. Reinfection disease is considered to include post-primary progression, reinfection, and superinfection; acute forms of the disease, if not treated, may be progressive and fatal. The chronic forms may persist for years with exacerbations, remissions, and relapses.[2]

Lesions of tuberculosis are highly diverse in appearance, and their manifestations are numerous. No single system of classification can give information that completely describes the lesions. Certain classifications and descriptions are used, however, for records and statistical purposes. A detailed discussion of the subject can be found in the *Diagnostic Standards and Classification of Tuberculosis* prepared by the American Thoracic Society, Medical Section of the National Tuberculosis Association.[3] Locally, it may be desirable to modify the generally used classifications and descriptions to serve their special purposes.

The term "form of tuberculosis" has two main groupings—pulmonary and extrapulmonary. The basis for classification of pulmonary tuberculosis includes: extent of disease (minimal, moderately advanced, far advanced), status of clinical activity, bacteriologic status, therapeutic status, exercise status. In addition, there are certain optional classifications that can be used to give supplementary information. Classification of extrapulmonary tuberculosis is listed by sites of the disease. Hematogenous (miliary tuberculosis), respiratory passages, serous membranes, cardiovascular system, chest wall, lymphatic system, gastrointestinal system, spleen, urinary tract, genital organs, bones and joints, central nervous system (meningitis), eye, endocrine system, skin.

TRENDS IN TREATMENT

Hospital treatment. Before the introduction of modern drug therapy in the nineteen forties the major therapeutic tool in managing clinical tuberculosis was general and localized physical rest.[4] When pulmonary cavities failed to close, surgical procedures generally known as "collapse therapy" were followed. Surgical procedures such as pneumothorax, pneumoperitoneum, thoracoplasty, and paralysis of the diaphragm provided rest for the diseased lung on either a temporary or permanent basis. Physical immobilization of the patient by "bed rest" for a year or more was common.[5]

In recent years surgical treatment has become much more selective. Excisional surgery to remove infected areas of lungs is performed, when indicated, in connection with chemotherapy. Collapse therapy is done infrequently and periods of complete physical rest have been drastically shortened, being reserved for those patients who are toxic, febrile, or actively bleeding, or who have bacilli resistant to drugs. The amount of physical activity permitted the patient may be related more to the patient's exercise capability and physical tolerance and, in general hospitals, to the demands for isolation rather than to the fact that he has tuberculosis.

Formerly, these therapeutic approaches required long periods of hospitalization, which contributed greatly to the shortage of beds available for new cases. Thus, many states had long lists of patients waiting to be hospitalized. Hospitals and sanatoria were often located in isolated areas far from population centers in accordance with the then-prevalent theory that an abundance of fresh air and complete isolation from the stresses and strains of urban living were necessary in the treatment of the disease.

Collapse therapy, an operative immobilization of the diseased lung in the treatment of pulmonary tuberculosis, was introduced in the last century and continued in general use well into the fifth decade of this century. James Carson (1772–1843) in 1821 [6] was the first to clearly express the fundamental principles of collapse therapy. He wrote, "It has long been my opinion that if ever this disease (phthisis) is to be cured, and it is an event of which I am by no means disposed to dispair, it must be accomplished by mechanical means, or in other words by a surgical operation." Marked improvement in a person's condition that occasionally followed a spontaneous pneumothorax, suggested its possible therapeutic application, and it was first made in 1882 by Carlo Forlanini (1847–1918), an Italian physician,[7] and in the United States independently by John Benjamin Murphy (1857–1916) in 1898.[8] Forlanini's original attempt was followed by the development of various surgical procedures to collapse the lung (pneumothorax, oleothorax, pneumonolysis, pneumoperitoneum, phrenic nerve interruption, thoracoplasty), which led to the use of excisional surgery of the lung proper (segmental wedge resection, lobectomy, and pneumonectomy). Each of these procedures had its advocates and periods of popularity.

In present-day treatment stress is laid on keeping patients in the hospital at least until they have achieved a noninfectious state.[9] Sputum conversion, the process by which positive sputum containing infectious tubercle bacilli becomes negative and is no longer infectious, under adequate and appropriate chemotherapy, can occur within one to two months after initiation of therapy. Laboratory methods used in the past required 6 to 8 weeks to confirm this change, and at times, prolonged hospitalization. Recently developed laboratory techniques, which shorten the time necessary to demonstrate conversion, appreciably reduce the hospitalization period for patients responsive to conventional drug regimen.[10]

Chemotherapy has also changed the character of hospital care for the tuberculous because the patient becomes ambulatory much sooner and is capable of pursuing a variety of recreational and educational activities within the hospital. Potent chemotherapeutic agents have become most effective treatment tools in tuberculosis and antibiotics have revolutionized medical practice.[11] Their origin began with the study of immunology when Élie Metchnikoff (1845–1916) uncovered phagocytosis, the scavenger role of white blood cells, and Paul Ehrlich (1854–1915) found salvarsan to be a specific remedy against the syphilis microorganism *T. pallidum*. This use of special chemical compounds against specific causative organisms of disease inaugurated modern chemotherapy. With the discovery in the 1930's of the sulfonamides and numerous derivatives, chemistry made its greatest contribution towards conquering disease. In the discipline of biochemistry, antibiotics, substances originating from living organisms such as molds that are antagonistic to bacteria, were discovered in the 1940's. Sir Alexander Fleming (1881–1955) discovered penicillin. Selman A. Waksman (1888–) [12] and his associates discovered the potent antimicrobial agent streptomycin in 1943–44. In 1944–45, W. H. Feldman (1892–) and H. C. Hinshaw (1902–) demonstrated the specific effect of streptomycin in inhibiting tuberculosis.[13] Although streptomycin has limitations due to a certain degree of toxicity and resistance to it will develop rapidly by the infecting organism, the difficulties have been overcome by reducing the amount and frequency of the dosage and by combining streptomycin with PAS (para-aminosalicylic acid) and INH (isonicotinic acid hydrazide) in the treatment of tuberculosis. The introduction of isoniazid (INH) in 1952, the most important modern drug in the therapy of tuberculosis, came about with simultaneous discovery of its efficacy in the United States and Germany.[14]

Antibiotics are largely bacteriostatic agents or inhibitors of growth, although some are bactericidal or bacteriolytic. *Mycobacterium tuberculosis* strains which were originally sensitive to antibiotics may develop resistance to drugs, but a culture of an organism that has become resistant to one antibiotic still may remain sensitive to others. This biological phenomenon gives rise to the rationale of multiple drug treatment in tuberculosis. Streptomycin, isoniazid, and para-aminosalicylic acid, primarily in combination, are the most widely used drugs. Other drugs, somewhat more toxic, are employed in treating tuberculosis patients whose organisms are resistant to one or more of the three mentioned above.[15]

Shorter periods of hospitalization and decreased incidence rates have reduced the demand for tuberculosis hospital beds. Though physicians sometimes treat patients at home, initial treatment in a hospital is still recommended. The selection of the proper drug combination, isolation of the patient, and his education about the disease are best carried out within the hospital under the close supervision of a medical staff. Hospitalization is mandatory for patients with tuberculosis caused by drug-resistant organisms. Their treatment with potentially highly toxic drugs requires skilled professional supervision and the laboratory services of a modern hospital. In addition, such patients frequently need surgical procedures to supplement their specialized drug treatment program.[16]

The tuberculosis patient, faced with having to spend approximately six months in the hospital, frequently experiences a host of social, economic, and psychological problems. Alcoholism among tuberculosis patients, for example, is a major institutional problem requiring skillful management. Though the definition of alcoholism varies from one institution to another, some tuberculosis hospitals report that as many as 30 percent of their adult male patients and 10 percent of adult female patients are alcoholic. Many of these, especially the males, are drawn from skid row populations and are single and homeless. Special medical and social services are necessary if these patients are to be persuaded to remain under treatment. Alcoholism among hospital patients is not a new phenomenon. However, the problem is a fairly recent one for tuberculosis hospitals and sanatoria, which now accept more readily the "hard core cases," who previously would have been rejected for disciplinary reasons when tuberculosis beds were scarce. Rehabilitation services, including recreational, diversional, and educational programs, are of considerable value for all long-term patients. Vocational counseling and prevocational exploration can also be utilized to advantage.

Out-of-hospital services. The Arden House Conference on Tuberculosis in 1959 recognized that the elimination of tuberculosis is a realistic objective in the United States.[17] To this end, it recommended a program for the widespread application of chemotherapy, as a public health measure, in order to prevent further spread of tubercle bacilli by persons currently suffering from active tuberculosis and to prevent reactivation and spread of the disease by persons who previously had active disease and were inadequately treated. The conference also recommended that state and local health authorities assume responsibility for insuring adequate treatment and rehabilitation of all patients with tuberculosis.

Continuity of inpatient and outpatient care is of critical importance if the patient is not to reactivate his disease. The increasing proportion of patients who now receive the bulk of their treatment after leaving the hospital underscores the importance of accurate record keeping and long-term surveillance.[18] In addition to the diagnostic and treatment services provided through outpatient clinics, collaborative arrangements are occasionally developed with community agencies to offer supporting services to the patient and his family, for example, rehabilitation services, home nursing, social services, homemaker services, occupational guidance, and income maintenance. Health department physicians are being called upon increasingly to assume responsibility for supervision of clinical programs and, in some instances, to provide clinical care and related services. Specific efforts, therefore, must be made to keep these physicians abreast of the latest methods of treating tuberculosis.

Relaxation of restrictions on hospital and clinic use, of residence requirements, and of the "means test," which determines the patient's ability to pay for his medical care and treatment, has also occurred in some states as tuberculosis beds have become generally available.

Chronic nontuberculous pulmonary diseases. The growing proportion of patients in tuberculosis hospitals who are being treated for chronic nontuberculous respiratory diseases may be a factor in the future role of some of these institutions. Information prepared by the Veterans Administration illustrates what probably will emerge as a well-defined trend in most states. The data suggest that within a few years the number of veterans hospitalized for chronic nontuberculous respiratory diseases will equal or exceed the number of hospitalized tuberculosis patients. In 1954, the number of patients hospitalized in Veterans Administration hospitals for tuberculosis was approximately six times the number hospitalized for chronic nontuberculous respiratory disease. By 1961, this relationship had decreased to two times. Later estimates suggest that there might have been an equal number of each type of patient shortly thereafter. Although a decline in the number of tuberculosis patients is partly responsible for this change, there has been a corresponding or greater absolute increase in the number of other chronic pulmonary patients seeking treatment.

A certain number of these patients, with nontuberculous pulmonary disease, have always been treated in tuberculosis hospitals. Thus, the trend evidenced by the Veterans Administration data is probably also the situation, in some degree, in many state and local tuberculosis hospitals today. However, the extent of the effect of such patients on the occupancy rates of most tuberculosis hospitals and sanatoria will probably be slight because of their generally shorter periods of hospitalization, the specialized treatment required, and the fact that most of them will be treated in general hospitals.

Chemoprophylaxis. The value of preventive treatment for tuberculosis with the drug isoniazid (INH) has been established by the U. S. Public Health Service trials. Current follow-up results of these prophylaxis trials confirm the undiminished effectiveness of isoniazid over the ten years since the trials were started in 1956–57. When isoniazid was taken continuously for one year it decreased the frequency of tuberculosis by at least 75 percent during the year of medication, and by 50 percent each year thereafter. Apparently, use of isoniazid was able to nullify the tuberculous infection and thereby destroy the potential for infection to progress into clinical disease in half of the infected population. Because all infected persons are today at considerably higher risk of developing active disease than are the uninfected in the population, the indications for chemoprophylaxis can now be expanded to include all persons known to have had a tuberculous infection. The identification and treatment of tuberculous infection is not a substitute for treatment of patients with active and inactive disease and of contacts, which remain the first priority in community tuberculosis programs.[19]

BCG vaccine. BCG (*Bacillus Calmette Guérin*), a vaccine against tuberculosis, is an attenuated live vaccine that offers some protection to those who have never been infected. The vaccine offers no protection to those already infected, among whom the majority of cases arise in this country. It has limited application in the present-day control of tuberculosis in the United States.[20]

BCG was developed by Albert Calmette (1863–1933),[21] a French bacteriologist, and Alphonse F. M. Guérin (1816–95), a Paris surgeon. Calmette introduced BCG in France in 1921. The vaccinating procedure met with relatively little acceptance in the United States until 1940 when studies by Dr. Joseph D. Aronson (1889–1958) [22] and Dr. Sol R. Rosenthal (1903–   ) [23] showed that under certain conditions it had value. Only a small fraction of the children in this country have been vaccinated with BCG. It is estimated that probably fewer than 60,000 vaccinations with BCG were performed each year in the early 1950's, and these were mostly of hospital staffs and close "contacts" of patients with active disease.[24]

Use of BCG vaccination in the United States has been debated for several decades. In 1966, an international panel of tuberculosis specialists, reviewed epidemiologic information relating to the status of tuberculosis in this country, as well as field trials of BCG not only in the United States, but also in Great Britain and other countries. They were fully cognizant of the past positions of the Public Health Service as well as the current views in other countries and of the World Health Organization. In view of the favorable epidemiologic, medical, and socioeconomic conditions prevailing in this country and the effectiveness of chemoprophylaxis, the panel of experts concluded that there was no indication for the use of BCG on a group or community basis in the United States. The recommendations of this committee were approved by the surgeon general of the U.S. Public Health Service.

CASEFINDING

Tuberculosis casefinding surveys in this country have had their periods of popularity; formerly, in many cities they were the principal activity of antituberculosis agencies.[25] At a time when there was a great deal of tuberculosis which would normally not be discovered until it became manifest diesease, chest X-ray surveys of the general population were a necessary and important function of health departments. Assistance was given by the Public Health Service to many communities throughout the United States in the conduct of chest X-ray screening programs. Aid was provided through the loan of X-ray equipment and by technical personnel for demonstration and pilot-program purposes, as well as through the assignment of PHS chest X-ray teams to facilitate full-scale casefinding services. By June 1953 approximately 11.8 million X-ray films were taken in connection with local tuberculosis programs which utilized the Public Health Service casefinding resources.[26]

The impact of these programs was substantial and they stimulated similar surveys throughout the country. In community chest X-ray surveys conducted from 1947 to 1953 the number of persons with active tuberculosis found in large city surveys ranged from 0.3 to 3.1 cases per 1,000 people examined. Since then, the yield from such surveys of previously unknown and therefore unreported tuberculosis cases has decreased, and the cost of conducting such surveys has increased. Consequently, they are done less frequently or limited to areas where there is a high prevalence of tuberculosis. In many large cities, routine admission chest X-ray programs in municipal general hospitals find a much higher proportion of new active cases per 1,000 persons examined than do community-wide chest X-ray surveys. Although the reported number of films taken is incomplete and excludes X-rays taken by federal agencies, Table 2.1 shows the estimated number of chest X-rays taken for tuberculosis casefinding in the United States from 1946 to 1960. Since then there has been a drop in these totals. Regardless of their casefinding value, X-ray surveys were responsible for introducing the concept of screening examinations to the American public and popularized the idea of X-ray examination for tuberculosis.

A number of studies have shown that the search for unrecognized tuberculosis can be most profitable when casefinding targets are those segments of the infected population which are known to produce the greatest amount of tuberculous disease and which can be found with

efficiency as part of the routine procedures of health department tuberculosis activities. This thesis is substantiated by statistics compiled from
state and local special tuberculosis project areas which receive grants
from the Public Health Service.[27] Among 30,011 household contacts
(people known to have been in close association with cases of clinically
active tuberculosis) examined from January to June 1967, 875 new
cases of clinically active tuberculosis were found or a rate of 29 cases
per 1,000 household contacts. On the other hand, among 36,555 nonhousehold contacts (individuals who were less intimately associated
with the active disease cases), 170 cases were found or 5 new active

Table 2.1   Chest X-rays taken for
             tuberculosis casefinding:
             United States, 1946-60
             (not including X-rays
             taken by federal agencies)

Year	Chest X-rays reported
1946	6,000,000
1947	8,700,000
1948	11,345,000
1949	13,837,000
1950	14,794,000
1951	12,539,000
1952	13,466,000
1953	15,546,000
1954	16,233,000
1955	17,598,000
1956	18,280,000
1957	17,655,000
1058	13,612,000
1959	13,204,000
1960	13,592,000[a]

[a]In addition to the 13,592,000 films
taken in chest X-ray casefinding activities reported by the states,
4,424,000 films were taken by the
Army, Navy, Air Force, and Veterans
Administration, making a total of
over 18,000,000 films in 1960.

cases per 1,000 nonhousehold contacts examined. In another group of
24,762 persons who were suspected for a variety of reasons of having
tuberculosis, including unexplained chest X-ray findings, a diagnosis of
tuberculosis was established in 2,704 instances or at a rate of 109 cases
per 1,000 people examined. Other examples can be cited to show that
selective casefinding can be a highly productive public health procedure. The foregoing casefinding rates for selected groups represent
averages for the combined project areas and should not be interpreted
to be standards. Specific rates will vary widely from place to place.

HOSPITAL ADMISSION CHEST X-RAY PROGRAM

Routine chest X-rays of people receiving service from hospitals can uncover much tuberculosis, because persons who suffer from other illnesses have higher rates of the disease than whose who are well. This proportion has been found to be especially true for both inpatients and outpatients of large city public hospitals. For example, during 1967 in nineteen municipal general hospitals in New York City 245,281 persons were given chest X-rays on admission and 699 were found to have active pulmonary tuberculosis (2.8 per 1,000 examined) not previously registered with the city health authorities; in fourteen voluntary general hospitals 69,173 admission X-rays were taken and 31 new cases found (0.4 per 1,000 examined). The new active tuberculosis case rates for the thirty-three institutions were: inpatients, 3.4; outpatients, 1.5; employees and others, 1.2.

The potential benefits to be derived from this type of program can be envisaged from the fact that in 1967, 7,172 registered hospitals of all types, both federal and nonfederal, reported 29,361,424 inpatient admissions; and 148,229,113 outpatient visits in 6,121 hospitals which reported the number of visits.[28] Even though the net total would be less when tuberculosis hospitals and other special or very small institutions were excluded for a variety of reasons and duplications were eliminated, the opportunity to examine so many people provides an established method to discover people with tuberculosis who might otherwise not be diagnosed for some time as having active disease, with consequent delay in medical treatment.

Routine hospital admission chest X-ray programs can have other benefits in addition to finding unsuspected tuberculosis. These programs uncover much nontuberculous chest disease (cancer, heart conditions, silicosis, histoplasmosis, and so forth). The program also provides an opportunity to focus attention on other health problems within the household of the tuberculous patient as a result of home visits after an active case of disease is reported to the health department for further epidemiologic follow-up.

FACILITIES FOR TUBERCULOSIS CARE

The exact number of institutions in the United States with beds for the tuberculous prior to 1900 is uncertain. During the latter part of the nineteenth century the following were established: Channing Home (Boston, 1857), House of the Good Samaritan (Boston, 1861), Cullis

Consumptives Home (Boston, 1864), the Home for Consumptives at Chestnut Hill (Philadelphia, 1876), Mountain Sanitarium for Pulmonary Diseases (Asheville, North Carolina, 1876, Dr. J. W. Gleitsmann), Adirondack Cottage Sanitarium (Saranac, New York, 1884, Dr. Edward Livingston Trudeau), Sharon Sanatorium (Sharon, Massachusetts, 1891, Vincent Y. Bowditch). Other sanatoria organized during this period were: Los Angeles County General TB Ward (1878), Brooklyn Home for Consumptives (1881), Cook County TB Sanitarium (Dunning, Illinois, 1898), Sanitarium Gabriels (1895) and Loomis Sanatorium (upstate New York, 1896), Massachusetts State Sanatorium (Rutland, 1898), Ft. Bayard for Army personnel and Ft. Stanton as a Public Health Service Marine Hospital (New Mexico, 1899). James Blake, F.R.C.S., of San Francisco, following the "Gold Rush" treated consumptives in a summer, tentless camp in the Coastal Range (1855) and in 1876 he set up a short-lived sanatorium on Monte Sol near Livermore, California. According to Godias J. Drolet (1882–1968), in 1895 there were 19 tuberculosis sanatoria or hospitals with a capacity of 1,450 beds; in 1900, 34 institutions with 4,485 beds (*Am. Rev. Tuberc.*, vol. 14, 1926). *The National Tuberculosis Association Tuberculosis Hospital and Sanatorium Directory* (1954 edition) states that in 1904, there were 9,107 beds for tuberculous patients exclusive of beds in state mental and penal institutions.

Early in this century, sanatoria played an important function in tuberculosis control by providing direct medical care and by isolating patients who would otherwise be sources of infection in a community. Most of the sanatoria in the United States were privately owned, but by mid-century the great majority of such institutions were under municipal, county, or state control, and the character of these institutions was more that of a hospital than a sanatorium. In 1900 there were approximately 4,500 beds for tuberculosis patients; by 1954 the rated bed capacity for tuberculosis was 111,715 in federal and nonfederal hospitals, exclusive of beds in mental and penal institutions (see Table 2.2). In 1967 the total rated capacity fell to 43,069 beds.[29]

Every state has some facility or arrangement to provide hospital and clinic care for tuberculosis patients. The extent and character of these differ in that the facilities available may be under private, state, county, city, or other administrative auspices. In addition, the Veterans Administration, the Armed Forces, and the U.S. Public Health Service provide tuberculosis hospitalization for their respective legal beneficiaries. In 1967, federal facilities accounted for 23 percent of the hospital facilities for the care of tuberculosis and for 14 percent of the rated bed capacity.

Because of the changing modes of care and treatment and the decline in the amount of tuberculosis, the number of institutions assigned exclusively for hospitalization of the tuberculous has decreased. A picture of the trend from 1925 to 1953, a period for which details are available for both public and private institutions, is given in Table 2.3. During the period from 1927 through 1937, there were about 500 public and private tuberculosis hospitals in the United States. Although this number declined gradually to 420 in 1953, the number of beds in such institutions rose meanwhile, particularly after World War II. A more

Table 2.2   Federal and non-federal hospital facilities for the care of tuberculosis, rated capacity, beds occupied: United States, 1954, 1961, 1963, 1965, 1967

Agency[a]	1954	1961	1963	1965	1967
Federal and non-federal					
Number of hospitals	669	432	409	387	348
Rated bed capacity	111,715	67,634	60,363	52,781	43,069
Beds occupied	95,239	48,856	43,086	36,619	30,028
Non-federal					
Number of hospitals	552	345	314	297	267
Rated bed capacity	91,640	57,922	51,817	45,332	37,208
Beds occupied	76,819	40,820	36,084	30,798	25,172
Federal[b]					
Number of hospitals	117	87	95	90	81
Rated bed capacity	20,075	9,712	8,546	7,449	5,861
Beds occupied	18,420	8,036	7,002	5,821	4,856

Source: U. S. Department of Health, Education, and Welfare, Tuberculosis Beds In Hospitals and Sanatoria, Tuberculosis Program, National Communicable Disease Center, Public Health Service, Public Health Service publication, No. 801, series since 1946.

[a]Data are for hospitals with 10 or more beds for tuberculosis.
[b]1963, 1965, and 1967 figures for federal institutions include all tuberculosis beds.

recent picture of the downward trend in the number of tuberculosis hospitals and their use is evident in the data relating to nonfederal institutions in Table 2.3. Within the brief period of one decade from 1956 to 1967 the number of such institutions and their use was cut by more than half. Of the 105 nonfederal hospitals in 1967, the states controlled 42, counties controlled 45, other nonfederal governmental agencies ran 9, and 9 were controlled by nongovernmental agencies, principally voluntary nonprofit institutions. The federal government had only two tuberculosis hospitals. Details regarding the type of control of tuberculosis hospitals within the period 1942 to 1953 are set forth in Appendix Table A.1. The trend is toward shorter periods of hospitalization.

Table 2.3   Tuberculosis hospitals, beds, admissions, and average daily census:
            United States - public and private hospitals, 1925-53; non-federal
            hospitals, 1946-67   (numbers for beds, admissions, and average daily
            census are in thousands)

Year	Public and private				Non-federal			
	Hospitals[a]	Beds	Admissions	Average daily census	Hospitals[b]	Beds	Admissions	Average daily census
1925	466	49	----	40	----	----	----	----
1927	508	63	----	51	----	----	----	----
1928	508	62	----	----	----	----	----	----
1929	502	61	----	51	----	----	----	----
1930	515	66	----	56	----	----	----	----
1931	509	66	81	56	----	----	----	----
1932	512	70	93	60	----	----	----	----
1933	497	71	84	60	----	----	----	----
1934	495	70	82	60	----	----	----	----
1935	496	70	86	61	----	----	----	----
1936	506	74	99	63	----	----	----	----
1937	508	77	102	65	----	----	----	----
1938	493	76	101	66	----	----	----	----
1939	480	76	91	65	----	----	----	----
1940	479	78	91	67	----	----	----	----
1941	477	82	101	71	----	----	----	----
1942	468	82	102	70	----	----	----	----
1943	455	80	92	65	----	----	----	----
1944	453	80	88	63	----	----	----	----
1945	449	79	86	60	----	----	----	----
1946	450	83	100	62	412	75	85	55
1947	441	81	99	63	411	70	94	55
1948	438	82	106	66	409	76	112	66
1949	444	83	113	69	414	78	128	66
1950	431	86	113	72	398	72	79	62
1951	430	88	107	74	399	73	83	62
1952	428	90	110	75	391	73	76	62
1953	420	88	108	75	384	72	77	62
1954	----	----	----	----	368	74	89	61
1955	----	----	----	----	347	70	87	56
1956	----	----	----	----	315	66	76	53
1957	----	----	----	----	280	62	71	49
1958	----	----	----	----	261	57	69	44
1959	----	----	----	----	254	57	79	45
1960	----	----	----	----	238	52	68	39
1961	----	----	----	----	222	49	65	36
1962	----	----	----	----	203	45	60	33
1963	----	----	----	----	186	39	55	29
1964	----	----	----	----	187	40	62	28
1965	----	----	----	----	178	37	52	26
1966	----	----	----	----	156	31	45	21
1967	----	----	----	----	105	18	26	12

Sources: Bureau of the Census, Historical Statistics of the United States,
Colonial Times to 1957, Series B215, 216, 267, 268, Washington, D. C. 1961;
Hospitals, Journal of the American Hospital Association, Guide issue, August 1968.

[a]Data relate to hospitals as defined by the American Medical Association.
[b]Data relate to hospitals as defined by the American Hospital Association.

About half the patients occupying tuberculosis beds on June 30, 1960, were in the hospital less than six months. On the other hand, approximately 25 percent of all patients had been in the hospital continuously for one or more years. An indication of the trend is provided by Table 2.4, which shows the average length of stay in nonfederal tuberculosis hospitals from 1945 through 1967. From a high of almost 300 days of stay per person in 1952, the average dropped irregularly to a low of 165 days in 1964.

Table 2.4   Average length of stay in days, non-federal tuberculosis hospitals: United States, 1945-67

Year	Average length of stay in days	Percent change from previous year
1945	255.7	...
1946	236.2	- 7.6
1947	213.6	- 9.6
1948	215.7	+ 1.0
1949	188.2	-12.7
1950	286.5	+52.2
1951	272.7	- 4.8
1952	298.6	+ 9.4
1953	293.9	- 1.6
1954	250.2	-14.9
1955	234.9	- 6.1
1956	255.2	+ 8.6
1957	251.9	- 1.3
1958	232.8	- 7.6
1959	207.9	-10.7
1960	209.9 -	+ 1.0
1961	202.2	- 3.7
1962	200.8	- 0.7
1963	192.5	- 4.1
1964	164.8	-14.4
1965	182.5	+10.7
1966	170.3	- 6.7
1967	168.5	- 1.1

Sources: U. S. Department of Health, Education, and Welfare, Medical Care, Financing, and Utilization, Health Economics Series, No. 1, Public Health Service Publication No. 947, 1962; and Hospitals, Journal of the American Hospital Association, Vol. 42, No. 15, Part 2, August 1, 1968.

Outpatient care plays an increasingly important role in present day treatment of tuberculosis. In 1960, almost 1,200 tuberculosis clinics were operating within the United States according to agencies reporting to the National Tuberculosis Association (see Table 2.5). Of such agencies, over two thirds were in state and local health departments, over one sixth were attached to a tuberculosis hospital, and the rest were variously distributed.

Decline in the demand for tuberculosis beds has created problems of converting unneeded tuberculosis hospitals to other health uses or closing them. Many in the tuberculosis field at first failed to recognize the immensity of the impact the new drugs would have on the future of tuberculosis hospitals and were reluctant to convert or close unneeded facilities. Communities sometimes objected to the expected loss of income or employment or were concerned about the type of facility that might replace the hospital. Nevertheless, between 1954 and 1961, some 227 hospitals partially converted the unused portion of their facilities for the care of nontuberculous patients or discontinued all treatment of tuberculosis. By 1968 there was a further reduction in the rated

Table 2.5   Tuberculosis clinics in the United States, 1960

Agency operating clinics	Number of clinics	Percent distribution
Total reporting	1,037	100.0
Total clinics	1,176	...
Health department		
Local	427	41.2
State	164	15.8
Local and state	120	11.6
Tuberculosis hospital	182	17.6
General hospital	58	5.6
Tuberculosis association	47	4.5
Other	38	3.7
Not stated	1	...

Source: Bailey, M. V., Census of Tuberculosis Clinics, National Tuberculosis Association, 1962.

bed capacity of hospitals providing care for tuberculous patients. Major reasons for the changes were the lessened demand for tuberculosis beds, the higher per diem costs of patient care, and the growing pressure on states and communities to provide facilities for the chronically ill, the mentally ill and retarded, and the aged (see Table 2.6).

Nationwide statistics on the type of tuberculosis patients cared for are limited and conclusions must be based on newly reported active cases, a large proportion of whom receive their initial treatment in a hospital. Since 1953, as shown elsewhere in this monograph, the stage of pulmonary tuberculosis of new active cases first reported to health departments, has shown only minor variations in the overall pattern for the country.

In various hospital reports in which the severity of tuberculous disease is specifically given, it appears that about 80 percent of the patients admitted to most institutions have moderately or far advanced tuberculosis. Of these, 70 percent have positive sputums on admission and are therefore infectious cases. The majority of patients with positive sputum when admitted to a hospital for the first time are infected with tubercle bacilli which are susceptible to treatment with "first line" drugs. However, approximately one third of all tuberculous patients admitted to hospitals are readmissions. These patients have had various degrees and quality of treatment during their earlier hospitalization. In this group, the majority of patients with positive sputum have organisms that are resistant to either or both streptomycin and isonia-

Table 2.6   Reasons for closure or conversion of non-federal
             tuberculosis hospitals: United States, 1954-61

Reasons for closure or conversion	Number of reasons reported[a]		Percent distribution	
	Total	Primary reasons	Total	Primary reasons
Total	438	218	100.0	100.0
Low tuberculosis occupancy rate	172	151	39.3	69.3
Difficulties of maintaining a qualified staff	39	4	8.9	1.8
Withdrawal of or inadequate financial support	34	6	7.8	2.8
Increased cost of operation	68	7	15.5	3.2
Unsatisfactory physical condition of facility	29	3	6.6	1.4
Failure to meet licensure standards	15	3	3.4	1.4
The availability of tuberculosis facilities elsewhere	45	30	10.3	13.8
All other reasons	36	14	8.2	6.4

Source: U. S. Department of Health, Education, and Welfare, Area-wide planning of facilities for tuberculosis services, Public Health Service Publication No. 930-B-4, 1963.

[a]Excluding Colorado.

zid. Treatment of these patients therefore becomes a much more difficult medical matter.

HOSPITALIZATION COST

In spite of the facts that the average hospital stay for tuberculosis patients is lessening and that the number of tuberculosis hospitals and beds for patients with the disease has decreased sharply, hospitalization is still a major item of public and private expense. According to Table 2.7, the total expenses of nonfederal tuberculosis hospitals was in the area of about $200 million annually from 1955 to 1961, with a decline to $94 million in 1967. Meanwhile, the cost per patient-day in nonfed-

Table 2.7   Payroll and other expenses, non-federal tuberculosis hospitals: United States, 1945-67

Year	Total hospital expenses (payroll and other)				Hospital expenses							
					Payroll				Other			
	Dollars in millions	Percent of total	Per patient-day	Per bed[a]	Dollars in millions	Percent of total	Per patient-day	Per bed[a]	Dollars in millions	Percent of total	Per patient-day	Per bed[a]
1945	$ 81	100.0	$ 4.03	$1,125	$ 42	51.9	$ 2.09	$ 583	$39	48.1	$1.94	$ 542
1950	162	100.0	7.22	2,250	91	56.2	4.06	1,264	71	43.8	3.16	986
1955	208	100.0	10.13	2,971	133	63.9	6.48	1,900	75	36.1	3.65	1,071
1958	195	100.0	12.08	3,421	128	65.6	7.91	2,246	67	34.4	4.17	1,175
1959	208	100.0	12.80	3,650	139	66.8	8.54	2,439	69	33.2	4.26	1,211
1960	192	100.0	13.37	3,693	128	66.7	8.92	2,462	64	33.3	4.45	1,231
1961	192	100.0	14.72	3,918	129	67.2	9.89	2,633	63	32.8	4.83	1,285
1962	182	100.0	15.22	4,044	124	68.1	10.38	2,756	58	31.9	4.84	1,288
1963	158	100.0	15.13	4,051	108	68.4	10.31	2,769	50	31.6	4.82	1,282
1964	163	100.0	15.72	4,075	112	68.7	10.78	2,800	51	31.3	4.94	1,275
1965	165	100.0	17.39	4,459	116	70.3	12.20	3,135	49	29.7	5.19	1,324
1966	147	100.0	19.16	4,742	102	69.4	13.36	3,290	45	30.6	5.80	1,452
1967	94	100.0	21.36	5,222	65	69.1	14.66	3,611	29	30.9	6.70	1,611

Sources: U. S. Department of Health, Education, and Welfare, Medical care, financing, and utilization, Health Economics Series, No. 1, Public Health Service. Data for 1961 to 1967 based on August issues, Part 2, Hospitals, Journal of the American Hospital Association.

[a]Expenses per bed gives an annual cost for providing care, and is a convenient tool for projecting future hospital costs, since it is divorced from volume of admissions and changes in length of stay.

eral tuberculosis hospitals rose from $7.22 in 1950 to $22.48 in 1967, notwithstanding a declining case load. Over two thirds of the total cost in 1967 was for payroll expenses. The 1967 cost per patient-day represents an average of a wide range, because costs vary not only from one area to another but in different hospitals within a community. Indicative are data for the tuberculosis units of the New York City Department of Hospitals, where the average cost per patient-day in 1967 was $57.11 but ranged from $42.16 to $118.66. The outpatient average cost per visit for these institutions was $11.29, with a range from $6.75 to $22.47. Since then, especially for care in general hospitals, the cost of hospitalization has risen.

Construction of new tuberculosis hospitals has become rather rare, but renovation of old or outmoded facilities is a continuing expense. In the 15 years from 1946 to 1961, the Hill-Burton hospital projects provided 7,142 beds for tuberculosis patients at a total cost of $70,148,-000, about 37 percent of which came from federal funds. Of the total beds, 3,366 were in new facilities, costing $37,294,000; 3,776 beds were provided by additions or alternations at a cost of $32,854,000. It was estimated that in 1962 the total cost of tuberculosis hospitalization for the United States was $335,800,000, including care in federal and nonfederal mental, penal, and general hospitals. By 1967, with the reduction of tuberculosis incidence and shorter average hospital stay the cost of hospitalization was estimated to be around $250 million.[30]

REPORTING AND REGISTRATION OF TUBERCULOSIS CASES

The success achieved by the application of public health measures is ultimately reflected in the morbidity and mortality rates of a community. Traditionally, the collection and analysis of morbidity and mortality data have been a basic part of public health policy because the government, through its public health agencies, whether local, state, or national, is responsible for the control of contagious diseases. Control of communicable diseases can be accomplished best when the incidence and prevalence information is up to date and there is reasonably good and prompt reporting by the attending physician.

A basic plan for reporting and registration of cases which was adopted by the New York City Board of Health in 1893 was not fully implemented for several years. At about that time other cities began to experiment with similar reporting systems. Public awareness of the importance of systematic recording of tuberculosis as a disease was stimulated by a few individuals who recognized the public health importance and urgent need of this type of recordkeeping. Reporting and registration of tuberculosis cases for the entire United States have been attained comparatively recently. Even though the notification of tuberculosis was mandatory in some cities since the early years of the century, there have been, meanwhile, differences from state to state in standards of reporting practice.[1]

The primary purposes of tuberculosis reporting are: case supervision, to assure continued medical attention, treatment, isolation, and follow-up of all known cases as long as may be necessary to prevent spread of the disease; contact supervision, to assure the examination of contacts of all known active cases; program management, to provide information for use in determining the extent and characteristics of the community tuberculosis control problem and in evaluating the effectiveness of tuberculosis control measures.

A comprehensive tuberculosis register would contain information on all aspects of tuberculosis care and control in the community. It would take into account changes occurring in the different classes of patients by clinical status and whether under private physicians' care, clinic supervision, or hospital care. When considered no longer in need of intensive medical attention, persons would be continued under surveillance in the records system for varying lengths of time. Records would include categories of individuals suspected of being at risk of developing disease, contacts of active cases, tuberculin reactors or recent converters, and others. Although such data are provided and reported upon by state health authorities in general terms, the constant internal changes in registers are difficult to keep up to date. Consequently, it is not possible at present to retrieve information for the total United States. One solution would be to utilize modern computer retrieval systems, which can handle large masses of data with a high degree of efficiency and speed. In a mobile population, a nationwide system to keep track of tuberculous persons as they move from state to state would be an invaluable public health tool. This could also provide a timely inventory of tuberculosis in this country.

In connection with its special tuberculosis projects activities, the Tuberculosis Program of the Public Health Service receives semiannual statistical reports from about one thousand reporting areas, which submit data on various aspects of their tuberculosis control programs. One of the computer programs developed in 1966 based on these reports provided current data on school tuberculin testing surveys in 500 counties throughout the country, giving detailed results of the tests and characteristics of the major types of techniques used by health agencies.[2]

Because registration of tuberculosis cases is the responsibility and administrative function of local and state health authorities, the published statistics for the earlier years reflected a variety of interpretations as to what constituted a "case." Both active and inactive, new and previously known cases were often included in statistical summaries. Lack of standardization made comparison of data between communities difficult. Development of a standard definition for statistical reporting was a matter of evolution. At present this task has been undertaken by the U.S. Public Health Service. One of the complications in establishing a statistical standard for the entire country was that, since about 1925, there were periodic changes in the clinical classification of tuberculosis.[3]

The more recent practice of using new active tuberculosis cases as an index of incidence provides a reasonable measure that presents less variation in definition and gives a more consistent basis for compari-

son, both geographic and chronological.[4] Although this index of incidence appears to be adequate for statistical purposes it does not ex-
clude entirely the possibility of bias or error. Differences in clinical
interpretations as to what constitutes active disease do occur. The National Tuberculosis Association's diagnostic standards and classification of tuberculosis have been adopted widely and provide a basis for
achieving relative uniformity.

In 1961 the U.S. Public Health Service recommended that all public
health departments require, as a minimum, the reporting of active
cases of tuberculosis. Since some health departments may request more
than the reporting of new active cases, it was recommended that in such
circumstances record keeping be set up so that the health department
can identify the active cases among the total cases that are reported.

The following were to be included in the term, "new active tuberculosis cases": (1) diagnosed cases with tubercle bacilli demonstrated (all
forms: pulmonary and extrapulmonary, both primary and reinfection
tuberculosis); (2) diagnosed cases without tubercle bacilli demonstrated but where there is X-ray or histological evidence consistent with
active tuberculosis (all forms: pulmonary and extrapulmonary, both
primary and reinfection tuberculosis); (3) unexplained pleurisy with
effusion.

Primary cases with X-ray evidence of tuberculous involvement, as
well as those with tubercle bacilli demonstrated, were counted in the
"active" category. However, tuberculin converters and infant reactors,
without X-ray evidence of tuberculous involvement and without tubercle bacilli demonstrated, were to be excluded. The sequence in which
reporting of tuberculosis by the physician and registration of the case
by the health department occurs often affects the interpretation of the
statistics, as in the case of reporting before or after death.[5]

To implement public policy in health matters certain procedures are
followed in transmitting vital statistics data. The physician who makes
a diagnosis of tuberculosis or attends a person at death must, by law,
report this fact to the local or state health authorities. The local health
department makes an official record of this fact as part of its registration of communicable diseases and deaths and in turn notifies the state
health authorities who transmit the statistics to the U.S. Public Health
Service. Only part of the original information is reported from one
jurisdiction to the next. It is becoming obvious that much more vital
data must be available to national health authorities than is possible
with current practices if country-wide planning for tuberculosis control

and eradication is to function effectively. As suggested earlier, a national tuberculosis register service center is one means whereby coordination might be achieved. Feasibility of such a central statistical repository of tuberculosis data which would make possible better administrative management of tuberculosis on a local, state, and national basis is being explored by the U.S. Public Health Service.

SIZE OF THE TUBERCULOSIS PROBLEM

New active cases of tuberculosis provide an index of the impact of the disease in the United States, and deaths are an index of its ultimate toll. However, neither new cases nor deaths adequately reveal the overall size of tuberculosis as a community health problem. Although tuberculosis deaths represent much unnecessary waste of human life, they do not entirely reflect the seriousness of the situation as in days when they were the inevitable sequelae of most cases affected with the disease. New active cases reported each year, the measure commonly used now, do not include relapses of previously reported inactivated cases which are estimated to add another six to seven thousand cases to the total annual incidence.

A more appropriate measure of the size of the tuberculosis problem is the number of people who are directly affected by tuberculosis during a given year. Therefore, a realistic assessment of the overall extent of the tuberculosis problem in a community should take into account new active cases reported during the year, persons in whom the disease has reactivated, all other active cases currently in need of treatment or supervision, inactive cases, young children who had recently been infected, individuals with suspicious X-ray findings, as well as others who are considered to be at special risk of developing active disease. Thus, the number affected by tuberculosis in 1963 would have been at least a total of 610,000 persons (110,000 known active cases, an estimated 250,000 inactive cases, and a like number of contacts to newly reported cases).

Tuberculosis death statistics, as usually tabulated and published, represent only those persons who were reported to have died from tuberculosis. Other persons may have died with tuberculosis, but had another condition assigned as the principal or underlying cause of death on the death certificate. A study of multiple causes of death in the United States for the year 1955 showed that tuberculosis was mentioned on 21, 331 death certificates: 14,779 times as the underlying or primary cause of death and 6,552 times as a contributory cause of death.

Another area of concern is the large number of people who are well but still at some risk of developing tuberculosis. An estimated 25 million people in the United States today are believed to have been infected with the tubercle bacillus. An important part of tuberculosis control is to select those tuberculin reactors who are at greatest risk and provide appropriate public health measures to minimize and, if possible, prevent the development of active tuberculosis. Chemoprophylactic use of the drug isoniazid can lower the occurrence of the disease in such cases.

Each of the 50 states conducts a tuberculosis control program and has data available on the number of persons under active care or supervision. Local and state tuberculosis registers usually contain records not only of the new active cases reported and currently under care but also of persons whose disease activity has not been determined and of inactive cases under supervision. Because policies and recordkeeping practices differ among states, reports summarizing the type of care received vary widely or are often inadequate, so that a strict comparison between communities is not always possible. However, statistics are reported for a substantial segment of the population in sufficient detail to give an adequate ground for estimates for the United States.

During 1967, 45,647 new active tuberculosis cases were reported to state health departments. About 1,600 persons were first reported to public health authorities as new cases of tuberculosis at time of death; other tuberculosis cases were found a relatively short time prior to death. Former patients, whose disease had been inactive for years, returned for additional medical care because their tuberculosis reactivated. These figures are given merely to suggest the complex dynamics of tuberculosis registers. The net result of the many changes that took place throughout the nation during the year is reflected in the tuberculosis statistics of December 31, 1967. It is estimated that on the last day of 1967 there were 315,000 cases on all state and local tuberculosis registers, with 77,000 persons classified as having active tuberculous disease. On that day 32,000 of the active disease cases were in hospitals, and 45,000 people with active tuberculosis were under the care or supervision of clinics and private physicians. Many patients with active tuberculosis, who were under medical supervision "at home" at the end of the year, had already completed a recommended short period of hospitalization during the year (see Table 3.1). Therefore, these register statistics refer to the status of patients on a specific day and they accordingly represent "point prevalence" figures. In December 1967, about 32,000 or 71 percent of the active cases who were under care "at home" were receiving some form of chemotherapy for tuberculosis. In addition, of the 238,000 "other than active disease cases," 83,000 or 35 percent were on drug therapy or chemoprophylaxis.

TRENDS IN TUBERCULOSIS MORBIDITY

In 1930, a total of 124,940 new tuberculosis cases, both active and inactive, were reported to state health authorities in the United States. The number reported fluctuated from year to year, reaching a high of 137,006 in 1948 (see Table 3.2). It was recognized that these annual figures (active and inactive), which were incomplete in some instances,

Table 3.1   Estimated number of cases on tuberculosis registers: United States, December 31 of specified year

Type of case	1960	1961	1962	1963	1964	1965	1966	1967
Total[a]	330,000	330,000	330,000	320,000	320,000	325,000	320,000	315,000
Active disease	120,000	115,000	110,000	105,000	105,000	100,000	90,000	77,000
Hospitalized	58,000	52,000	46,000	44,000	42,000	40,000	37,000	32,000
Not hospitalized	62,000	63,000	64,000	61,000	63,000	60,000	53,000	45,000
All other cases[b]	210,000	215,000	220,000	215,000	215,000	225,000	230,000	238,000

[a]Tuberculosis registers include records of the active cases currently under care, the cases for which disease activity has not been determined, and inactive cases under supervision. Also retained on health department rolls are records of people who fail to respond to treatment or who have received inadequate or interrupted treatment.
[b]Cases with activity undetermined and inactive cases under current supervision.

were necessarily a crude index of incidence. Under the guidance of the Public Health Service the practice of reporting previously unknown new active cases separately was initiated in 1952 as a better way of measuring incidence of the disease. The suggested definition of new active cases was generally accepted and a more uniform standard of practice was thereby established. However, the year 1953 was chosen as a start of analysis for the United States, because it is the first for which data on new active cases were recorded for the entire country with a reasonable semblance of completeness. For the years 1953 through 1961 newly reported active tuberculosis cases include clinically active and probably active pulmonary, nonpulmonary, and unexplained pleurisy with effusion cases. As already indicated, the Public Health Service revised its recommendations on the reporting of tuberculosis in

Table 3.2   Newly reported tuberculosis
cases (active and inactive)
and deaths: Continental
United States[a], 1930-61

Year	New cases		Deaths	
	Number	Rate	Number	Rate
1930	124,940	101.5	87,509	71.1
1931	124,858	100.7	84,679	68.3
1932	121,961	97.7	78,390	62.8
1933	114,412	91.1	74,842	59.6
1934	113,020	89.4	71,609	56.7
1935	111,856	87.9	70,080	55.1
1936	107,086	83.6	71,527	55.9
1937	112,394	87.2	69,324	53.8
1938	107,021	82.4	63,735	49.1
1939	103,922	79.4	61,609	47.1
1940	102,984	78.0	60,428	45.8
1941	105,567	79.3	59,251	44.5
1942	117,204	87.5	57,690	43.1
1943	120,253	89.6	57,005	42.4
1944	126,294	95.0	54,731	41.2
1945	114,931	86.8	52,916	39.9
1946	119,256	85.2	50,911	36.4
1947	134,946	94.1	48,064	33.5
1948	137,006	93.8	43,833	30.0
1949	134,865	90.7	39,100	26.3
1950	121,742	80.4	33,959	22.4
1951	118,491	77.3	30,863	20.1
1952	109,837	70.5	24,621	15.8
1953	106,925	67.5	19,544	12.3
1954	100,540	62.4	16,392	10.2
1955	98,860	60.2	14,940	9.1
1956	90,465	54.1	14,061	8.4
1957	86,861	51.0	13,324	7.8
1958	82,266	47.4	12,361	7.1
1959	75,029	42.6	11,429	6.5
1960	70,124	39.2	10,832	6.0
1961	66,984	36.8	9,892	5.4

[a]48 states and the District of Columbia.

1961. The new recommendations were adopted by some of the states in 1961 and have been followed by all since 1962, although there was some evidence that not all of the new recommendations were applied uniformly. Obviously the modifications in classification of new active cases recommended by the Public Health Service in 1961 tend to impair comparability of data over time.

During the period from 1953 through 1961 the new active cases averaged 77 percent of all new cases reported, both active and inactive, with a yearly range from 76 to 79 percent. New active tuberculosis cases reported annually for the 50 states of the nation (including the District of Columbia) declined from 84,304 in 1953 to 45,647 in 1967 a decrease of 45.9 percent (see Table 3.3). The new active case rate,

Table 3.3   Trend in new active tuberculosis cases and deaths: United States[a], 1953-67

Year	New active cases				Tuberculosis deaths			
	Number	Change in cases (%)	Rate	Change in rate (%)	Number	Change in deaths (%)	Rate	Change in rate (%)
1953	84,304	...	53.0	...	19,707	...	12.4	...
1954	79,775	− 5.4	49.3	− 7.0	16,527	− 16.1	10.2	− 17.7
1955	77,368	− 3.0	46.9	− 4.9	15,016	− 9.1	9.1	− 10.8
1956	69,895	− 9.7	41.6	− 11.3	14,137	− 5.9	8.4	− 7.7
1957	67,149	− 3.9	39.2	− 5.8	13,390	− 5.3	7.8	− 7.1
1958	63,534	− 5.4	36.5	− 6.9	12,417	− 7.3	7.1	− 9.0
1959	57,535	− 9.4	32.5	− 11.0	11,474	− 7.6	6.5	− 8.5
1960	55,494	− 3.5	30.8	− 5.2	10,866	− 5.3	6.0	− 7.7
1961	53,726	− 3.2	29.4	− 4.5	9,938	− 8.5	5.4	− 10.0
1962	53,315	− 0.8	28.7	− 2.4	9,506	− 4.3	5.1	− 5.6
1963	54,042	+ 1.4	28.7	0.0	9,311	− 2.1	4.9	− 3.9
1964	50,874	− 5.9	26.6	− 7.3	8,303	− 10.8	4.3	− 12.2
1965	49,016	− 3.7	25.3	− 4.9	7,934	− 4.4	4.1	− 4.7
1966	47,767	− 2.5	24.4	− 3.6	7,625	− 3.9	3.9	− 4.9
1967	45,647	− 4.4	23.1	− 5.3	(6,560)[b]	− 14.0	(3.3)[b]	− 15.4
Decrease from 1953 to 1967								
Difference	38,657	...	29.9	...	(13,147)	...	(9.1)	...
Percent	45.9	...	56.4	...	(66.7)	...	(73.4)	...
Average annual decrease	...	4.2	...	5.7	...	(7.5)	...	(8.9)

Source: U. S. Department of Health, Education, and Welfare, Reported Tuberculosis Data-1967, Tuberculosis Program, National Communicable Disease Center, Public Health Service Publication No. 638, 1969.

[a]Including Alaska and Hawaii.
[b]Provisional.

which was 53.0 per 100,000 population in 1953, dropped by 56.4 percent to a rate of 23.1 in 1967. The year-to-year changes in the number of cases reported within the period 1953 to 1967 range from 0.8 percent to 9.7 percent. There was a small increase in cases reported for 1963, but a downward trend was again evident in the four succeeding years. Table 3.4 shows, in comparison with Table 3.2, the number of new cases for the conterminous United States during each year from 1952 to 1967; in comparison with Table 3.3 there is shown the number of newly reported cases, both active and inactive, for the 50 states and the District of Columbia during each year from 1951 to 1961. A ready view of the trend of the new active case rate for tuberculosis compared with that of its death rate is shown in Figure 3.1.

A recent picture of the distribution of tuberculosis according to its form and extent is provided by the data in Table 3.5. Of the 45,647 new active tuberculosis cases reported in 1967, 89 percent (40,699) were cases of pulmonary disease, and 4,415 of the latter were classified as primary tuberculosis. This group of active primary cases, which comprised one tenth of all new active cases reported for the country,

Table 3.4   Newly reported tuberculosis cases:
              United States, 1951-67

Year	Active and inactive cases Total United States[a] Number	Rate	Active cases Conterminous United States[b] Number	Rate
1951	119,631	77.7	---	...
1952	111,413	71.2	85,607	55.0
1953	108,285	68.1	83,250	52.6
1954	102,006	63.0	78,592	48.8
1955	100,341	60.8	76,245	46.4
1956	91,986	54.7	68,866	41.2
1957	88,031	51.4	66,437	39.0
1958	83,158	47.8	63,000	36.4
1959	75,841	42.8	56,951	32.3
1960	70,843	39.4	54,977	30.7
1961	67,745	37.0	53,167	29.2
1962	---	...	52,698	28.5
1963	---	...	53,526	28.5
1964	---	...	50,256	26.4
1965	---	...	48,434	25.1
1966	---	...	47,361	24.3
1967	---	...	45,189	23.0

[a]Including Alaska and Hawaii, and the District of
Columbia.
[b]Excluding Alaska and Hawaii.

are mainly children with X-ray evidence of tuberculosis involvement or
those with tubercle bacilli demonstrated.

Stage of pulmonary disease was reported for 34, 205 cases: minimal,
7,034 (20 percent); moderately advanced, 15,245 (45 percent); and far
advanced, 11,926 (35 percent). For the entire country there has been
no significant change in these proportions during the period from 1953
through 1967, notwithstanding the change in definition of new active
cases introduced in 1961 (see Table 3.6). However, these are nation-

Table 3.5   Form and extent of disease of new active
              tuberculosis cases: United States, 1967

Form and extent of disease	Number		Percent	
Total new active cases	45,647	100.0	...	...
Pulmonary	40,699	89.2	100.0	...
With extent specified	34,205	...	84.0	100.0
Minimal	7,034	...	...	20.5
Moderately advanced	15,245	...	...	44.6
Far advanced	11,926	...	...	34.9
Extent not specified	2,079	...	5.1	...
Primary	4,415	...	10.9	...
Nonpulmonary	4,213	9.2	...	100.0
Unexplained pleurisy	693	...	...	16.4
Other	3,520	...	...	83.6
Form not specified	735	1.6	...	...

Figure 3.1. New active tuberculosis case rate and death rate, United States, 1953–67.

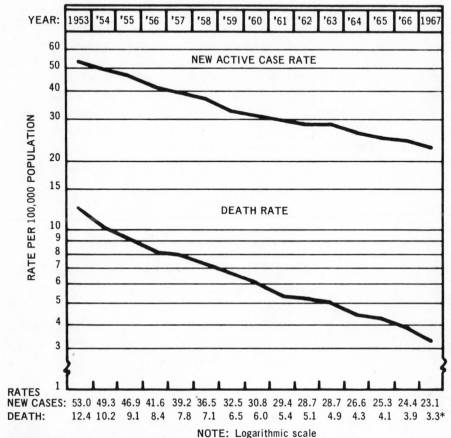

NOTE: Logarithmic scale

*Provisional death rate based on National
 Center for Health Statistics ten percent sample

wide averages; the proportions vary considerably from one state to another.

NEW ACTIVE TUBERCULOSIS CASES BY AGE, COLOR, AND SEX
Almost half of the new active tuberculosis cases reported in the United States during 1967 were persons 45 years or older (see Table 3.7a). Available evidence indicates that several generations earlier the age profile of tuberculosis in this country was different from that for 1967 in that a larger proportion of the active cases occurred at younger periods of life. Of special public health concern is the fact that, in 1967,

over 20 percent of the new cases occur in younger people and children under 25 years of age, the group among whom the disease is generally considered to be most readily preventable; in 1953, the corresponding proportion was less than 19 percent. Although the total number of new active cases of tuberculosis has decreased, the age distribution for the country as a whole has been about the same each year since 1963. The proportion of nonwhites among the new active tuberculosis cases is rising rapidly, from 26 percent in 1953 to 37 percent in 1967. The ratio of male to female cases is about 2 to 1 for the whites and 1.7 to 1 for nonwhites; for each color category, the proportion of males among the new cases increased somewhat from 1953 to 1967.

It will be noted in Table 3.7a that the number of new cases at ages

Table 3.6   Percent of new active pulmonary tuberculosis cases by stage of disease: United States, 1953-67[a] (total for year = 100.0 percent)

Year	Minimal	Moderately advanced	Far advanced
1953	22.6	40.7	36.7
1954	22.4	40.6	37.0
1955	22.4	42.1	35.5
1956	22.2	42.4	35.4
1957	21.8	42.6	35.6
1958	21.7	42.3	36.0
1959	21.4	43.1	35.5
1960	21.1	43.1	35.8
1961	20.5	43.5	36.0
1962	20.7	43.9	35.4
1963	21.2	43.3	35.5
1964	21.4	43.8	34.8
1965	21.2	43.6	35.2
1966	20.8	44.1	35.1
1967	20.5	44.6	34.9

[a]Based on areas for which extent of pulmonary tuberculosis was specified.

under 15 years increased from 1961 to 1963. In part, this may be attributed to improved reporting practices. Figures for the more recent years in this table undoubtedly reflect more accurately the incidence of active primary tuberculosis than the earlier figures. In 1967, almost half of the new active cases of tuberculosis at ages under 15 years were among nonwhites; the proportion fell somewhat to over two fifths at ages 15–44 years, and to over one fourth at ages 45 and over. Tuberculosis becomes increasingly a male problem with advance in age. Whereas males constituted one half of the new active cases at ages under 25 in 1967, their proportion rose to 69 percent at ages 65 and over. From 1953 to 1967, nearly one half of all new active cases of tubercu-

Table 3.7a New active tuberculosis cases; number and case rate by age: United States, 1953-67

Year	Total	Age					
		Under 5	5-14	15-24	25-44	45-64	65 and over
				Number of cases			
1953	84,304	2,719	2,525	10,412	31,488	25,838	11,322
1954	79,775	2,679	2,654	9,585	28,663	24,642	11,552
1955	77,368	2,976	2,603	8,725	27,094	24,307	11,663
1956	69,895	2,621	2,470	7,515	23,757	22,123	11,409
1957	67,149	2,405	2,213	6,866	22,308	21,934	11,423
1958	63,534	2,469	2,352	6,178	20,449	20,988	11,098
1959	57,535	2,209	2,113	5,281	18,364	19,063	10,505
1960	55,494	2,198	2,190	4,950	17,217	18,470	10,469
1961	53,726	2,429	2,457	4,596	16,240	17,737	10,267
1962	53,315	3,044	2,992	4,806	15,522	17,182	9,769
1963	54,042	3,080	3,405	4,733	15,097	17,496	10,231
1964	50,874	2,827	3,269	4,538	14,282	16,434	9,524
1965	49,016	2,748	3,142	4,549	13,500	15,721	9,356
1966	47,767	2,551	3,077	4,193	13,000	15,650	9,296
1967	45,647	2,247	2,794	4,315	12,517	14,996	8,778
White							
male	19,400	584	729	1,201	4,357	7,867	4,662
female	9,446	595	688	1,190	2,572	2,336	2,065
Nonwhite							
male	10,614	539	685	946	3,488	3,545	1,411
female	6,187	529	692	978	2,100	1,248	640
				Percent distribution of cases			
1953	100.0	3.2	3.0	12.4	37.4	30.6	13.4
1967	100.0	4.9	6.1	9.5	27.4	32.9	19.2
				Case rate per 100,000 population			
1953	53.0	15.4	9.1	49.5	67.7	79.9	82.9
1954	49.3	14.9	9.1	45.5	61.2	75.0	81.9
1955	46.9	16.1	8.6	41.0	57.6	72.8	80.0
1956	41.6	13.8	7.8	35.0	50.3	65.2	76.1
1957	39.2	12.4	6.8	31.3	47.2	63.5	74.0
1958	36.5	12.5	7.0	27.1	43.4	59.9	70.1
1959	32.5	11.0	6.1	22.5	39.1	53.5	64.7
1960	30.8	10.8	6.1	20.5	36.8	51.1	62.9
1961	29.4	11.8	6.6	18.5	34.7	48.3	60.4
1962	28.7	14.7	8.0	18.2	33.3	46.1	56.4
1963	28.7	14.9	9.0	17.1	32.4	46.2	58.2
1964	26.6	13.7	8.5	15.6	30.6	42.7	53.3
1965	25.3	13.4	8.0	15.0	29.0	40.3	51.5
1966	24.4	12.9	7.7	13.4	28.0	39.6	50.4
1967	23.1	11.7	6.8	13.4	26.8	37.3	46.7
White							
male	22.8	7.1	4.1	8.6	21.5	45.0	62.7
female	10.6	7.6	4.0	8.4	12.3	12.4	20.9
Nonwhite							
male	91.8	33.7	23.0	46.9	139.7	195.1	212.8
female	50.0	33.6	23.3	46.4	72.7	61.6	79.4
				Percent decline in case rate			
1953-67	56.4	24.0	25.3	72.9	60.4	53.3	43.7

losis reported in the United States have been contributed by white males, predominantly those at the older ages.

In contrast to numbers, new case rates for the nonwhite population are markedly higher than for the white population and particularly so in the case of females. Moreover, the ratio of nonwhite to white case rates is increasing, notwithstanding the downward trend in these rates for each color-sex category. In other words, the pace of decline in these rates has been greater for whites than for nonwhites; from 1953 to 1967, the white population benefited by a 62.3 percent drop in their case rates compared with 45.3 percent for the nonwhite population, as shown in Table 3.7b. A graphic view of the trend in case rates according to color and sex is given in Figure 3.2. For each color category, the rate of decline was somewhat greater for females than for males. In

Table 3.7b New active tuberculosis cases; number and case rate by color and sex: United States, 1953-67

Year	White Male	White Female	Nonwhite Male	Nonwhite Female
	Number of cases			
1953	41,159	21,055	13,056	9,034
1954	38,774	19,440	12,809	8,752
1955	37,167	18,913	12,510	8,778
1956	33,599	16,718	11,783	7,795
1957	32,700	15,648	11,470	7,331
1958	30,404	14,442	11,472	7,216
1959	27,363	13,043	10,489	6,640
1960	26,396	12,499	10,285	6,314
1961	25,139	11,957	10,265	6,365
1962	24,325	11,687	10,526	6,777
1963	24,160	11,888	11,083	6,911
1964	22,623	10,988	10,596	6,667
1965	21,455	10,269	10,595	6,697
1966	20,751	10,136	10,505	6,375
1967	19,400	9,446	10,614	6,187
	Percent distribution of cases			
1953	48.8	25.0	15.5	10.7
1967	42.5	20.7	23.2	13.6
	Case rate per 100,000 population			
1953	59.0	29.4	156.2	102.2
1954	54.4	26.6	149.1	96.3
1955	51.2	25.5	141.6	94.2
1956	45.5	22.1	129.1	81.5
1957	43.6	20.3	123.3	74.6
1958	39.9	18.5	120.2	71.6
1959	35.3	16.4	107.2	64.2
1960	33.6	15.5	102.6	59.6
1961	31.5	14.6	100.1	58.7
1962	30.1	14.0	100.4	61.0
1963	29.4	14.1	103.4	60.8
1964	27.3	12.8	96.8	57.3
1965	25.6	11.8	94.7	56.4
1966	24.5	11.5	92.4	52.6
1967	22.8	10.6	91.8	50.0
	Percent decline in case rate			
1953-67	61.4	63.9	41.2	51.1

Figure 3.2 New active tuberculosis case rates by race and sex, United States, 1953–67.

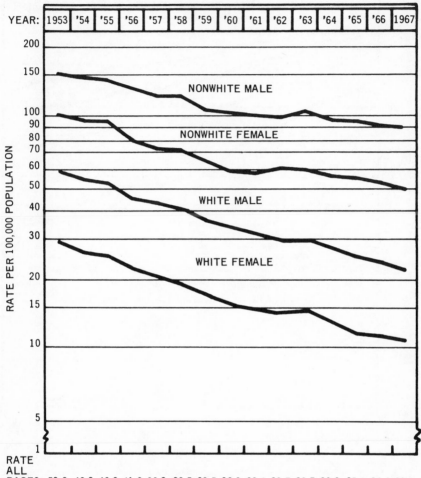

NOTE: Logarithmic scale

1967, the ratio of nonwhite to white rates was 4.0 to 1 for males and 4.7 to 1 for females.

The reduction in new active case rates from 1953 to 1967 was slow at ages under 15 years, where the rates were already at a relatively low level. The pace of improvement was most rapid at ages 15–24 years, the rate for 1967 being 72.9 percent under that for 1953. However, the percent decline fell off with advance in age, amounting to only 43.7 percent at ages 65 and over (see Fig. 3.3).

Figure 3.3. New active tuberculosis case rates by age, United States, 1953–67.

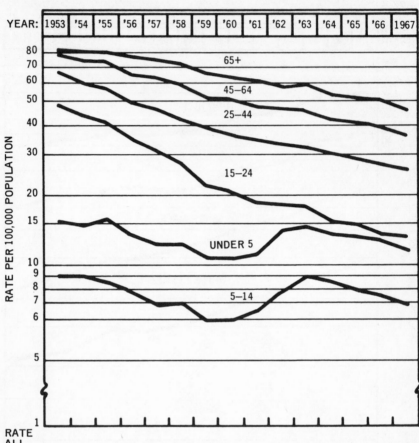

NOTE: Logarithmic scale

A more penetrating insight into age variations in the numbers and rates for new active tuberculosis cases according to color and sex is shown in Table 3.8a. These data were prepared through the cooperation of state and city public health authorities, who submitted individual cards for each new tuberculosis case reported during the year 1959, 1960, and 1961 to the Tuberculosis Program of the U.S. Public Health Service for statistical analysis. Cards were received from all states but it was possible to use data only from 30 states and the District of Columbia; they represented 136,664 cases, or 81 percent of the total cases reported for the United States for the three-year period 1959–61. These were distributed according to color and sex on the basis of ratios devel-

Table 3.8a New active tuberculosis cases by age, color, and sex:
United States, 1959-61

Age	Number of cases						
	Total	White			Nonwhite		
		Both sexes	Male	Female	Both sexes	Male	Female
All ages	166,755	116,397	78,898	37,499	50,358	31,039	19,319
Under 20	19,429	11,164	5,398	5,766	8,265	3,828	4,437
Under 1	491	269	154	115	222	116	106
1	1,620	843	435	408	777	400	377
2	1,931	1,068	546	522	863	433	430
3	1,566	867	442	425	699	343	356
4	1,228	720	379	341	508	258	250
5	1,051	596	298	298	455	216	239
6	952	557	290	267	395	189	206
7	795	467	233	234	328	146	182
8	699	399	200	199	300	139	161
9	599	352	179	173	247	118	129
10	531	301	142	159	230	99	131
11	516	274	106	168	242	104	138
12	512	306	137	169	206	99	107
13	510	305	138	167	205	84	121
14	595	340	137	203	255	100	155
15	770	455	176	279	315	117	198
16	1,017	552	233	319	465	198	267
17	1,139	702	326	376	437	203	234
18	1,349	831	399	432	518	200	318
19	1,558	960	448	512	598	266	332
Under 5	6,836	3,767	1,956	1,811	3,069	1,550	1,519
5- 9	4,096	2,371	1,200	1,171	1,725	808	917
10-14	2,664	1,526	660	866	1,138	486	652
15-19	5,833	3,500	1,582	1,918	2,333	984	1,349
20-24	8,994	5,320	2,674	2,646	3,674	1,743	1,931
25-29	10,580	6,181	3,117	3,064	4,399	2,168	2,231
30-34	12,565	7,476	4,088	3,388	5,089	2,756	2,333
35-39	14,379	9,087	5,655	3,432	5,292	3,247	2,045
40-44	14,297	9,624	6,639	2,985	4,673	3,176	1,497
45-49	14,761	10,602	7,974	2,628	4,159	3,027	1,132
50-54	14,683	11,019	8,734	2,285	3,664	2,791	873
55-59	13,748	10,512	8,570	1,942	3,236	2,507	729
60-64	12,078	9,459	7,594	1,865	2,619	1,942	677
65-69	11,033	8,880	6,812	2,068	2,153	1,614	539
70-74	8,977	7,491	5,400	2,091	1,486	1,086	400
75-79	6,084	5,155	3,476	1,679	929	661	268
80-84	3,358	2,917	1,857	1,060	441	304	137
85-89	1,336	1,148	689	459	188	134	54
90-94	380	305	185	120	75	46	29
95 and over	73	57	36	21	16	9	7

Source: Based on a sample for 30 states and the District of Columbia
(135,664 cases or 81 percent of the total cases reported in the United States)
for the three-year period 1959-61. Distribution was based on individual ratios
developed for whites to nonwhites, and for males to females for each specific
age group. These ratios were computed separately for each of the three years.

oped for each specific age group, treating each of the years 1959, 1960, and 1961 separately. Table 3.8a presents for the first time for the entire country a distribution of new active tuberculosis cases and case rates by color and sex for single years under age 20, in five-year age groups up to 95 years and older. Another important feature of this table is that these new case rates for the 1959–61 period, are based on the population in the 1960 census and may be considered, accordingly, to have greater precision than rates based on estimates of the population for other years. The pattern of the new active case rates for single ages under 20 years according to color and sex is shown in Figure 3.4 and the like rates for five-year age groupings are in Figure 3.5.

The new active tuberculosis case rates for each color-sex category reach a low point at ages 10–14 years. As these children reach the late teens and the young adult ages, they move increasingly in a widening environment so that the relative risk of becoming infected with tubercle bacilli and of developing active disease grows. This is reflected in rising case rates up to age 30, after which the grade continues upward at a slower pace to the extreme ages of life (see Table 3.8b).

At ages under 5 years, the new active tuberculosis case rates are practically identical for males and females in the case of both the white and nonwhite populations. This changes to somewhat higher rates for females at ages 5–19, but thereafter the rates are consistently higher for males. The relative margin between the sexes rises with advance in age so that the ratio of male to female rates reaches a maximum of 4.5 to 1 at ages 60–64 years for white persons and 3.0 to 1 for nonwhite persons. At ages 65 and over, the sex ratio is of the order of 3 to 1.

The ratio of nonwhite to white case rates changes appreciably with advance in age. Under age 35 the case rate for nonwhites is fully five times that for the white population. This ratio falls to 3 to 1 at ages 55–59 years and continues to decrease to a little over 2 to 1 at ages 80–89 years.

If current trends continue, it seems that tuberculosis will be reduced by relatively the greatest amount first among children. Not only are case rates and incidence rates of infection much lower for children than for adults, but the total amount of serious disease being found among children in recent years is becoming progressively smaller.

GEOGRAPHIC DISTRIBUTION
Variations in the incidence and prevalence of tuberculosis among the states and their political subdivisions arise not only from differences in

Figure 3.4. New active tuberculosis case rates, by age, color, and sex, children under twenty years of age, United States, 1959–61.

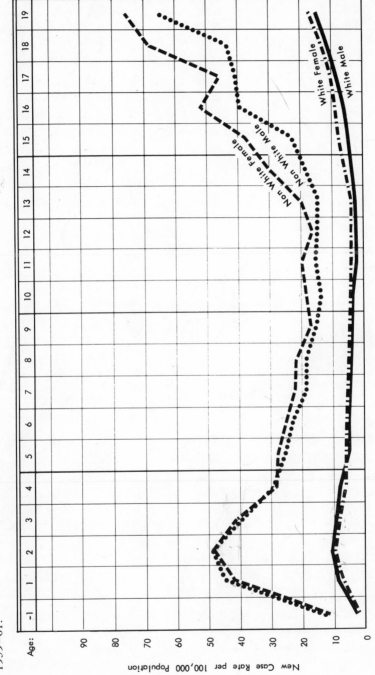

Figure 3.5. New active tuberculosis case rates, by age, color, and sex, United States, 1959–61.

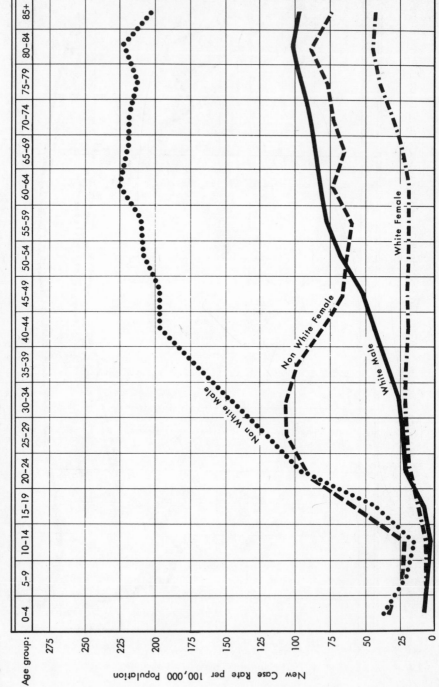

Table 3.8b   New active tuberculosis case rates by age, color, and
              sex: United States, 1959-61

Age	Total	White Both sexes	Male	Female	Nonwhite Both sexes	Male	Female
All ages	31.0	24.4	33.6	15.5	81.9	103.8	61.2
Under 20	9.4	6.2	5.9	6.5	29.6	27.4	31.7
Under 1	4.0	2.6	2.9	2.2	12.1	12.6	11.4
1	13.2	8.0	8.1	7.9	43.0	44.4	41.7
2	15.7	10.2	10.2	10.1	48.4	48.5	48.4
3	13.0	8.4	8.4	8.4	40.2	39.4	40.9
4	10.3	7.0	7.3	6.8	29.5	29.9	29.1
5	8.9	5.9	5.7	6.0	26.9	25.5	28.2
6	8.3	5.7	5.8	5.5	24.6	23.6	25.6
7	7.0	4.8	4.7	4.9	20.9	18.6	23.1
8	6.4	4.2	4.1	4.3	20.2	18.7	21.7
9	5.7	3.9	3.9	3.9	16.9	16.1	17.7
10	5.1	3.3	3.1	3.6	16.1	13.8	18.4
11	5.0	3.0	2.3	3.8	17.5	15.0	20.0
12	4.8	3.3	2.9	3.7	15.6	14.9	16.2
13	4.8	3.3	2.9	3.7	17.0	13.9	20.0
14	7.2	4.8	3.8	5.8	24.0	18.9	29.1
15	9.3	6.3	4.8	7.9	30.1	22.4	37.8
16	12.1	7.4	6.2	8.8	46.0	39.2	52.7
17	13.3	9.3	8.5	10.0	43.2	40.4	46.1
18	17.8	12.4	12.0	13.0	56.2	43.9	68.1
19	22.8	16.1	15.2	16.8	70.9	65.6	75.8
Under 5	11.2	7.2	7.4	7.1	34.5	34.9	34.2
5- 9	7.3	4.9	4.9	5.0	22.1	20.7	23.4
10-14	5.3	3.4	3.0	4.0	17.8	15.2	20.4
15-19	14.7	10.1	9.0	11.1	48.3	41.2	55.2
20-24	27.8	18.7	19.2	18.3	92.1	92.7	91.4
25-29	32.4	21.6	22.0	21.1	111.6	118.2	105.9
30-34	35.1	23.5	26.1	21.0	124.7	146.3	106.2
35-39	38.4	27.2	34.6	20.1	131.6	171.1	96.3
40-44	41.1	30.8	43.2	18.8	132.3	189.4	80.7
45-49	45.2	36.1	55.1	17.7	126.7	190.4	66.8
50-54	51.0	42.2	67.9	17.3	133.9	207.3	62.8
55-59	54.4	45.9	76.6	16.6	134.2	209.6	60.0
60-64	56.4	48.1	81.1	18.1	147.5	225.0	74.2
65-69	58.8	51.6	84.6	22.6	138.4	217.9	66.1
70-74	63.1	56.9	89.2	29.4	142.4	216.9	73.7
75-79	66.4	60.6	92.3	35.4	141.9	211.6	78.3
80-84	70.8	65.7	99.9	41.0	148.1	221.4	85.4
85-89	63.9	58.9	89.7	38.9	128.8	202.9	67.5
90-94	68.8	60.2	100.2	37.2	171.9	260.1	112.2
95 and over	50.4	48.2	90.7	27.1	63.1	87.0	46.7

population size but also from differences in their composition according to age, sex, color, and other demographic characteristics. There are, in addition, a multiplicity of social and environmental influences, differing from one community to another, that bear upon the size of a local tuberculosis problem. Because of these sources of variation—demographic, social, and economic—direct comparisons of the tuberculosis situations between aggregates of population must be tempered.

For many years, case rates for individual states were deemed adequate for planning overall programs designed to control tuberculosis. This traditional use of state case rates is no longer appropriate because they obscure problems of specific areas within a state or even a county where the disease may be concentrated. Although case rates are suited for the statistical analysis of a widespread disease, in planning programs for tuberculosis control, it is necessary to pinpoint the actual number of cases that occur in a small geographic area in order to obtain an operating basis to ascertain needed clinic and hospital facilities as well as many other health and welfare services.

As an example of the wide range of the tuberculosis problem among the states, some data for 1967 may be cited. In that year, the number of new active tuberculosis cases ranged from 5,069 in New York State to only 31 in Wyoming (see Appendix Table A.2). The eight states with the largest numbers—New York, California, Illinois, Pennsylvania, Texas, Michigan, Florida, and Ohio—accounted for more than half of the total for the country. Collectively, during 1965–67 the states of the north central region had proportionately fewer new active cases than the number of people, as shown in Figure 3.6. On the other hand, the states of the south as a unit accounted for the highest proportion of new cases, namely 39 percent, but for only 31 percent of the population.

The active tuberculosis case rates among the states in 1967 ranged from a high of 45.7 per 100,000 population in Hawaii to a low of 5.5 in Iowa. The national average case rate was 23.1; eight states had rates less than 10, and two states and the District of Columbia had rates of 40 or more. Alaska classified more than half of its new pulmonary active cases as minimal and somewhat less than that proportion were so classified by Hawaii, Utah, and Montana (see Appendix Tables A.3 and A.4). On the other hand, well over half of the new pulmonary active cases were considered far advanced by Idaho and Iowa.

Beginning in 1962, data on new active tuberculosis cases were reported to the Public Health Service for over 3,000 counties. Table 3.9 shows that, in 1965, no new active cases of tuberculosis were found or reported to health departments in 614 counties with 2.9 percent of the nation's population. These figures should not suggest that there was no tuberculosis present among the 5.7 million persons in these counties, nor can it be assumed that no tuberculosis developed during the year.

Figure 3.6. Percent distribution by region, new active tuberculosis cases and population, United States, average 1965−67.

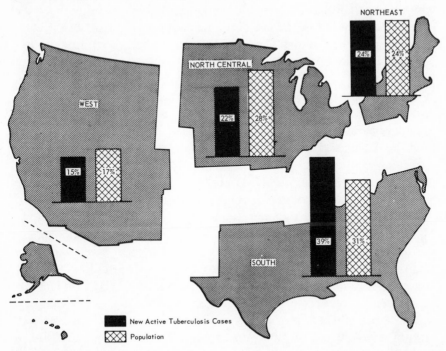

Old inactive cases that reactivated and developed into active tuberculosis during the year were not recorded in the new case figures if they had been officially reported as "new cases" in earlier years. The 614 counties, with no new cases in 1965, are scattered throughout the nation, but most of them are located in the north central, plains, and Rocky Mountain states. In a few, the number of residents was relatively large, but generally their population was small. It should be emphasized that the above figures refer to 1965 only and that cases of tubercu-

Table 3.9   Range of new active tuberculosis cases by counties: United States, 1965

Range of new cases in county	Counties		Population 1965(est.)		New cases reported		
	Number	Percent	Number	Percent	Number	Percent	New case rate
All counties	3,084[a]	100.0	193,795,000	100.0	49,016[b]	100.0	25.3
0	614	19.9	5,655,000	2.9	0	0.0	0.0
1−9	1,721	55.8	41,153,000	21.2	6,194	12.8	15.1
10−99	670	21.7	72,585,000	37.5	17,406	35.9	24.0
100−499	70	2.3	29,894,000	25.7	13,977	28.8	28.0
500+	9	0.3	24,508,000	12.7	10,931	22.5	44.6

[a]Includes areas corresponding to counties, but having no organized county government.
[b]Includes 508 cases in miscellaneous administrative areas.

losis were reported in many of the counties in earlier and following years. Over half the new cases in 1965 were located in 79 counties, each with at least 100 such cases; these counties, which include all of the major cities and conurbations, contained almost two fifths of the total population of the country. The wide geographic variation in the number of new active cases reported among the counties is shown in Figure 3.7.

The combined data for 1962 through 1965 provided a reasonably reliable base for computing representative county case rates for the four-year period (see Fig. 3.8 and Appendix Table A.5). For this purpose, it was necessary to use population estimates prepared mainly by state and local agencies because there is no national source for estimates covering all counties in the country. Very high new case rates will be noted for many counties containing Indian reservations in those parts of Appalachia designated as poverty areas and in areas along the Mexican border. Although their rates are high and many of these counties are small in population and the numbers of new active cases are small, they do present important problems for tuberculosis control. However, in general the new active case ratio tends to rise with increasing concentration of population. Thus, in 1965 the new active case rate was 45.4 per 100,000 population in cities of 500,000 or more, 31.5 in cites of 250,000 to 500,000 population, 28.8 in cities of 100,000 to 250,000, and 19.4 in all other areas. On the other hand, these residual areas contained over half of the new active cases in 1965, and the cities of 500,000 or more had somewhat less than one third of the total.

The wide range in size and varying demographic characteristics of counties and cities and the great differences in the number of cases emphasizes the need for adjusting tuberculosis control programs to specific requirements of local conditions. This geographic pattern of tuberculosis was established decades ago and shows very little prospect of being changed without an accelerated and intensified effort to eliminate the remaining seedbeds of infection and disease. One particular type of program may not necessarily be appropriate for all communities even if they are of similar size.

The number of cases and the rates in Appendix Table A.2 show that each state benefited by a reduction in its tuberculosis problem from 1952 to 1967. However, care should be taken in interpreting state morbidity changes from one time to the next because occasionally the data are affected by and may reflect increased casefinding activities.

Figure 3.8. New active tuberculosis case rates by county, average 1962–65.

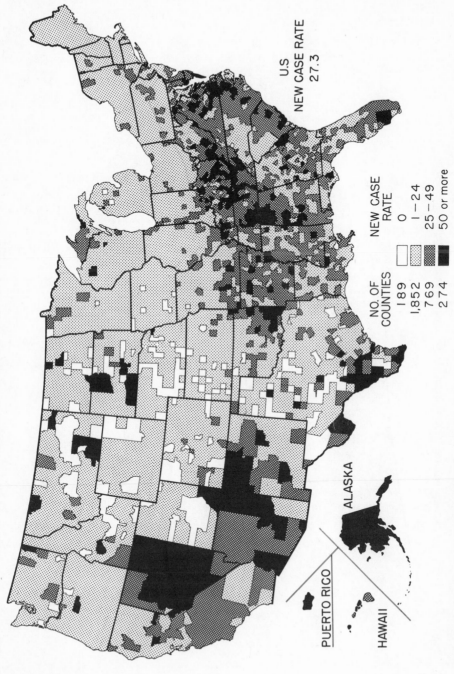

U.S
NEW CASE RATE
27.3

NO. OF COUNTIES		NEW CASE RATE
189		0
1,852		1 – 24
769		25 – 49
274		50 or more

ALASKA

PUERTO RICO

HAWAII

RATE PER 100,000 POPULATION

Figure 3.7. Tuberculosis cases reported: counties and large urban areas, United States, 1965.

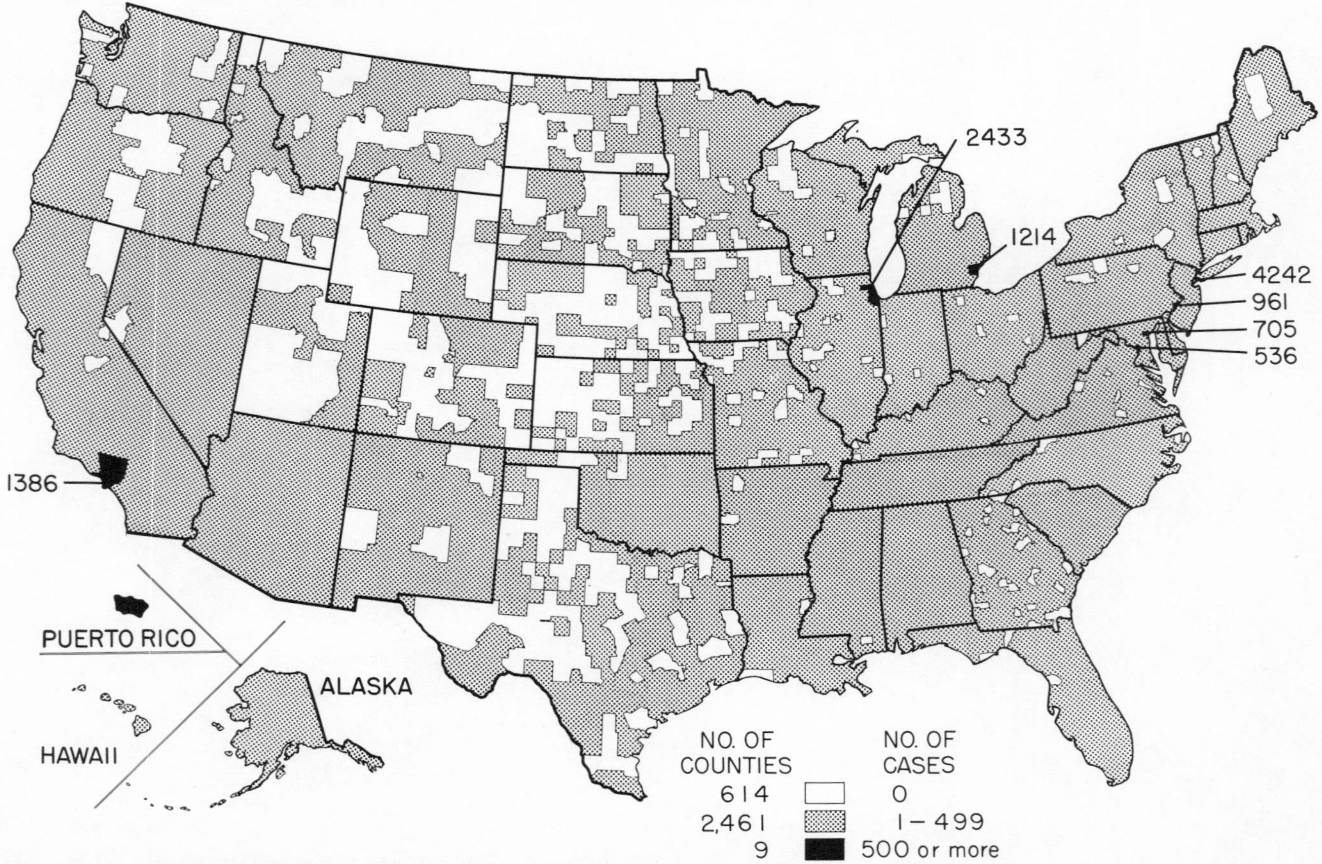

Figure 3.9. Tuberculosis in the United States, 1966 (total pop. 195,936,000).

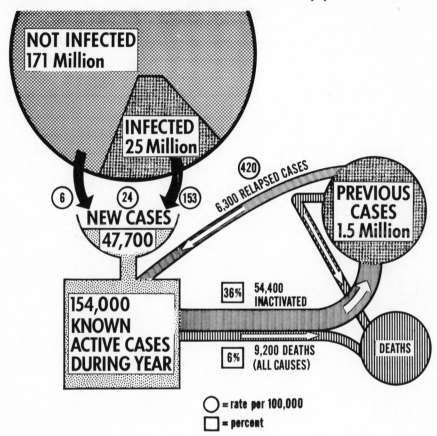

DYNAMICS OF TUBERCULOSIS

In the dynamics of tuberculosis, a continuous flow of persons infected with tubercle bacilli develop active disease and enter the pool of active cases; this pool is also fed by relapses of previous cases. As shown in Figure 3.9, these two groups are cumulative and during 1966 became a part of the 154,000 patients with active disease. About 90,000 patients were on health department tuberculosis registers on any one day. The flow into the pool of active cases from the infected population, from the uninfected, and from the pool of previous cases is at very different rates. The overall annual rate of new cases was 24 per 100,000 population. Four fifths of these new cases came from the 25 million persons who were infected sometime during their lifetime, producing a rate of

153 per 100,000 infected. This was in contrast to a rate of 6 per 100,000 among the 171 million persons who were uninfected at the beginning of the year. On the other hand, a rate of 420 per 100,000 was found among those who had a history of previous tuberculosis, a figure for the risk of developing active disease (relapse in these cases) appreciably different from those for the uninfected and the infected. Included in the infected group of 25 million persons are those who had previous disease and in some instances were not officially reported as cases.

The pool of known active cases is diminished in two ways: deaths and inactivation of the disease. The outflow of deaths could be reduced radically by adequate treatment. Treatment can also rapidly increase the outflow of inactive cases and, if continued for a sufficient length of time, reduce markedly the flow of relapses.[6]

TUBERCULOSIS MORTALITY SINCE 1900

Reduction of the tuberculosis death rate in the United States reflects in a very tangible way the gains being made in lifesaving through the direct application of emerging medical knowledge and new techniques in treatment, in addition to benefits due to the general rise in the standard of living and improved environment. During the nineteenth century the death rate was the most common index used to measure the trend of tuberculosis, because nationwide registration of morbidity data did not exist. Reporting of "cases" was very limited in scope and a matter of local option, often done with a high degree of individuality. Also, there is some evidence to suggest that deaths due to tuberculosis were often ascribed to other causes in order to circumvent social stigma that was then attached to familial association.

With more complete understanding of tuberculosis as an infectious disease in the early 1900's and with the eventual development of reporting systems for communicable diseases, the quality of public health statistics began to improve.[1] However, since 1950 the importance of tuberculosis as a cause of death has become more difficult to evaluate. Published mortality statistics reflect only the primary or underlying cause of death recorded on a death certificate and do not show the significant part often played by tuberculosis as a contributing cause of mortality. In effect, persons with long-standing tuberculous disease may die "with" but not "from" tuberculosis, and thus the official record for a given community can be an understatement of the problem. There is need, therefore, of a better index reflecting "lethality" as well as "mortality." For example, in 1955 when there were 14,940 deaths in the United States with tuberculosis as the underlying cause, the disease was actually mentioned 21,331 times on death certificates.[2]

In 1966 the tuberculosis death rate for the United States was 3.9 per 100,000 population, only one fiftieth of its level in 1900 when it was 194.4 in the death registration states and 201.9 in the death registration area. It is estimated that at the beginning of this century approximately 150,000 people died each year from tuberculosis in the continental United States compared to 7,625 in 1966 in the 50 states (see Table 4.1). The annual rate of decline of the tuberculosis death rate during the early years of this century was consistent but relatively slow until the period of World War I. Following the influenza pandemic in

Table 4.1   Tuberculosis mortality in the United States since 1900[a]

Year	Death registration states[b] Deaths	Rate per 100,000 Respiratory	Other forms	All forms	Death registration area Deaths	Rate per 100,000 Respiratory	Other forms	All forms	Estimated tuberculosis deaths entire U.S.[c]
1900	38,820	174.5	19.9	194.4	61,888	180.5	21.4	201.9	153,800
1901	38,434	169.4	20.5	189.9	61,599	174.5	22.4	196.9	153,200
1902	35,859	154.4	19.9	174.2	58,938	162.6	21.9	184.5	146,800
1903	37,102	155.6	21.5	177.2	61,487	164.9	23.6	188.5	153,100
1904	40,125	165.8	22.3	188.1	66,797	176.2	24.5	200.7	166,000
1905	39,168	157.1	22.9	179.9	65,352	166.7	25.6	192.3	161,700
1906	59,393	153.3	22.6	175.8	75,512	155.6	24.6	180.2	154,500
1907	60,194	152.0	22.2	174.2	76,650	154.3	24.2	178.5	156,500
1908	62,628	140.1	22.0	162.1	78,289	144.0	23.6	167.6	149,600
1909	69,105	134.9	21.3	156.3	81,720	139.3	21.5	160.8	146,000
1910	73,028	133.2	20.6	153.8	86,309	136.0	24.3	160.3	147,600
1911	83,663	134.2	20.9	155.1	94,205	132.7	26.5	159.2	149,000
1912	79,734	125.9	19.5	145.4	90,360	125.0	24.7	149.7	142,600
1913	83,434	123.7	19.7	143.5	93,421	123.0	24.8	147.8	142,800
1914	86,359	123.0	18.7	141.7	96,903	123.5	23.7	147.2	144,000
1915	86,726	122.6	17.5	140.1	98,194	123.5	22.8	146.3	145,000
1916	92,688	121.0	17.4	138.4	101,396	119.9	22.2	142.1	143,100
1917	100,789	126.2	17.3	143.5	110,285	124.6	22.5	147.1	150,200
1918	118,334	132.9	16.9	149.8	122,040	128.6	21.4	150.0	155,400
1919	104,486	111.3	14.4	125.6	106,985	107.5	18.1	125.6	132,300
1920	97,366	99.8	13.4	113.1	99,916	97.0	17.0	114.0	121,500
1921	85,739	84.5	13.2	97.6	88,135	85.6	13.3	98.9	107,100
1922	88,385	83.3	12.0	95.3	90,452	84.3	12.1	96.4	105,500
1923	88,788	80.4	11.4	91.7	90,732	81.3	11.5	92.8	103,700
1924	87,346	76.5	11.4	87.9	89,724	78.0	11.7	89.7	101,900
1925	86,510	74.1	10.7	84.8	89,268	75.9	10.8	86.7	99,900
1926	88,740	74.9	10.5	85.5	91,568	76.6	10.7	87.3	101,400
1927	85,194	70.1	9.5	79.6	87,567	71.4	9.5	80.9	95,700
1928	89,007	69.3	9.0	78.3	90,659	70.3	9.0	79.3	94,700
1929	86,885	67.0	8.3	75.3	88,352	67.6	8.4	76.0	92,400
1930	83,352	63.0	8.1	71.1	84,741	63.4	8.1	71.5	88,000
1931	80,129	60.4	7.4	67.8	81,395	60.7	7.4	68.1	84,500
1932	74,267	56.1	6.4	62.5	75,509	56.4	6.4	62.8	78,500
1933	74,842	53.7	5.9	59.6					
1934	71,609	51.2	5.5	56.7					
1935	70,080	49.9	5.2	55.1					
1936	71,527	50.8	5.1	55.9					
1937	69,324	49.2	4.7	53.8					
1938	63,735	44.7	4.4	49.1					
1939	61,609	43.1	4.0	47.1					
1940	60,428	42.2	3.7	45.9					
1941	59,251	40.8	3.7	44.5					
1942	57,690	39.6	3.5	43.1					
1943	57,005	39.0	3.4	42.4					
1944	54,731	38.2	3.0	41.2					
1945	52,916	36.9	3.0	39.9					
1946	50,911	33.5	2.8	36.4					
1947	48,064	31.0	2.5	33.5					
1948	43,833	27.7	2.3	30.0					
1949	39,100	24.2	2.1	26.3					
1950	33,959	20.6	1.9	22.5					
1951	30,863	18.4	1.7	20.1					
1952	24,621	14.4	1.4	15.8					
1953	19,544	11.3	1.1	12.3					
1954	16,392	9.3	0.8	10.2					
1955	14,940	8.3	0.8	9.1					
1956	14,061	7.8	0.6	8.4					
1957	13,324	7.3	0.6	7.8					
1958	12,361	6.6	0.5	7.1					
1959	11,474	6.0	0.4	6.5					
1960	10,866	5.6	0.4	6.0					
1961	9,938	5.0	0.4	5.4					
1962	9,506	4.7	0.4	5.1					
1963	9,331	4.6	0.4	4.9					
1964	8,303	4.0	0.3	4.3					
1965	7,934	3.8	0.3	4.1					
1966	7,625	3.6	0.3	3.9					
1967[d]	(6,560)	(3.0)	(0.3)	(3.3)					

[a]The annual collection of mortality statistics by the Bureau of The Census began with the calendar year 1900. The national death – registration area for 1900 consisted of 10 states, the District of Columbia, and a number of cities in non-registration states. This area grew gradually by the addition of more states until in 1933 it included the entire continental United States. Death – registration states (which include the District of Columbia) are exclusive of registration cities in non-registration states.

[b]Includes Alaska and Hawaii beginning 1959.

[c]Computed by applying death rate in registration area to population of entire continental United States.

[d]Provisional.

1918, and into the nineteen forties, there was some acceleration in the decline of tuberculosis death rates. With the introduction of antibiotics in 1947 and chemotherapeutic agents in 1952, the tuberculosis death rate began to decrease dramatically as compared with the new active tuberculosis case rate. However, by the mid-fifties the annual changes in the death rate began to stabilize.[3]

For both white and nonwhite males the decline of the tuberculosis death rates was such that their level in 1965 was only about three percent of that in 1910; for females, the ratio was a little over one percent (see Table 4.2 and Fig. 4.1). Since 1950, the decline in the female mor-

Table 4.2   Tuberculosis death rates by age, sex, and color: expanding death registration states, 1900-1965

Year, sex, color	Total	Age under 1	1-4	5-14	15-24	25-34	35-44	45-54	55-64	65-74	75-84	85 & over
					Death rates							
Total												
1900	194.4	311.6	101.8	36.2	205.7	294.3	253.6	215.6	223.0	256.1	279.3	204.5
1910	153.8	212.9	84.6	29.7	152.0	217.6	214.9	188.1	192.9	203.5	189.2	115.8
1920	113.1	106.5	45.4	22.4	136.1	164.9	147.4	137.2	141.3	163.8	157.7	132.3
1930	71.1	51.6	25.9	11.9	77.3	102.8	92.4	93.2	97.0	111.7	115.5	76.9
1940	45.9	24.6	12.3	5.5	38.2	56.3	59.4	66.3	75.8	81.5	80.1	63.9
1950	22.5	8.5	6.3	1.8	11.3	19.1	26.1	35.9	47.4	58.2	63.2	47.7
1959-61	6.0	0.9	0.7	0.1	0.6	2.3	5.0	9.2	15.4	23.2	32.2	38.6
1965	4.1	0.7	0.3	0.1	0.3	1.1	3.1	5.7	10.6	16.7	24.4	37.4
White male												
1914	146.9	182.6	64.3	19.6	119.5	196.8	230.0	218.5	221.3	201.3	173.6	103.5
1920	104.1	108.3	43.9	14.7	86.0	142.5	147.8	154.7	164.7	178.8	159.9	120.0
1930	63.4	46.0	20.4	6.7	40.3	77.3	93.1	108.5	118.1	124.0	114.9	74.5
1940	44.7	18.0	8.9	2.9	17.0	40.2	59.2	83.6	103.0	102.3	90.8	67.9
1950	25.0	5.1	4.4	1.1	4.3	11.4	25.4	45.4	68.6	84.8	85.7	67.4
1959-61	7.6	0.6	0.4	0.1	0.2	1.2	3.8	11.1	22.5	36.7	43.8	56.0
1965	5.2	0.5*	0.1*	0.0*	0.2	0.5	2.3	6.2	14.9	26.1	38.8	55.0
White female												
1914	112.9	136.7	57.9	26.7	134.7	169.9	144.1	111.6	128.4	155.5	158.4	98.9
1920	94.8	87.7	38.4	19.1	129.7	145.7	115.8	94.0	101.4	133.9	146.3	127.3
1930	51.9	38.6	19.0	7.8	65.7	79.9	59.8	53.4	62.6	88.8	108.6	72.2
1940	28.3	17.6	8.8	3.4	27.7	39.8	33.3	28.7	36.4	55.1	69.2	57.4
1950	10.8	5.7	4.9	1.2	6.6	12.0	13.0	11.5	15.0	25.9	41.0	31.9
1959-61	2.6	0.4	0.5	0.1	0.3	1.2	2.6	3.6	4.2	7.7	15.9	23.0
1965	1.7	0.3*	0.2*	0.0*	0.1*	0.4	1.4	2.2	3.1	5.1	10.7	22.9
Nonwhite male												
1914	417.8	551.5	234.2	125.5	493.6	515.2	516.4	451.9	534.0	515.0	543.4	205.3
1920	255.4	204.8	92.4	55.7	362.4	384.8	326.5	295.6	285.2	336.6	256.6	337.0
1930	194.3	128.4	77.0	40.3	235.8	319.1	275.0	239.6	199.2	243.3	219.1	115.7
1940	139.1	76.7	38.6	18.6	141.8	201.2	215.2	227.7	189.1	169.8	132.3	93.2
1950	74.7	32.1	21.2	5.4	46.3	84.2	107.1	153.8	168.4	164.5	129.8	80.4
1959-61	18.2	3.6	2.1	0.3	1.8	11.7	25.4	41.0	60.9	73.5	91.8	114.8
1965	13.1	1.6*	0.6*	0.3*	1.2	7.0	15.4	29.7	46.3	74.2	76.7	95.1
Nonwhite female												
1914	374.0	334.1	234.7	183.4	545.3	497.0	390.4	326.7	266.6	262.8	241.5	258.2
1920	269.6	198.0	88.0	95.3	431.3	408.1	291.9	254.9	220.6	226.7	238.6	126.1
1930	189.8	122.6	71.9	58.7	300.0	298.8	209.8	167.5	150.1	147.8	140.3	107.2
1940	117.2	72.1	33.9	26.6	189.1	191.9	134.7	107.7	93.1	72.2	50.1	73.6
1950	50.6	26.5	16.2	7.7	63.5	82.0	68.6	61.8	60.9	59.2	49.8	49.8
1959-61	8.5	2.6	1.9	0.5	3.3	10.5	16.0	13.8	17.9	21.9	29.0	39.7
1965	5.6	3.2*	1.7	0.2*	1.7	4.2	11.9	10.5	12.5	16.3	23.3	37.0
					Number of deaths, 1959-61							
Total	32,276[a]	110	322	141	397	1,600	3,631	5,668	7,188	7,647	4,476	1,075
White male	17,963[a]	33	88	40	75	355	1,219	3,031	4,626	5,178	2,752	556
White female	6,191[a]	20	92	40	95	356	866	1,008	927	1,259	1,165	363
Nonwhite male	5,450[a]	33	75	23	75	436	909	1,204	1,254	913	413	108
Nonwhite female	2,672[a]	24	67	38	152	453	637	425	381	297	146	48

[a]Includes age not stated.

Figure 4.1. Tuberculosis death rates, by color and sex, United States, since 1910.

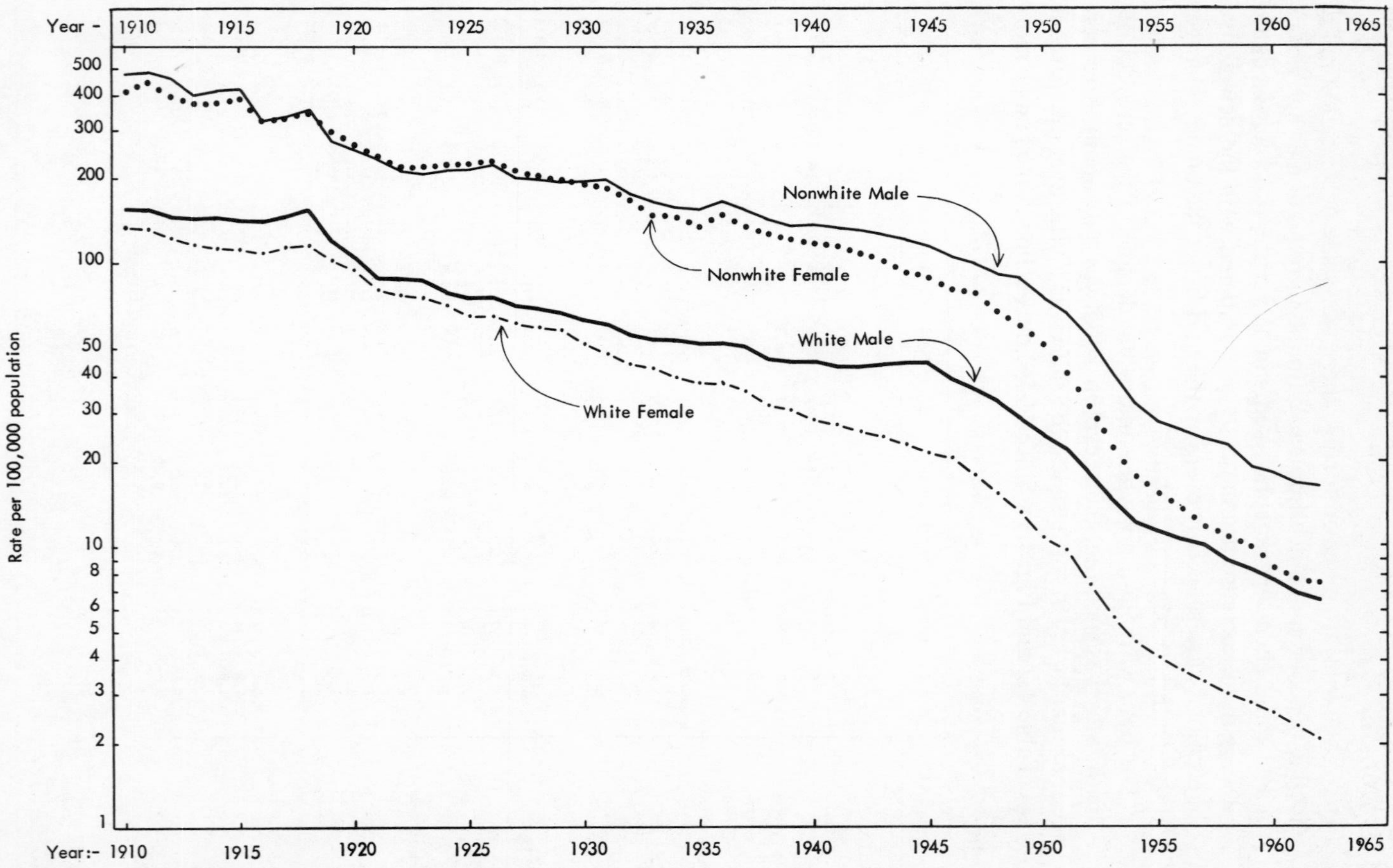

tality has been at a somewhat greater rate than for males. Over the longer period from 1910, nonwhite mortality from tuberculosis had declined more rapidly than that for the white population. As a result, the ratio of nonwhite to white death rates fell from 3.0 to 1 in 1910 to 2.5 to 1 in 1965. Reduction in death rates since 1900 has been at a much greater rate in early adult life than in midlife and later for males and females, as is evident in Table 4.2 and Figures 4.2 and 4.3. In place of the peaks in the curves in early adult life for males in 1900 and 1910, and for females up to 1950, the 1960 curves show a steady rise with advance in age. All areas of the country have shared in the reductions of mortality from tuberculosis, as is apparent from the data for each state over selected years from 1952 to 1965 shown in Appendix Table A.6.

In 1900, and several years thereafter, tuberculosis was the leading cause of death in the United States, but by 1965 it was reduced to twentieth place in the list of causes (see Table 4.3). In this connection, it is worth discussing in detail the changed role of tuberculosis death rates in evaluating progress in tuberculosis control activities. In the past,

Table 4.3   Leading causes of death: United States, 1965

Rank	Cause of death[a]	Number of deaths			Death rate		
		Total	Male	Female	Total	Male	Female
	All causes	1,828,136	1,035,200	792,936	943.3	1,088.4	803.3
1	Diseases of heart	712,087	412,831	299,256	367.4	434.0	303.2
2	Malignant neoplasms	297,588	161,422	136,166	153.6	169.7	138.0
3	Vascular lesions, central nervous system	201,057	93,520	107,537	103.7	98.3	108.9
4	Accidents	108,004	74,062	33,942	55.7	77.9	34.4
5	Influenza and pneumonia	61,903	34,973	26,930	31.9	36.8	27.3
6	Certain diseases of early infancy	55,398	32,504	22,894	28.6	34.2	23.2
7	General arteriosclerosis	38,102	17,299	20,803	19.7	18.2	21.1
8	Diabetes mellitus	33,174	13,588	19,586	17.1	14.3	19.8
9	Other diseases, circulatory system	27,279	16,209	11,070	14.1	17.0	11.2
10	Other bronchopulmonic diseases	26,518	21,155	5,363	13.7	22.2	5.4
11	Cirrhosis of liver	24,715	15,984	8,731	12.8	16.8	8.8
12	Suicide	21,507	15,490	6,017	11.1	16.3	6.1
13	Congenital malformations	19,512	10,375	9,137	10.1	10.9	9.3
14	Other hypertensive disease	11,667	5,942	5,725	6.0	6.2	5.8
15	Homicide	10,712	8,148	2,564	5.5	8.6	2.6
16	Chronic unspecified nephritis	10,595	5,893	4,702	5.5	6.2	4.8
17	Ulcer, stomach and duodenum	10,424	7,361	3,063	5.4	7.7	3.1
18	Hernia, intestinal obstruction	10,003	4,668	5,335	5.2	4.9	5.4
19	Infections of kidney	9,813	4,652	5,161	5.1	4.9	5.2
20	Tuberculosis	7,934	5,789	2,145	4.1	6.1	2.2
	Other (remaining) causes	130,144	73,335	56,809	...	...	...

[a]Rank order for total. Seventh Revision of the International Lists, 1955 (numerals refer to category digits in international classification): (1) Diseases of heart, 400-402,410-443, (2) Malignant neoplasms, including neoplasms of lymphatic and hematopoietic tissues, 140-205, (3) Vascular lesions affecting central nervous system, 330-334, (4) Accidents, E800-E962, (5) Influenza and pneumonia, except pneumonia of newborn, 480-493, (6) Certain diseases of early infancy, 760-776, (7) General arteriosclerosis, 450, (8) Diabetes mellitus, 260, (9) Other diseases of circulatory system, 451-468, (10) Other bronchopulmonic diseases, 525-527, (11) Cirrhosis of liver, 581, (12) Suicide, E963, E970-E979, (13) Congenital malformations, 750-759, (14) Other hypertensive disease, 444-447, (15) Homicide, E964, E980-E985, (16) Chronic and unspecified nephritis and other renal sclerosis, 592-594, (17) Ulcer of stomach and duodenum, 540, 541, (18) Hernia and intestinal obstruction, 560, 561, 570, (19) Infections of kidney, 600, (20) Tuberculosis, all forms, 001-019.

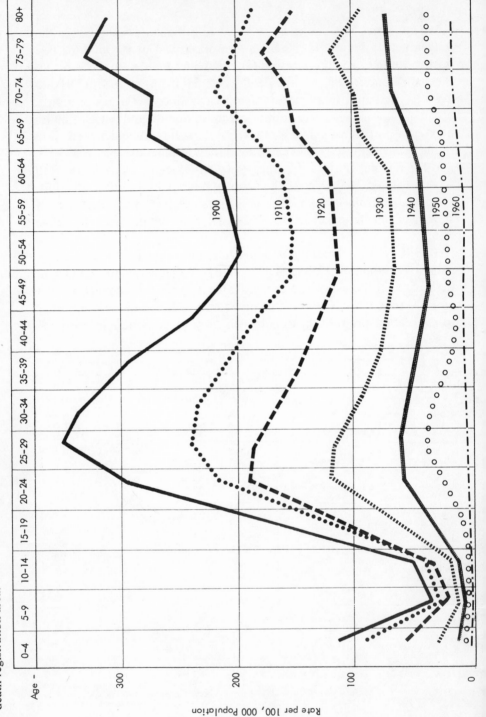

Figure 4.2. Male tuberculosis death rate by age, years 1900, 1910, 1920, 1930, 1940, 1950, 1960, United States (expanding) death registration area.

Lowell, Edwards, Palmer: TUBERCULOSIS

Figures on pages 72 and 73 are mislabeled. The figure on page 72 is for females, and the figure on page 73 is for males.

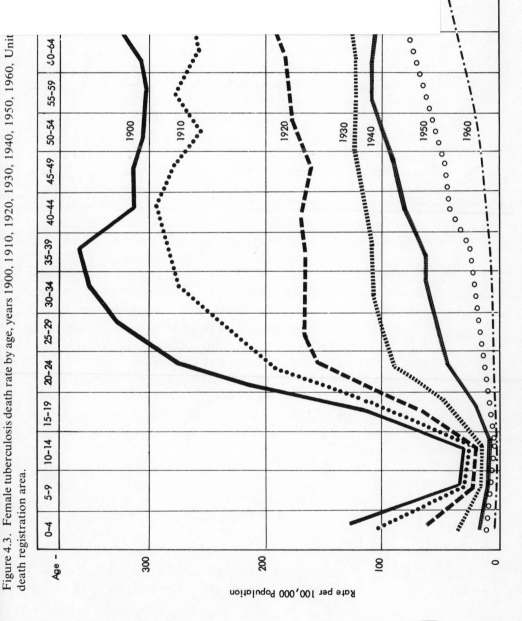

Figure 4.3. Female tuberculosis death rate by age, years 1900, 1910, 1920, 1930, 1940, 1950, 1960. Unit death registration area.

when nationwide indices of tuberculosis incidence and prevalence were not available, or when there was some doubt about the validity of the reported morbidity statistics, tuberculosis mortality served as a useful, even if crude, administrative device for the purpose. However, with the rapid reduction in tuberculosis deaths since World War II, mortality rates are used less frequently to measure the progress being made against the disease. Greater reliance is now placed on several types of morbidity data in planning national and local antituberculosis activities. Incidence of infection with tubercle bacilli, the number of active cases reported annually and the number of active and inactive tuberculosis cases present in a community are considered to be better indices than deaths when estimates of tuberculosis prevalence are needed for program planning. The revolution in the care, treatment, and prevention of active tuberculosis brought about by chemotherapy and chemoprophylaxis have modified traditional viewpoints as to what can be done to control and eradicate tuberculosis. More complete and, in some respects, different types of morbidity statistics must be available to tuberculosis control officers. These statistics should reflect the status of the disease among the living and make possible the rational application of new epidemiologic concepts as they apply to tuberculosis control.

To draw inferences as to the epidemiology of tuberculosis based only upon the number of deaths recorded or from changes in death rates might easily lead to misinterpretation and unwarranted conclusions. Death rates are still important indices that can be used to evaluate the impact of tuberculosis as a specific cause of death in relation to other causes. However, in many parts of the United States the number of tuberculosis deaths is now so small that it becomes increasingly difficult to use mortality exclusively as a measure of the importance of tuberculosis as a community health problem. Many places that have a great deal of tuberculosis requiring medical care and treatment report few or no tuberculosis deaths.

TUBERCULOSIS AMONG CHILDREN

By 1966, deaths from tuberculosis among children had become rare. During that year, in the entire United States only 102 such deaths were recorded for children under 15 years of age and these constituted less than 0.1 percent of deaths from all causes at that stage of life. Nearly three fourths of these deaths were at ages under five years. Nonwhites accounted for a disproportionately large share of the deaths from tuberculosis under 15 years of age, namely 53 percent. In contrast to this situation, there were 1,601 deaths from tuberculosis at ages under 15 years in the United States (including Alaska and Hawaii) in 1950, and as many as 6,648 in the Death Registration Area of 1900, when they comprised 3.5 percent of deaths from all causes in this age group. An indication of the shift of tuberculosis deaths away from childhood is seen in the reduction of the proportion of deaths from this cause reported for ages under 15 years to the number for all ages; this rate fell from 11 percent in 1900 to 1.3 percent in 1966.

Tuberculous meningitis is still a serious complication among children, especially among the very young. In 1966, meningitis was responsible for 54 deaths or 53 percent of all tuberculosis deaths among children under 15 years of age. Whereas tuberculous meningitis was practically always fatal to the child before the advent of chemotherapy, at present the prognosis for recovery can be favorable even when associated with miliary tuberculosis. Figure 4.4 shows the progress made in reducing tuberculosis mortality, particularly meningeal, among children during the first half of the twentieth century in New York City, one of the most highly congested urban communities in the country.

Perhaps the advantage that has accrued to children is due at least in part to the fortunate circumstances that not only are fewer children being infected nowadays but chemoprophylaxis can prevent progression to active tuberculosis. Also, when disease occurs, specific medical therapy is available to prevent a fatal outcome. It is, therefore, urgent not only that infection of children be prevented but also if it does occur that this event be known to public health departments at the earliest possible moment.[4]

TUBERCULOSIS MORTALITY, 1959–61

An opportunity to observe tuberculosis mortality in detail is provided by the extensive tabulations of death rates derived from recorded deaths for the period 1959–61, using the 1960 census of population as a base.[5] The essential results are summarized in Tables 4.4 and 4.5. Death rates for this period according to age, sex, and color are shown in Table 4.2.

Form of tuberculosis. During the three year period 1959–61, over thirty-two thousand deaths from tuberculosis were recorded in the United States. Of this total, 93 percent were attributed to the respiratory system, 2 percent to the meninges and central nervous systems, less than 1 percent to the bones and joints, and the rest to other organs and

Figure 4.4. Tuberculosis death rate, children under fifteen, New York City, since 1898.

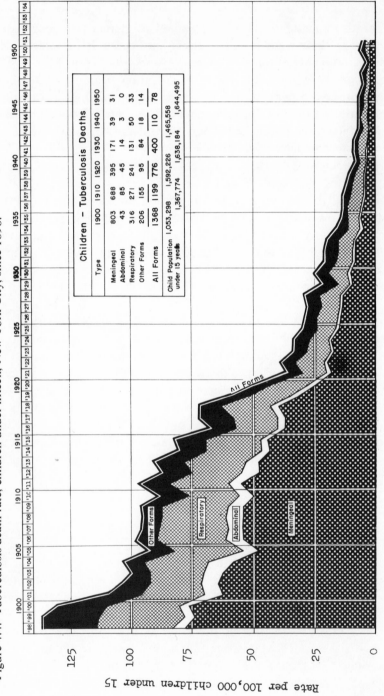

Children — Tuberculosis Deaths					
Type	1900	1910	1920	1930	1940	1950
Meningeal	803	688	395	171	39	31
Abdominal	43	85	45	14	3	0
Respiratory	316	271	241	131	50	33
Other Forms	206	155	95	84	18	14
All Forms	1368	1199	776	400	110	78
Child Population under 15 years	1,053,298	1,367,774	1,592,226	1,638,184	1,465,558	1,644,495

Rate per 100,000 children under 15

All Forms

Other Forms

Respiratory

Abdominal

Meningeal

Compiled from reports of Bureau of Records and Statistics, Department of Health, City of New York, by G. J. Drolet and A. M. Lowell, New York Tuberculosis and Health Association.

systems (see Table 4.4). For Negroes, about 3 percent of the total deaths for tuberculosis were attributed to the meninges and central nervous system, but for Indians the proportion was over 7 percent. The crude death rate for this form of tuberculosis was relatively high among Indian females, namely 2.9 per 100,000.

For each race category, the crude death rate for the total of all forms of tuberculosis was appreciably higher for nonwhites than for whites, the levels reached being 26.1 per 100,000 for the Chinese, 24.3 for In-

Table 4.4 Tuberculosis deaths and death rates by type of disease, according to race and sex: United States, 1959-61

Race and sex	All forms	Respiratory system	Meninges and central nervous system	Intestines, peritoneum, mesenteric glands	Bones and joints	Other organs and systems	Disseminated
			Number of deaths				
Total	32,276	29,922	725	170	242	533	684
Male	23,413	22,071	385	86	138	313	420
Female	8,863	7,851	340	84	104	220	264
White							
Male	17,963	17,147	220	44	101	227	224
Female	6,191	5,590	180	47	79	166	129
Negro							
Male	5,001	4,533	148	37	31	72	180
Female	2,429	2,074	133	35	21	44	122
Indian							
Male	192	153	14	3	4	7	11
Female	176	130	24	2	2	7	11
Chinese							
Male	106	98	–	1	1	3	3
Female	9	6	1	–	–	–	2
Japanese							
Male	61	59	–	–	1	1	–
Female	10	8	–	–	–	2	–
Other							
Male	90	81	3	1	–	3	2
Female	48	43	2	–	2	1	–
			Death rates per 100,000 population				
Total	6.0	5.6	0.1	0.0	0.0	0.1	0.1
Male	8.8	8.3	0.1	0.0	0.0	0.1	0.2
Female	3.3	2.9	0.1	0.0	0.0	0.1	0.1
White							
Male	7.6	7.3	0.1	0.0	0.0	0.1	0.1
Female	2.5	2.3	0.1	0.0	0.0	0.1	0.1
Negro							
Male	18.3	16.6	0.5	0.1	0.1	0.3	0.7
Female	8.3	7.1	0.5	0.1	0.1	0.2	0.4
Indian							
Male	23.4	18.6	1.7	0.4	0.5	0.9	1.3
Female	21.3	15.9	2.9	0.2	0.2	0.8	1.3
Chinese							
Male	26.1	24.1	...	0.2	0.2	0.7	0.7
Female	2.9	2.0	0.3	...	...	...	0.7
Japanese							
Male	9.0	8.7	...	...	0.1	0.1	...
Female	1.4	1.1	...	...	...	0.3	...
Other							
Male	13.2	11.9	0.4	0.2	...	0.4	0.3
Female	9.6	8.6	0.4	...	0.4	0.2	...

dians, 18.3 for Negroes, 9.0 for the Japanese, and 7.6 for the white population.

Because tuberculosis of the respiratory system constitutes a very large proportion of the total deaths from tuberculosis, further discussion of the 1959–61 data will be restricted to the latter. Also, nonwhites will be considered as a group, because only 8 percent of them are other than Negro.

Nativity. In 1959–61, the age-adjusted deaths for tuberculosis for the white foreign born were appreciably higher than for the white native born, the excess mortality amounting to 11 percent for males and 29 percent for females (see Table 4.5). Although this pattern is evident at ages under 15 years, it is not consistent at the higher ages. Thus, foreign-born males show to advantage at ages 15–64 years, and foreign-born females at ages 65 and over.

Marital status. Irrespective of age, sex, or color, death rates from tuberculosis among the unmarried are appreciably higher than for the married. For example, among white males, the age-adjusted death rates for ages 15 and over for the single and the widowed are almost four times that for the married (see Table 4.5). The ratios are not quite as high for nonwhite males, and for each color category they are somewhat lower for females. The data for the divorced will not be commented upon, because the quality of reporting of their marital status on the death certificate and the census is uncertain.

These data suggest that many single persons with a tuberculous condition stay out of marriage. The relatively high mortality from tuberculosis among the widowed may reflect the consequences of a reduced standard of living. It is also possible that many of these deaths are the result of acquisition of the disease from the deceased spouse.

Geographic division. Among white persons, mortality from tuberculosis was by far the lowest in the West North Central states and highest in the East South Central area of the country. The same picture will be noted, in Table 4.5, for each sex at ages 15–64 years and again at ages 65 and over. This is a situation which is very likely to reflect the relative position of the standards of living in these two areas.

Because the data for the nonwhites include Indians, Chinese, and Japanese, who are concentrated in the Mountain and Pacific Coast states, this comparison will be restricted to the other geographic divisions in which the nonwhites are largely Negro. In these other divisions, the death rates for the nonwhites are outstandingly high in the Middle Atlantic states, an area with a large contingent of recent Negro mi-

Table 4.5   Age-adjusted death rates for tuberculosis, all forms, by color, sex, and broad age groups according to geographic division, type of residence, marital status, and nativity (for white only): United States, 1959-61 (ISC codes 001-019)

Color; geographic division; type of residence; nativity; and marital status	Male				Female			
	All ages	Under 15	15-64	65 and over	All ages	Under 15	15-64	65 and over
White								
United States	6.7	0.2	5.7	40.6	2.1	0.2	2.0	10.4
Native born	6.5	0.2	5.6	38.8	2.1	0.2	1.9	10.6
Foreign born	7.2	1.8*	5.1	48.0	2.7	1.9*	2.2	10.1
Single	23.0[a]	...	16.5	87.9	5.7[a]	...	4.7	15.0
Married	5.8[a]	...	3.4	29.3	2.2[a]	...	1.5	8.7
Widowed	21.9[a]	...	18.0	61.4	4.4[a]	...	3.7	11.2
Divorced	37.5[a]	...	29.8	114.2	5.1[a]	...	4.5	11.5*
New England	6.8	0.1*	5.8	41.3	1.8	0.2*	1.7	9.0
Middle Atlantic	8.1	0.2*	7.0	47.7	2.2	0.1*	2.3	9.0
East North Central	5.8	0.0*	4.8	36.9	1.8	0.2*	1.7	8.5
West North Central	4.2	0.0*	3.6	25.2	1.4	0.0*	1.4	6.6
South Atlantic	6.1	0.2*	5.2	37.0	2.0	0.2*	1.7	11.7
East South Central	9.9	0.4*	8.3	60.8	4.3	0.5*	3.2	29.3
West South Central	8.6	0.6*	7.3	50.5	3.0	0.4*	2.7	15.5
Mountain	8.1	0.2*	6.7	50.6	2.6*	0.2*	2.7	9.9
Pacific	5.4	0.2*	4.6	32.7	1.8	0.2*	1.8	7.5
Metropolitan counties	7.3	0.2	6.1	45.2	2.1	0.2	2.1	9.1
With central city	7.9	0.2	6.8	47.0	2.2	0.2*	2.2	9.3
Without central city	5.0	0.0*	3.7	35.8	1.8	0.1*	1.8	7.8
Nonmetropolitan counties	5.8	0.3*	4.9	34.4	2.2	0.2*	1.9	12.5
Nonwhite								
United States	21.2	1.0	22.7	79.8	9.5	1.0	11.1	24.4
Single	58.3[a]	...	50.4	136.5	23.7[a]	...	23.5	25.7
Married	18.8[a]	...	14.6	60.7	9.1[a]	...	8.2	17.3
Widowed	65.9[a]	...	61.9	105.5	19.5[a]	...	18.7	27.0*
Divorced	61.6[a]	...	53.6	141.0	17.7[a]	...	16.4	30.5*
New England	21.0*	...	20.6	102.0*	9.8*	0.5*	11.5*	27.2*
Middle Atlantic	34.9	1.0*	39.1	117.5	13.8	1.2*	17.0	27.8*
East North Central	23.1	0.9*	23.2	103.5	8.4*	1.1*	9.3*	25.7*
West North Central	19.2*	0.9*	19.7*	80.7*	8.6*	1.8*	10.4*	15.0*
South Atlantic	18.3	0.7*	20.0	65.4	8.5	0.7*	9.9	22.9
East South Central	20.0	1.2*	22.3	65.4	10.1	1.2*	12.1	22.3
West South Central	17.5	0.9*	19.4	59.6	8.5	0.7*	9.9	23.2
Mountain	28.7*	6.5*	22.4	172.6	22.7*	5.3*	22.2*	91.0*
Pacific	14.4*	0.5*	11.7	91.6	6.2*	0.5*	6.3*	26.1*
Metropolitan counties	24.2	0.8*	25.7	94.7	10.0	1.0*	11.9	24.3
Nonmetropolitan counties	15.9	1.2*	16.7	61.2	8.5	1.0*	9.6	24.5

[a]Age-adjusted death rate for ages 15 and over.

grants from the South and now living in slum conditions. The same situation may also account for the high nonwhite mortality from tuberculosis among nonwhite males in the East North Central states. Relative to other areas, the nonwhites (largely Negro) of the West South Central states have a favorable mortality record.

The large Indian population in the Mountain states is undoubtedly the contributing factor to the high nonwhite mortality from tuberculosis in that area. In like fashion, the low mortality among nonwhites in the Pacific Coast states reflects the high proportion of Japanese among them.

The numbers of deaths and the age-adjusted death rates in 1959–61 for each state according to color and sex are shown in Appendix Table A.7. Deaths and death rates in each state by age, but not color or sex, will be found in Appendix Tables A.8 and A.9. Tuberculosis mortality data for standard metropolitan statistical areas are shown in Appendix Tables A.10 and A.11.

Type of residence. The prefatory note to this monograph explains what is meant by "metropolitan" and "nonmetropolitan" counties. The latter are essentially rural in character. Metropolitan counties without a central city are suburban in nature for the most part, and those with a central city typify agglomerations of population.

For white persons at all ages, the adjusted death rate for tuberculosis is lowest in metropolitan counties without a central city (that is, the suburbs); this advantage is evident in Table 4.5 for females in each age group and for males under 65 years. Among males, mortality is highest in the counties with central cities, but in the case of females there is little difference at ages under 65 between these cities and rural areas.

For nonwhites at all ages combined, tuberculosis death rates are much lower in rural areas than in metropolitan counties; most of the nonwhites in metropolitan counties are in central cities. Among nonwhite males, the rate for metropolitan counties is more than 50 percent above that of nonmetropolitan counties; for nonwhite females the excess is only 18 percent.

Children in nonmetropolitan counties had slightly higher tuberculosis death rates than children in metropolitan counties. Because death rates for other causes of death among children are also higher in nonmetropolitan than in metropolitan counties, it has been suggested that availability of adequate and easily accessible medical facilities, as well as appropriate early care and treatment for serious disease may explain, in part, the difference in mortality. In the case of tuberculosis, the small number of deaths in children from this cause and the lack of sufficient collateral information regarding these deaths makes it difficult to reach such a conclusion with any degree of certainty. Public health clinics for children, tuberculosis units of health departments, large municipal hospitals with tuberculosis wards, and other centers with modern facilities such as medical schools are generally located in cities. Presumably excellent medical care for tuberculosis is available to those patients and their families who may want to take advantage of the help offered by these health agencies either to prevent or treat the disease. This has not always been the case in rural areas of the country.

CHANCES OF DEATH FROM TUBERCULOSIS

The relatively low mortality from tuberculosis in 1959–61, compared with that of earlier decades, is also evident in the results of computations for the chances of eventual death from the disease. For example, if mortality conditions of 1939–41 had continued without change, the chance, at birth, of eventually dying from tuberculosis was 31.26 per 1,000; this dropped to only 6.79 in 1959–61 (see Table 4.6). For nonwhite males, these chances fell from 75.74 to 16.21 over the same time interval. White females of each color not only had smaller chances of eventual death from tuberculosis than their male

Table 4.6   Chances per 1,000, at birth, of eventually dying from tuberculosis, by sex and color: United States, 1939-41, 1949-51, and 1959-61

Period	White		Nonwhite	
	Male	Female	Male	Female
1959-61	6.79	2.70	16.21	7.93
1949-51	20.10	9.61	52.47	33.42
1939-41	31.26	21.17	75.74	62.58

counterparts but they also benefited by more rapid reductions in these chances.

In 1959–61, the chances of eventual death from tuberculosis did not vary much from birth to age 50 for white males, to age 40 for nonwhite males, to age 30 for white females, and to age 25 for nonwhite females. The declines after these ages accelerated with advance in age, but the chances were still relatively appreciable at age 65 (see Table 4.7).

Because deaths from tuberculosis in 1959–61 were only about one half of 1 percent of the deaths due to all causes, its elimination as a cause of death adds only a fraction of a year to the average length of life of the general population. Thus, its elimination in 1959–61 would have added only 0.10 years to the expectation of life at birth for white males, 0.05 years for white females, 0.29 years for nonwhite males, and 0.19 years for nonwhite females (see Table 4.7). This situation is much different from that of 1920, when the toll of tuberculosis

Table 4.7   Chances of eventually dying from tuberculosis and
average years of life gained by its elimination as a
cause of death, by age, sex, and color:
United States, 1959-61

Age	Chances per 1,000 of eventual death from tuberculosis				Years of life gained by eliminating tuberculosis			
	White		Nonwhite		White		Nonwhite	
	Male	Female	Male	Female	Male	Female	Male	Female
0	6.79	2.70	16.21	7.93	.10	.05	.29	.19
5	6.97	2.74	17.03	8.20	.10	.05	.30	.19
10	6.99	2.74	17.07	8.20	.10	.05	.30	.19
15	7.00	2.74	17.12	8.19	.10	.05	.30	.19
20	7.04	2.74	17.21	8.14	.10	.05	.30	.18
25	7.08	2.73	17.31	7.93	.10	.05	.30	.17
30	7.09	2.70	17.20	7.59	.10	.04	.29	.15
35	7.07	2.63	16.81	7.07	.10	.04	.27	.13
40	7.02	2.54	16.19	6.40	.09	.04	.24	.11
45	6.92	2.42	15.42	5.81	.09	.03	.21	.09
50	6.73	2.29	14.54	5.42	.08	.03	.18	.07
55	6.41	2.16	13.47	5.04	.07	.02	.15	.06
60	5.98	2.06	12.24	4.71	.06	.02	.12	.05
65	5.46	1.96	11.15	4.35	.05	.02	.10	.04
70	4.81	1.84	10.50	4.01	.03	.01	.08	.03
75	4.03	1.68	9.52	3.76	.02	.01	.06	.02
80	3.26	1.46	8.53	3.44	.02	.01	.04	.02
85	2.55	1.17	7.69	3.19	.01	.00	.03	.01

was such that its elimination as a cause of death would have added 1.9 years to the expectation of life at birth for white persons.[6]

SEASONAL VARIATION IN MORTALITY

The excess mortality from influenza and pneumonia during epidemic outbreaks of influenza is accompanied by an excess in mortality attributed to other causes, including tuberculosis. The monthly rates for 1963, a year of influenza epidemic, showed peaks in February and March for all causes of death, the major cardiovascular-renal diseases, and tuberculosis (see Fig. 4.5). The unusually high seasonal increase in the death rate for tuberculosis during these months slowed down but did not interrupt the downward trend that prevailed during the preceding years.

Figure 4.5. Death rates for influenza and pneumonia and for tuberculosis, by month: United States, 1959–63.

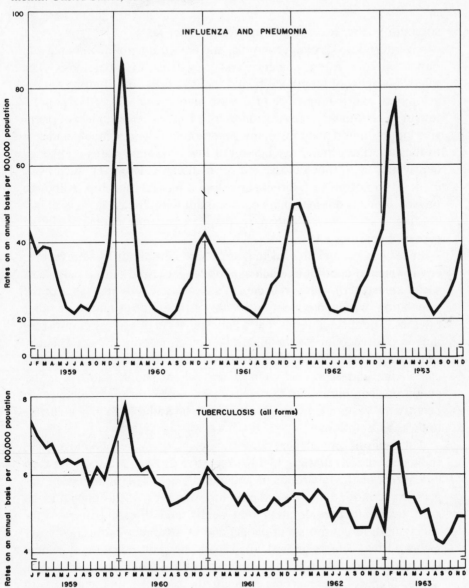

Source: National Center for Health Statistics, *Monthly Vital Statistics Report, Provisional Statistics, Annual Summary for the United States, 1963,* vol. 12 (July 1, 1964).

SOCIOECONOMIC AND ENVIRONMENTAL FACTORS

Many interrelated social, economic, and environmental factors play an important role in the incidence and prevalence of tuberculosis. The relative weights of these factors and the way they contribute to the development and maintenance of disease among enclaves of the population or in certain segments of communities have been a subject of intensive inquiry and debate for many generations. There is much evidence to illustrate the general association of low economic status and social deprivation with tuberculosis and other diseases. However, such associations do not prove a direct cause and effect relationship. Although poverty alone is not inevitably concomitant with disease in general, according to some evidence there is an apparent strong association in the case of tuberculosis.[1]

Belief has been expressed that stress brought about by unfavorable environmental conditions, such as those experienced during periods of social upheaval or war, is reflected in a weakened body resistance of the population, with consequent outbreaks of tuberculosis and some other diseases. The speculation is that a concatenation of such circumstances may in part account for the high tuberculosis rates in the newer countries formed after World War II, which are undergoing drastic political, social, and economic changes and where people still live under conditions comparable to those which prevailed during the nineteenth century in Western Europe. Evidence can be adduced to give credence to these assumptions.[2]

Tuberculosis prevalence rates and selected socioeconomic indices show correlations that are highly suggestive of an association between conditions of the environment and the disease. This relationship appears to be more than a casual one. Interpretation of this phenomenon must take into consideration that health and disease patterns vary widely in different groups of people and in dissimilar cultural environments. Urban centers in the United States have attracted many people from agricultural areas in this country as well as from other parts of the world. Some of these people brought the seeds of tuberculosis with them, and others were infected with tubercle bacilli after reaching new homes, that often fostered conditions that ultimately led to disease.[3]

To demonstrate the association of socioeconomic conditions and tuberculosis prevalence, indices describing housing conditions, relative levels of income, and predominant color or race stock in an area have been used, because such data are usually compiled in census reports for the smaller statistical subdivisions of cities. These statistical parameters make it feasible to work out relationships for relatively homogeneous groups of people or selected communities. Using this technique, a study of tuberculosis in relation to socioeconomic indices was made for New York City, taking advantage of its subdivision into several hundred health areas for each of which details on demographic characteristics and tuberculosis prevalence and other health data were compiled at the time of the 1950 census of population.[4]

The New York City study showed that, during 1949–51, tuberculosis prevalence rates in New York City were generally highest in those

Table 5.1   Coefficients of correlation between tuberculosis, "poor" housing, family income, and race indices[a] in health areas: New York City, 1949–51

Pairs of indices	Borough[b]				New York City
	Manhattan	Bronx	Brooklyn	Queens	
Tuberculosis and poor housing	+ .64	+ .53	+ .78	+ .09	+ .71
Tuberculosis and income	− .56	− .79	− .70	− .48	− .57
Tuberculosis and race	− .66	− .86	− .64	− .36	− .71
Poor housing and income	− .52	− .47	− .76	− .33	− .56
Poor housing and race	− .39	− .36	− .61	− .18	− .52
Income and race	+ .51	+ .77	+ .60	+ .35	+ .56

Source: Lowell, A. M., Socio-Economic Conditions and Tuberculosis Prevalence, New York City, New York Tuberculosis and Health Association, New York, 1956.

[a]Indices: Tuberculosis (average annual prevalence rate) 1949–51; "poor" housing (proportion of dwelling units in dilapidated contition or with inadequate plumbing in 1950); income (median family income in 1949); race (proportion of population white, excluding Puerto Ricans, 1950).

[b]Coefficients for The Borough of Richmond are not shown due to small number of health areas, but figures are included in the New York City total.

sections of the city where a large proportion of the housing was classified as grossly dilapidated; for the city as a whole, the coefficient of correlation was + .71 (see Table 5.1). Although the association between levels of tuberculosis prevalence rates and the index expressing the physical state of housing was striking, some health areas departed from the general pattern. In a few parts of the city a large number of poor housing facilities were located in areas where tuberculosis rates were comparatively low, whereas in other areas with very high tuberculosis rates most of the homes and apartments were in good condition. In one such area with good housing located in the lower part of Manhattan almost all the tuberculosis was concentrated in a very small part of it adjoining a slum district where many cases of the disease were found among transient homeless men. Similar relationships were found for indices of median family income, welfare status, and color or race. Even within two parts of Manhattan very different in respect to demographic composition, namely the Central Harlem and Kips Bay–Yorkville Health Center districts, the smaller health area units confirmed the relationships being described.

Whereas the New York City studies were based on the prevalence of tuberculosis, a later study took into account new active case rates within the indicators. The indicators selected were: (1) a high percent of nonwhite population in the county—either 25 percent nonwhite or 10 percent Indian; (2) an area of low economic status—counties located in the Appalachian region or along the Mexican border; (3) a concentration of population—a county was classified in this category

Table 5.2   Selected factors associated with new active tuberculosis case rates; number and percent of counties within each case rate group: United States, 1962–65

Case rate[a] group	Total counties[b]		High proportion of nonwhite population		Low socio- economic areas		Large city in county		Combination of factors		Selected factors not present	
	Num- ber	Per- cent	Num- ber	Per- cent	Num- ber	Per- cent	Num- ber	Per- cent	Num- ber	Per- cent	Num- ber	Per- cent
All groups	3,070	100.0	421	13.7	295	9.6	50	1.6	217	7.1	2,087	67.9
Under 15	1,346	100.0	47	3.5	63	4.7	3	0.2	40	3.0	1,193	88.6
15.0–24.9	695	100.0	95	13.7	70	10.1	17	2.4	43	6.2	470	67.6
25.0–34.9	448	100.0	111	24.8	55	12.3	13	2.9	40	8.0	229	51.1
35.0–49.9	318	100.0	97	30.5	54	17.0	9	2.8	44	13.8	114	35.9
50.0 and over	263	100.0	71	27.0	53	20.2	8	3.0	50	19.0	81	30.8

[a]Rates for new active tuberculosis cases per 100,000 population.
[b]Three counties in the 35.0–49.9 rate group and eleven counties in the 50.0 and over group were excluded because they reflected extremes due to very small population.

if it contained a city of 250,000 or more people; (4) a combination of factors—a county was classified in this category if two or more of (1), (2), and (3) were identified with it.

In Table 5.2 the counties were grouped into five classes according to the level of their new active tuberculosis case rate during 1962–65. For each class, a count was made of the number of counties possessing the characteristics described by each of the indicators (1), (2), (3), and (4), with the results shown in the table. It is evident, from the table and from Figure 5.1, that the proportion of counties falling within the category of each indicator tends to rise as the level of the case rate increases, the sole exception being the counties with a high proportion of nonwhite population in the highest case rate group.

Low family income, limited education, lack of employment, and

Figure 5.1. Selected factors associated with tuberculosis, proportion of counties within each case rate group, 1962–65.

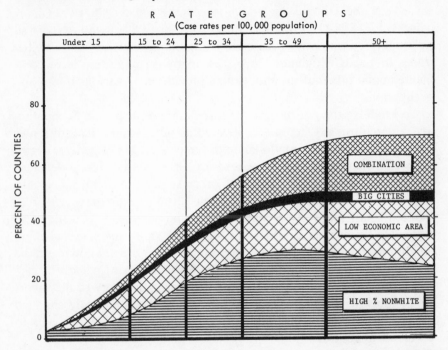

cheap, crowded, and substandard housing are socioeconomic circumstances conducive to tuberculosis. Although these are the conditions for large numbers in the white population, the proportion of nonwhites in these circumstances is inordinately large. These are reflected in the high case rates and death rates due to tuberculosis in the nonwhite population.

OCCUPATION

The fact that tuberculosis is highly prevalent among workers in certain occupations has been known for centuries.[5] In his *De Re Metallica* published in 1556, Georgius Agricola (1494–1555) discussed various diseases of the lungs in miners and noted the harmful effects of the dust inhaled. It is probable that, in addition to silicosis and possibly lung cancer, tuberculosis was involved in the conditions he described. The first monograph devoted to occupational diseases of mine and smelter workers, which appeared in 1567, was written by Aureolus Theophrastus Bombastus von Hohenheim (1493–1541), a Swiss chemist and physician, better known as Paracelsus. He recognized that work in certain mines gave rise to dyspnea, cough, and cachexia (which might have been due to tuberculosis) but thought that these symptoms were caused by the climate or "vapours" of the mines. Charles Turner Thackrah (1795–1833),[6] who died from tuberculosis, observed that pulmonary consumption was quite common among workers in textile trades in Leeds, England. Since then many other writers have commented upon tuberculosis and its high prevalence in various trades and occupations.[7]

To establish the reasons for the association of a specific occupation and tuberculosis is often a complicated matter, because in addition to the hazards of the occupational environment, effects of general socioeconomic conditions, age, race, and sex, the potential risk of developing active disease for a variety of other reasons must be taken into account. Although its connection with certain occupations was recognized, until relatively recently tuberculous disease was difficult to dissociate from other diseases that occurred under the same working conditions. Specific pathogenic microorganisms were unknown and the possibility of transmitting tuberculosis from person to person by airborne infection was questioned. Robert Koch's discovery of the tubercle bacillus in 1882 introduced a new era which completely changed philosophical viewpoints, and introduced the modern approach to tuberculosis control.

In the early part of this century an investigation of the conditions of women and child wage-earners in the United States,[8] made at the request of the United States Senate, brought out that, among operatives in the New England cotton mills of Fall River, Manchester, and Pawtucket, during 1905, 1906, and 1907, tuberculosis "showed an extraordinary excess," its death rate averaging annually 320 per 100,000. Among girls aged fifteen to twenty, the death rate was 219; among young women twenty to twenty-five years the rate was 304; among those twenty-five to thirty, it was 443; and in the age group thirty to thirty-five the tuberculosis death rate reached 473 per 100,000. Conditions peculiar to certain trades may cause disease which in turn predisposes to infection. For example, silicosis can lead to excessive disease and in sequence precipitate death from pulmonary tuberculosis.[9] Without being aware of it, persons with infectious disease can introduce tubercle bacilli into a previously disease-free working environment, thereby causing a local epidemic of pulmonary tuberculosis. Instances of bus drivers and school employees with active disease infecting school children have been recorded in the literature.

In the past, nurses were frequently exposed to tuberculosis in their hospital work, and medical students and laboratory workers are known to have contacted the disease in what were local epidemics. Such occurrences are relatively rare in recent years, but they underscore the need for constant vigilance, whatever the occupation.[10]

Under most circumstances the dissemination and spread of tuberculosis infection in a business organization or an industry can readily be prevented by applying ordinary hygienic precautions, including elimination of active tuberculosis from the environment through periodic screening of employees. A systematic procedure for examining those persons who are at special risk of developing tuberculosis would limit the number needing prolonged surveillance. This could be done by tuberculin testing the entire personnel, X-raying those who give a positive reaction to the test, and, if indicated, placing reactors on a regimen of chemoprophylaxis. Persons with lung lesions suspected of being tuberculous would be referred for further medical evaluation. In the long run preventive measures would be less disruptive of working routines and more acceptable to management. In essence, the public health measures needed for the control of tuberculosis in an industrial environment are not different from those appropriate for the general community.

The better-known studies of tuberculosis in relation to occupation during the first half of this century were based mainly on mortality statistics although, for a few occupations, investigations of prevalence and incidence of disease have been reported. The earliest large-scale investigations of deaths and occupations in the United States covered the occupational mortality experience of the Metropolitan Life Insurance Company among its industrial workers during the 1911–13 and 1922–24 periods.[11] A study by the National Tuberculosis Association based on reports of the U.S. Bureau of the Census for 1930 analyzed death rates, including tuberculosis, among occupied males in ten states.[12] An analysis published in 1965, by the National Center for Health Statistics of the U.S. Public Health Service, reviewed the 1950 mortality statistics for men according to occupation and industry.[13] In England and Wales a series of census reports provided somewhat similar data since 1921, and in Canada a report on occupational mortality rates was published in 1931.[14]

The 1950 study for the United States showed wide variations in mortality according to both industry and occupation. For example, Table 5.3 shows that males at ages 25–59 years in the mining industries had

Table 5.3   Tuberculosis mortality by industry among men 20-64 years of age: United States, 1950

Industry	Standardized mortality ratio[a]		Number of deaths by age groups							
	20-64	25-59	20-64	20-24	25-29	30-34	35-44	45-54	55-59	60-64
All Industries	100	100	15,839	555	873	1,138	3,463	4,751	2,635	2,424
Mining	163	157	654	14	25	26	126	206	132	125
Personal Services	158	163	752	33	48	49	160	227	120	115
Entertainment & Recreation Services	146	154	208	7	16	18	49	66	31	21
Transportation, Communication and Other Public Utilities	139	141	2,119	60	115	161	492	694	302	295
Construction	139	139	2,024	48	81	147	426	607	371	344
Business and Repair Services	112	116	500	7	30	42	145	150	74	52
Agriculture, Forestry and Fisheries	100	99	2,359	123	175	177	424	636	395	429
Wholesale and Retail Trade	91	91	2,375	71	106	162	549	774	382	331
Manufacturing	87	86	3,588	160	231	275	841	977	584	520
Public Administration	70	67	512	17	19	40	97	161	99	79
Finance, Insurance and Real Estate	67	70	308	5	3	14	69	105	68	44
Professional and Related Services	57	58	440	10	24	27	85	148	77	69

Source: U. S. Department of Health, Education, and Welfare, National Vital Statistics Division, Vital Statistics — Special Reports, Vol. 53, No. 4, September 1963.

[a]The standardized mortality ratio compares the tabulated number of deaths in an industrial group with the number to be expected had the death rate for the total male population with work experience prevailed in that industrial class.

Standardized mortality ratio = $\dfrac{\text{Tabulated deaths for an industrial-cause group}}{\text{Expected deaths for an industrial-cause group}} \times 100$

a death rate 57 percent in excess of that for all males of those ages with work experience. On the other hand, males in professional or related services had the advantage of a mortality only 58 percent of that for all males. According to Table 5.4, laborers (excepting farm) had an especially poor mortality record, particularly the nonwhites. Thus, for white laborers at ages 25–59 years, mortality was 66 percent in excess of that for all males of those ages with work experience, but for non-

Table 5.4   Tuberculosis mortality by occupation level among men 20-64 years of age and color: United States, 1950

Occupation level	Standardized mortality ratio[a]		Number of deaths by age group							
	20-64	25-59	20-64	20-24	25-29	30-34	35-44	45-54	55-59	60-64
All occupations	100	100	15,839	555	873	1,138	3,463	4,751	2,635	2,424
White	79	78	11,326	220	436	633	2,346	3,499	2,118	2,074
Nonwhite	312	316	4,513	335	437	505	1,117	1,252	517	350
Laborers, except farm	246	261	3,945	212	274	329	915	1,144	565	506
White	158	166	1,817	41	73	95	369	553	324	362
Nonwhite	469	476	2,128	171	201	234	546	591	241	144
Semi-skilled workers	121	124	4,303	133	236	329	1,038	1,354	656	557
White	103	104	3,233	71	135	202	743	1,043	550	489
Nonwhite	261	270	1,070	62	101	127	295	311	106	68
Agricultural workers	99	99	2,252	119	171	171	400	600	375	416
White	76	74	1,500	53	82	88	257	406	280	334
Nonwhite	258	259	752	66	89	83	143	194	95	82
Clerical, sales and skilled workers	74	72	4,401	81	150	251	923	1,352	859	785
White	69	67	3,930	50	113	194	814	1,222	802	735
Nonwhite	226	219	471	31	37	57	109	130	57	50
Technical, administrative and managerial, except farm	44	44	717	8	38	46	151	218	137	119
White	40	40	633	3	30	43	127	195	121	114
Nonwhite	171	180	84	5	8	3	24	23	16	5
Professional workers[b]	36	34	221	2	4	12	36	83	43	41

Source: U. S. Department of Health, Education, and Welfare, National Vital Statistics Division, Vital Statistics - Special Reports, Vol. 53, No. 5, September 1963.

[a]The standardized mortality ratio compares the tabulated numbers of death in an occupation group with the number to be expected had the death rate for the total male population with work experience prevailed in that occupation class.

Standardized mortality ratio = $\dfrac{\text{Tabulated deaths for an occupation-cause-color group}}{\text{Expected deaths for an occupation-cause-color group}}$ x 100

[b]Includes all races.

white laborers the excess was 376 percent. In fact, distinguished by color for each of the occupational groupings, in Table 5.4, mortality for nonwhites was considerably higher than that for whites.

A general conclusion is that tuberculosis rates are highest in those occupations or industries that engender detrimental working conditions tending to aggravate diseases which can lead to death. Associated with such occupational hazards are the deleterious effects of poor environment. Recruitment of employees in jobs that require few skills (pickup work, dishwashing, short-order cooking, and other similar ways of making a livelihood) is among individuals from poor socioeconomic environments. Many handicapped or chronically ill people take short-term employment because their illness does not permit them to work continuously in regular occupations. Obviously, in these circumstances the occupation is merely an incidental factor associated with the prevalence or incidence of disease in that occupation. On the other hand, the presence of persons with tuberculosis in such occupations constitutes a hazard to coworkers. The cause and effect relationships in a few occupations are more complex and therefore much more difficult to explain.

LEVEL OF EDUCATIONAL ATTAINMENT

Further insight into the relationship between tuberculosis mortality and socioeconomic factors is provided by the 1960 census–death certificate matching study conducted at the University of Chicago.[15] For the purpose of this study the basic procedure was to match a sample of deaths during May through August, 1960, with the returns for the same persons in the census of April 1, 1960. By this procedure it was possible to relate the social and economic characteristics of the decedents from the census returns to information on the death certificate, particularly the cause of death. This direct approach overcomes a difficulty present in the usual studies of occupational mortality in the general population. In these studies, the statements of occupation on the death certificate and in the census enumeration are taken as specified on each occasion, without regard to matching on individual cases. Furthermore, the statement of occupation for a decedent may differ from what he would have reported for himself in a census. Lastly, the death certificate in the United States asks for the usual occupations during a lifetime, whereas the census is concerned with the very recent occupation. These difficulties make the results of the 1960 census–death certificate matching study particularly pertinent for an insight into socioeconomic variations in mortality.

For their purpose, the authors of the 1960 census–death certificate matching study used the level of educational attainment reached by age 25 as a socioeconomic indicator. It has the advantage that, by age 25, the level is fixed for life for most persons, whereas occupation is subject to many shifts. Furthermore, occupation and income, both indicators of socioeconomic level, are generally highly correlated with level of educational attainment. The data from this study shown in Table 5.5 for tuberculosis mortality relate to white males only, because the numbers of white female deaths from this cause in the sample were too small for reliable inference; for purposes of comparison, corresponding mortality data are shown for the total of all causes.

The standard of comparison in Table 5.5 is a mortality index for persons who had completed one or more years of college. That index, computed separately for each educational attainment level is the ratio of the actual deaths for a specified cause to the number of expected in the educational category if it had experienced the corresponding age-specific death rates for the total United States in 1960. The findings

Table 5.5   Educational differentials in mortality from tuberculosis and from all causes of death for white males at ages 25 and over: United States, 1960

Years of school completed	Tuberculosis		All causes		
	Age 25 and over	Ages 25–64	Age 25 and over	Ages 25–64	Ages 65 and over
Fewer than 8 years	3.92	8.79	1.15	1.48	1.01
Elementary, 8 years	3.00	5.69	1.13	1.38	1.00
High school, 1–4 years	1.65	3.84	1.12	1.26	.98
College, one or more years	1.00	1.00	1.00	1.00	1.00

Source: E. M. Kitagawa and P. M. Hauser, "Educational Differentials in Mortality by Cause of Death," Demography, Vol. 5, 1968.

from this study confirm the socioeconomic patterns observed in the studies cited earlier in this chapter. The gradient of tuberculosis mortality with level of educational attainment was very marked, particularly for white males at ages 25–64 years. Thus, mortality from this cause for those with less than eight years of schooling was 8.79 times that of men with one or more years of college, but for all causes of death the ratio was only 1.48 to 1.

It is evident that the extent of the tuberculosis problem in a community is dependent not only on direct steps taken for its control but also upon efforts to improve the general social milieu. Control is easier in those communities that have already made the effort to improve the socioeconomic level of their population.

In most countries, the incidence, prevalence, and mortality from tuberculosis is very much higher than in the United States. Americans who reside for prolonged periods of time in countries where tuberculosis rates are very high are exposed to an increased risk of becoming infected with tubercle bacilli. Furthermore, the movement of United States military personnel, the Peace Corps, and other personnel on government assignment in many countries where tuberculosis is widespread presents additional health problems to the nation which must be anticipated and preventive action taken.

International comparisons of tuberculosis data are subject to many qualifications, particularly with regard to the completeness and accuracy of reporting the disease. Tables 6.1 and 6.2, which relate to countries of the western hemisphere, illustrate the questions to which the data give rise. Thus, the accuracy of the drop recorded for the new case rate for Jamaica from 39.1 per 100,000 population in 1960 to only 20.4 in 1962, much below the level for the United States in that year, may be questioned.

On the other hand, the rise in the new case rate for Mexico over this short period, during which its death rate remained stationary, may reflect improved reporting of the disease. Notwithstanding such qualifications, in most areas within the western hemisphere as shown in Tables 6.1 and 6.2, the new case rates and death rates for tuberculosis from 1960 to 1962 were consistently far above those for the United States; Canada is a notable exception. The upper left panel of Figure 6.1 shows, for selected countries in the western hemisphere, a rather consistent and rapid decline in death rates from tuberculosis since 1930, particularly following World War II.

Outside the English-speaking countries, the few areas in Africa, Asia, and Oceania, for which data are shown in Table 6.3, present a picture of case rates for tuberculosis appreciably above those for the western hemisphere. For example, case rates above 400 per 100,000 population in 1962 were recorded for the Coloured and Bantu population in the Union of South Africa and for Hong Kong and Japan. The rates were also very high for Singapore and the Maoris of New Zealand. A corresponding situation is most likely the case for the many densely populated areas of Asia for which no data are available. On the other hand, tuberculosis case rates approaching those of the United

Table 6.1   Tuberculosis new cases and case rates in countries of the western
hemisphere, 1960-62.

Country	New cases			New case rate		
	1960	1961	1962	1960	1961	1962
United States	55,494	53,726	53,315	30.8	29.4	28.7
Puerto Rico	1,938	1,812	1,816	82.0	75.2	73.8
Argentina	18,865	19,098	18,000[c]	90.0	90.6	84.0
Bolivia	1,136	1,244	1,714	32.8	35.5	48.3
Brazil (reporting areas)[a]	9,943	11,837	---	100.8	158.9	...
Canada[b]	6,345	5,966	6,284	35.5	32.7	33.8
Columbia (reporting areas)	14,392	13,961	14,362	106.5	101.5	105.2
Costa Rica	624	492	602	53.3	40.2	47.3
Cuba	1,856	2,625	2,725	27.3	37.8	38.6
Dominican Republic	2,122	1,197	1,060	70.8	38.5	32.9
Ecuador	5,223	5,660	5,115	119.1	125.1	112.7
El Salvador (reporting areas)	5,251	5,388	4,581	358.2	365.8	302.6
Guatemala	3,802	3,362	3,495	101.0	86.5	87.0
Haiti	2,860	3,332	3,875	68.8	78.4	89.2
Honduras	4,566	1,985	2,157	248.4	104.9	226.6
Jamaica	629	495	335	39.1	30.3	20.4
Mexico	12,417	13,801	16,242	35.5	38.2	43.6
Nicaragua	581	707	391[c]	39.3	46.3	24.8
Panama	1,487	1,104	1,423	137.8	99.5	124.9
Paraguay (reporting areas)	1,113	920	1,223	63.0	77.3	100.2
Peru (reporting areas)	23,915	21,503	24,011	407.8	441.0	466.0
Uruguay	1,928	2,044	1,836	68.2	71.4	63.0
Venezuela (reporting areas)	8,722	8,487	8,138	217.7	168.1	154.2
Antigua	8	6	2[c]	14.8	10.9	(3.4)
Bahama Islands	187	122	156	178.1	113.0	140.5
Barbados	43	47	74	18.5	20.3	31.9
Bermuda	12	22	10	27.3	48.9	21.7
British Guiana	186	172	212	32.9	29.6	35.5
British Honduras	72	54	58	79.1	58.1	60.4
Canal Zone	8	15	21	19.0	35.7	44.7
Cayman Islands	---	3[c]	3	...	37.5	37.5
Dominica	166	---	161	276.7	...	263.9
Falkland Islands	3	---	6	(150.0)	...	(300.0)
French Guiana	---	37	26	...	115.6	74.3
Grenada	45	37	29	50.6	41.1	32.2
Guadeloupe	241	106	208	89.3	37.4	72.0
Martinique	190	149	151	68.6	51.0	50.8
Montserrat	---	9	4	...	69.2	(30.8)
Netherlands Antilles	30	23	33	15.8	11.8	16.7
St. Kitts-Nevis-Anguilla	47	23	8	82.5	39.0	13.3
St. Lucia	67	59	53	77.9	67.8	55.8
St. Pierre and Miquelon	9	7	17	180.0	140.0	340.0
St. Vincent	35	---	---	43.8	...	...
Surinam	126	204[c]	143	46.7	(72.1)	46.6
Trinidad and Tobago	243	---	398	28.8	...	45.2
Turks and Caicos Islands	---	2	---	...	33.3	...
Virgin Islands (U. K.)	2	2	2	28.6	25.0	25.0
Virgin Islands (U.S.A.)	6	12	6	18.6	35.0	17.2

Source: Lowell, A. M., A view of tuberculosis morbidity and mortality fifteen
years after the advent of the chemotherapeutic era, 1947-1962; _Advances in Tuberculosis
Research_, Vol. 15, Karger, Basel, Switzerland, 1966.

[a]State of Guanabara and capitals of other states and territories, data not available
for Sao Paulo.
[b]Including Yukon and Northwest Territories.
[c]Provisional.

95

Table 6.2   Tuberculosis deaths and death rates in countries of the
western hemisphere, 1960-62

Country[a]	Deaths			Death rates		
	1960	1961	1962	1960	1961	1962
United States	10,866	9,938	9,506	6.0	5.4	5.1
Puerto Rico	689	633	566	29.2	26.3	23.0
Canada[b]	823	769	785	4.6	4.2	4.2
Chile	4,032	4,112	3,906	52.9	52.3	48.6
Colombia	4,074	4,066	4,260	28.8	28.2	28.8
Costa Rica	151	105	151	12.9	8.6	11.9
Dominican Republic	467	457	354	15.6	14.7	11.0
Ecuador	1,150	1,080	1,177	26.2	23.9	25.9
El Salvador	408	372	373	15.6	13.7	13.3
Guatemala	1,266	1,237	1,261	33.6	31.8	31.4
Haiti[c]	...	66	25	...	...	...
Honduras	265	236	271	14.4	12.5	13.9
Mexico	9,356	9,369	9,941	26.7	26.0	26.7
Nicaragua	123	97	128	8.3	6.4	8.1
Panama	288	233	252	26.7	21.0	22.1
Paraguay (reporting areas)	292	275	273	...	23.1	22.4
Peru (reporting areas)	3,083	3,137	3,164	77.0	80.8	71.8
Trinidad and Tobago	95	86	48	11.3	9.9	5.5
Venezuela	1,411	1,312	1,255	22.4	17.4	15.9

Source: Lowell, A. M., A view of tuberculosis morbidity and mortality fifteen years after the advent of the chemotherapeutic era, 1947-
1962; Advances in Tuberculosis Research, Vol. 15, Karger, Basel,
Switzerland, 1966.

[a] Tuberculosis deaths and death rates in 1962: Antigua 7 (12.1),
Bahama Islands 9 (8.1), Barbados 17 (7.3), Bermuda 1 (2.2), British
Guiana 36 (6.0), British Honduras 10 (10.4), Canal Zone 2 (4.3),
Dominica 19 (31.1), Grenada 11 (12.2), Guadeloupe 58 (20.1), Martinique
56 (18.9), Montserrat 2 (15.4), St. Kitts-Nevis and Anguilla 11 (18.3),
St. Lucia 15 (15.8), Surinam 6 (2.0), Virgin Islands (U.S.A.) 2 (5.6).
[b] For 1962 included are 75 deaths where underlying cause was reported as
inactive tuberculosis.
[c] Hospital deaths only.

States and Canada were reported for Australia, the Europeans in New
Zealand, and the white population in the Union of South Africa. In
fact, the crude death rates for tuberculosis in the first two of these countries were lower than those for the United States from 1960 to 1962,
and that for the third was somewhat higher (see Table 6.4). The Jewish
population of Israel also recorded a very low death rate for tuberculosis, but for all other areas in the table it was rather high. In the lower
right panel of Figure 6.1, it will be seen that Japan experienced a rising
death rate for tuberculosis from 1930 to the outbreak of World War II,
and Ceylon showed only a small improvement. Much better was the
prewar trend record for Australia, New Zealand, and the Union of
South Africa. The record since World War II is like that already noted
for the western hemisphere.

For most countries of Europe, the recorded new case rates for tuberculosis from 1960 to 1962 were higher than those of the United States
(see Table 6.5). The rates were especially high for such countries of
central Europe as Czechoslovakia, the Federal Republic of Germany,

Figure 6.1. Tuberculosis death rate (per 100,000 pop.) in various countries, between 1930 and 1953.

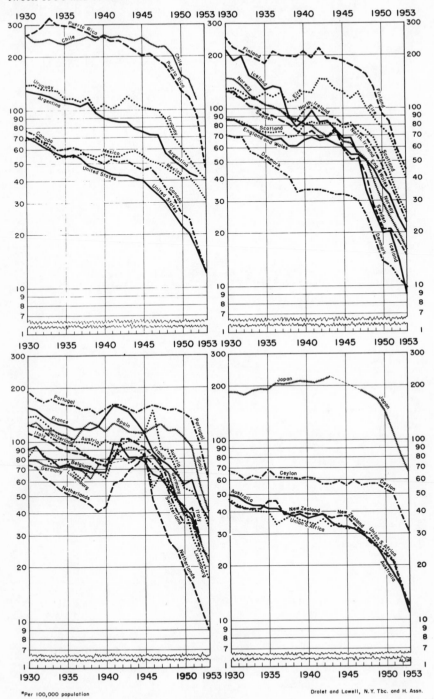

*Per 100,000 population

Drolet and Lowell, N.Y. Tbc. and H. Assn.

Table 6.3   Tuberculosis new cases and case rate in Africa, Asia, and Oceania, 1960-62

Country	New cases			New case rate		
	1960	1961	1962	1960	1961	1962
Africa						
South Africa						
White population	1,221	1,224	1,261	39.6	39.1	39.6
Asiatic population	896	1,055	969	188.6	216.9	194.7
Coloured population	7,896	6,979	7,419	526.8	450.4	464.4
Bantu population	50,224	49,233	53,801	461.4	442.3	472.4
Asia						
Ceylon	9,763	8,107	8,543	96.0	79.7	84.0
Hong Kong	12,425	12,584	14,263	416.8	396.0	419.4
Iraq	4,070	4,599	5,476	59.0	65.7	76.9
Japan	489,715	420,460	387,767	524.2	445.9	407.4
Singapore	5,057	6,299	5,773	309.4	373.4	333.1
Oceania						
Australia	4,057	3,570	3,825	39.4	34.0	35.7
Fiji (Colony)	648	566	560	161.6	141.1	139.6
New Zealand						
Europeans	939	848	797	42.3	37.5	34.4
Maoris	497	484	486	311.1	289.1	278.0

Source: Lowell, A. M., A view of tuberculosis morbidity and mortality fifteen years after the advent of the chemotherapeutic era, 1947-1962; Advances in Tuberculosis Research, Vol. 15, Karger, Basel, Switzerland, 1966.

Table 6.4   Tuberculosis deaths and death rates in Africa, Asia, and Oceania, 1960-62

Country	Deaths			Death rates		
	1960	1961	1962	1960	1961	1962
Africa						
Mauritius	76	80	69	11.9	12.2	10.1
South Africa:						
White population	219	208	188	7.1	6.6	5.9
Asiatic population	82	101	102	17.3	20.8	20.4
Coloured population	1,532	1,475	1,465	102.2	95.2	91.7
Bantu population	---	---	---	...	...	...
United Arab Republic (Egypt)	2,504	2,523	2,457	21.7	20.0	16.5[a]
Asia						
Ceylon	1,619	1,523	1,090	16.4	15.0	10.4
China: Taiwan	4,927	4,698	4,512	46.4	42.8	39.8
Hong Kong	2,085	1,907	1,881	69.9	60.0	55.3
Israel (Jewish population)	79	74	68	4.2	3.8	3.3
Japan	31,959	27,961	27,852	34.2	29.6	29.3
Singapore	646	645	654	39.5	38.2	37.7
Oceania						
Australia	489	447	475	4.8	4.3	4.4
Fiji (Colony) (five hospitals)	49	42	44	12.2	10.5	11.0
New Zealand:						
Europeans	84	95	88	3.8	4.2	3.8
Maoris	30	39	47	18.8	23.3	26.9

Source: Lowell, A. M., A view of tuberculosis morbidity and mortality fifteen years after the advent of the chemotherapeutic era, 1947-62; Advances in Tuberculosis Research, Vol. 15, Karger, Basel, Switzerland. 1966.

[a]For Health Bureau localities.

Table 6.5   Tuberculosis new cases and case rates in European countries, 1960-62

Country	New cases			New case rate		
	1960	1961	1962	1960	1961	1962
Belgium (Respiratory TB)	3,735	4,706	4,127	40.7	51.2	44.6
Czechoslovakia	18,124	14,291	13,747	132.7	103.7	99.2
Denmark	1,130	1,039	953	24.7	22.5	20.5
Eire	3,166	3,010	2,820	111.8	106.8	99.9
Finland	7,655	8.182	8,447	172.8	183.2	187.5
France[a]	38,108	34,606	31,022	84.0	75.8	66.7
Germany:						
Federal Republic	65,578	61,108	56,991	122.8	113.4	104.1
West Berlin[a]	4,689	3,932	3,534	212.7	178.4	161.7
Hungary	...	25,974	23,122	...	258.4	229.6
Iceland	79	78	79	44.9	43.6	43.4
Italy	58,644	51,117	51,518	114.6	101.0	100.6
Luxembourg	197	214	226	62.6	67.1	70.0
Malta	146	143	103	44.4	43.4	31.3
Netherlands	5,845	5,465	4,998	50.9	47.0	42.3
Norway (Bacillary TB)	1,152	964	805	32.2	26.7	22.1
Poland	80,541	77,784	80,561	271.2	259.6	265.7
Portugal	...	17,478	15,372	...	196.1	171.6
Spain	21,303	20,892	15,753	70.3	68.4	51.1
Sweden	4,194	3,996	3,777	56.1	53.1	49.9
Switzerland[b]	4,847	4,755	4,261	90.4	86.5	75.3
United Kingdom:						
England and Wales	24,557	22,783	21,535	53.7	49.4	46.1
Northern Ireland	921	835	730	64.9	58.6	50.9
Scotland	3,862	3,593	3,364	74.2	69.3	64.7

Source: Lowell, A. M., A view of tuberculosis morbidity and mortality fifteen years after the advent of the chemotherapeutic era, 1947-1962; Advances in Tuberculosis Research, Vol. 15, Karger, Basel, Switzerland, 1966.

[a]New cases registered by TB dispensaries.
[b]New cases registered by dispensaries of "Association Suisse Contra La Tuberculose."

Hungary, and Poland. In southern Europe (Italy and Portugal) the rates were consistently high; the sharp drop for Spain in 1962 may reflect a deterioration in the quality of reporting. Aside from the Netherlands and the Scandinavian countries, the only areas of Europe to show lower crude death rates for tuberculosis than the United States in 1962 are Iceland and Malta, both with very small populations (see Table 6.6). The upper right and lower left panels of Figure 6.1 trace the trend of death rates for tuberculosis in Europe from 1930 to 1953; these rates repeat the pattern already cited for the countries of the western hemisphere.

Apparently, the decline in tuberculosis death rates from 1930 to 1940 was practically worldwide. However, in no country of record was the rate of decline during that period comparable with that after World War II. The year 1947 virtually marks the division between two eras with different forms of treatment in tuberculosis. The period prior to 1947 was characterized by the general therapeutic practice of bed rest with long periods of sanatorium care and wide use of collapse ther-

Table 6.6   Tuberculosis deaths and death rates in European countries, 1960–62

Country	Deaths			Death rates		
	1960	1961	1962	1960	1961	1962
Austria	1,651	1,502	1,624	23.4	21.2	22.8
Belgium	1,565	1,334	1,335	17.1	14.5	14.4
Bulgaria	1,252	1,345	1,403	15.9	17.0	17.5
Czechoslovakia	3,435	2,989	3,220	25.2	21.7	23.2
Denmark	191	176	182	4.2	3.8	3.9
Eire	468	420	426	16.5	14.9	15.1
Finland	1,158	1,026	879	26.1	23.0	19.5
France	10,086	9,348	8,998	22.2	20.4	19.3
Germany:						
Federal Republic	8,658	7,703	7,488	16.2	14.3	13.7
West Berlin	565	497	517	25.6	22.6	23.7
Greece	1,381	1,508	1,368	16.6	17.9	16.2
Hungary	3,097	2,869	3,045	31.0	28.5	30.2
Iceland	5	2	5	2.8	1.1	2.7
Ireland	468	420	426	16.5	14.9	15.1
Italy	8,657	8,105	7,891	17.0	16.0	15.5
Luxembourg	42	39	52	13.3	12.2	16.1
Malta	22	17	14	6.7	5.2	4.3
Netherlands	325	316	296	2.8	2.7	2.5
Norway	229	216	202	6.4	6.0	5.6
Poland	11,602	11,950	12,474	39.1	39.9	41.1
Portugal	4,274	3,622	3,291	48.2	40.6	36.7
Spain	7,791	7,474	7,278	25.7	24.4	23.6
Sweden	461	403	327	6.2	5.4	4.3
Switzerland	662	613	624	12.3	11.2	11.0
United Kingdom:						
England and Wales	3,426	3,334	3,088	7.4	7.2	6.6
Northern Ireland	114	105	102	8.0	7.4	7.1
Scotland	509	481	434	9.8	9.3	8.4
Yugoslavia	9,789	8,452	8,531	53.2	45.4	45.3

Source: Lowell, A. M., A view of tuberculosis morbidity and mortality fifteen years after the advent of the chemotherapeutic era, 1947–1962; Advances in Tuberculosis Research, Vol. 15, Karger, Basel, Switzerland, 1966.

apy in those parts of the world where adequate medical facilities were available. The later period, which began around 1947, might be designated as the chemotherapeutic era, when tuberculosis care, treatment, and prevention include chemotherapy and universal use of antituberculosis drugs, selected excisional surgery in hospital treatment, and more recently the chemoprophylactic use of antituberculosis drugs. It is to be hoped that the eradication of tuberculosis on a worldwide basis will become a realistic objective in time; it is a matter requiring international cooperation.[1]

During the nineteenth century, state and city vital statistics consistently listed tuberculosis as the principal killing communicable disease, an invidious distinction held until the early part of the twentieth century. With assurance and with undue optimism, generation after generation of public health practitioners predicted that in a decade or two tuberculosis would no longer be a medical problem of consequence or that it would be of relatively minor importance. This notion was propagated by serious and knowledgeable men who had every reason to believe it, because the limited statistical evidence available to them, mainly mortality reports, seemed to provide a firm basis for their assumptions. In the light of the present understanding of tuberculosis epidemiology, current opinions are perhaps more tempered. Yet, in the third quarter of the twentieth century, tuberculosis is not only still present, but remains a serious disease which threatens the health, welfare, and economy of the nation. Furthermore, a document such as this is in itself evidence that a communicable disease that continues to kill thousands and disable tens of thousands each year should move the social conscience of the country to more aggressive action. Reluctantly, it must be concluded that, in spite of declining death rates and case rates, after more than sixty years of organized and unremitting effort, after discovery of many potent medical remedies and complicated biomedical techniques, and in the midst of unprecedented economic and social advances, the white plague of our forefathers is far from eradicated.

The nation's burden of human and fiscal costs of tuberculosis will continue to be great unless a concerted and rational effort is made to utilize to the best advantage public and private facilities, and expert medical, nursing, and paramedical manpower skilled in using the specific diagnostic, therapeutic, and preventive measures now available for tuberculosis. Resurgence of interest and activity in tuberculosis since 1963 has again raised the hope that the disease can be eradicated. Effective use of chemotherapy and chemoprophylaxis has added weight to the belief that there are practical ways of achieving this. From the example of virtual elimination of tuberculosis in cattle the inference may be drawn that this too can be done in the human population, admittedly with different and less drastic techniques. Epidemiologic evidence supports this point of view. As the more acute problem of serious disease declines, more attention will have to be given to the human, personal, and individual aspects of tuberculosis as it affects the lives of millions of Americans already infected with the tubercle bacillus.

New indices of infection, incidence, and prevalence of tuberculosis must also be developed as more sensitive measures of progress than the traditional death rates and case rates. The term "progress" may have different meanings to the administrator, clinician, and statistician. In a country with scores of state, county, and other local public health jurisdictions, which in many respects are administratively independent units, standardization of definitions in health matters is often difficult to achieve, although it is not impossible to do so. A universal set of generally acceptable indices and definitions is needed to serve as meaningful common denominators. To some extent this has been achieved for the clinical aspects of tuberculosis. As mentioned briefly in an earlier chapter, the Public Health Service has developed a computer program for a central Tuberculosis Records Service to serve the states as an efficient data processing center for current tuberculosis statistics.

To measure the full impact of tuberculosis in the country, a national tuberculosis reporting system for surveillance of all cases, whatever their public health status, has been proposed. It appears that if our statistics are to avoid the apparent demonstration of large epidemics in the future, because more than the new active cases are started on treatment, we will have to ask that anyone who is on treatment be recorded and then, for each patient, give the basis for that treatment and the clinical characteristics of the patient. The system would be keyed to report on every individual for whom antituberculosis therapy is recommended. The types of therapy, whether therapeutic or prophylactic, would be indicated and also whether or not there had been previous therapy or prophylaxis. This type of information would provide health authorities with a method to evaluate the total burden of tuberculosis on society in the form of public health and medical services.[1]

The broad geographic distribution of tuberculosis in the United States creates difficulties in implementing control programs which differ in details of application from area to area even though the underlying epidemiologic principles are the same. Although half of the tuberculosis cases in 1967 were concentrated in 79 metropolitan counties, the remaining half were scattered in 2,400 counties throughout the country. Hundreds of counties have inordinately high tuberculosis case rates. In many counties, even though the number of cases may be small in relation to the population, the tuberculosis situation may be very serious, for example, in certain counties in the Appalachian region, in the southwest, and in counties with predominately Indian population.

As in the past, a variety of medical, social, and economic ills in addition to tuberculosis plague the victims of this disease. Even though tuberculosis is partial to neither the rich nor the poor, poverty and social deprivation in their various manifestations are associated with a large proportion of tuberculous persons. A rough estimate suggests that about two thirds of these people are "poor or near poor." Solutions to the many aspects of the current tuberculosis problem are available. The question is not whether the ability or techniques to do what must be done is available but whether the zeal, initiative, and determination to expend the necessary effort is present among the people of the country.

Statistical Appendix

Table A.1 Tuberculosis hospitals, type of control, number of beds, and average daily census: United States, 1942-53

Type of control	All hospitals	Public agencies						Private				
		Public total	Federal	State	County	City	City-county	Private total	Church	Non-profit	Individual and partnership	Corporation general
Hospitals												
1942	468	323	18	75	184	30	16	145	20	82	27	16
1943	455	317	16	74	184	28	15	138	20	80	23	15
1944	453	318	18	76	182	26	16	135	20	82	20	13
1945	449	318	18	76	183	25	16	131	19	79	21	12
1946	450	320	23	77	180	25	15	130	21	79	20	10
1947	441	315	23	79	176	25	12	127	20	77	20	10
1948	438	319	24	82	174	25	14	119	18	76	17	8
1949	444	325	25	84	178	25	13	119	18	74	20	7
1950	431	323	25	84	177	25	12	108	15	69	18	6
1951	430	325	27	89	171	27	11	105	14	68	17	6
1952	428	327	28	92	169	27	11	101	13	67	14	7
1953	420	319	27	94	164	26	8	101	14	65	11	11
Beds												
1942	82,372	69,636	4,923	24,895	24,638	12,895	2,285	12,736	2,889	7,680	1,010	1,157
1943	79,860	67,389	4,257	24,681	23,946	12,256	2,249	12,471	2,546	7,857	942	1,126
1944	79,848	66,628	5,924	25,024	23,756	10,562	2,362	12,220	2,514	7,904	820	982
1945	78,774	67,190	6,180	24,696	23,434	10,531	2,349	11,584	2,419	7,430	838	897
1946	83,187	71,409	8,536	26,862	23,577	10,192	2,242	11,778	2,524	7,635	803	816
1947	81,328	71,041	8,858	26,184	22,629	10,155	2,215	11,310	2,400	7,229	850	831
1948	81,993	71,499	9,548	26,100	23,119	10,730	2,002	10,494	1,919	7,156	733	686
1949	83,470	73,032	10,213	26,028	24,241	10,669	1,881	10,438	1,943	7,128	842	525
1950	85,746	75,448	10,582	26,960	25,370	10,608	1,928	10,298	1,749	7,306	742	501
1951	88,379	78,645	11,624	29,349	24,739	11,171	1,762	9,734	1,615	6,911	708	500
1952	89,571	79,838	11,172	30,230	25,750	10,939	1,747	9,733	1,647	6,943	593	550
1953	88,406	78,436	10,326	30,654	25,300	10,651	1,505	9,970	1,729	7,027	479	735
Average census												
1942	70,005	60,008	4,309	21,451	20,845	11,448	1,955	9,997	2,319	6,015	729	934
1943	65,302	55,743	3,523	20,599	19,698	10,049	1,874	9,559	2,146	5,779	730	904
1944	63,025	53,852	4,550	20,225	18,824	8,485	1,768	9,173	2,148	5,620	663	742
1945	59,767	50,833	4,940	18,721	17,714	7,695	1,763	8,934	2,050	5,531	702	651
1946	61,931	52,635	6,253	18,612	17,704	8,395	1,671	9,296	2,222	5,793	655	626
1947	62,575	53,102	7,112	18,993	17,788	7,706	1,503	9,487	2,147	5,978	676	686
1948	66,484	57,828	8,274	20,200	19,023	8,617	1,714	8,656	1,691	5,715	604	630
1949	69,476	61,009	8,207	21,555	20,335	9,358	1,554	8,467	1,636	5,715	654	462
1950	72,370	63,868	8,228	22,529	21,913	9,654	1,544	8,502	1,494	5,968	588	452
1951	73,588	65,684	8,771	24,137	21,026	10,256	1,494	7,904	1,403	5,509	551	441
1952	75,253	67,487	8,657	25,131	22,184	9,961	1,554	7,766	1,468	5,426	439	433
1953	74,844	66,961	9,101	25,340	21,094	10,037	1,389	7,883	1,532	5,430	315	606

Source: Reports, Hospital Service in the United States, Council on Medical Education and Hospitals, American Hospital Association.

104

Table A.2   New active tuberculosis cases; number and case rate for each state: 1952, 1957, 1961, 1965, and 1967

State	Number of cases					Case rate per 100,000 population				
	1952	1957	1961	1965	1967	1952	1957	1961	1965	1967
United States	86,700	67,149	53,726	49,016	45,647	55.4	39.2	29.4	25.3	23.1
Conterminous United States	85,607	66,437	53,167	48,434	45,189	55.0	39.0	29.2	25.1	23.0
Alabama	1,375	1,547	1,313	1,417	1,379	44.5	48.7	39.5	40.6	38.9
Alaska	743	431	255	302	110	379.1	189.0	108.1	113.1	40.4
Arizona	1,409	841	694	573	436	167.1	75.6	48.6	36.4	26.5
Arkansas	1,481	822	905	649	497	79.5	45.8	50.2	33.4	24.9
California	8,232	6,288	4,916	4,577	4,171	69.9	44.2	30.0	24.9	22.1
Colorado	495	412	306	274	256	35.9	24.3	16.6	14.1	12.7
Connecticut	935	502	325	335	411a	45.6	21.8	12.7	11.8	14.1
Delaware	149	139	158	141	122	44.0	33.1	34.3	28.0	23.3
District of Columbia	1,217	655	513	536	423	151.0	84.4	65.9	66.8	52.4
Florida	2,002	1,716	1,359	1,521	1,601	64.2	40.4	25.9	26.2	26.5
Georgia	1,947	1,417	1,268	1,269	1,223	53.9	37.0	31.4	28.9	27.1
Hawaii	350	281	304	280	348	68.0	48.0	46.0	39.4	45.7
Idaho	173	91	82	52	55	29.7	14.2	12.0	7.5	7.8
Illinois	4,481	5,123	4,021	3,250	2,999	50.5	53.6	39.9	30.5	27.6
Indiana	1,683	1,419	1,152	1,119	1,069	40.6	31.3	24.5	22.9	21.3
Iowa	506	293	165	166	150	19.2	10.7	6.0	6.0	5.5
Kansas	461	429	240	242	223	23.4	20.2	10.9	10.8	9.8
Kentucky	2,276	1,800	1,257	1,193	1,071	77.7	61.2	41.1	37.6	33.4
Louisiana	1,748	1,298	1,055	931	966	61.4	41.6	32.2	26.2	26.3
Maine	380	224	159	142	120	41.8	23.8	16.1	14.4	12.2
Maryland	1,830	1,608	1,374	1,234	1,187	73.1	55.9	43.7	34.9	32.2
Massachusetts	1,723	1,600	1,275	969	910	37.3	32.8	24.8	18.1	16.8
Michigan	4,066	2,950	2,690	2,199	1,930	61.3	39.1	33.9	26.4	22.4
Minnesota	821	677	474	419	394	27.0	20.4	13.7	11.8	10.9
Mississippi	1,139	784	612	661	616	52.3	36.8	27.6	28.6	26.3
Missouri	2,086	1,561	1,092	1,043	882	52.0	36.7	25.2	23.2	19.2
Montana	192	244	103	133	109	32.2	36.9	14.7	18.9	15.6
Nebraska	225	210	160	141	121	17.2	15.1	10.9	9.7	8.4
Nevada	121	90	81	189	147	66.9	35.0	25.6	43.5	33.4
New Hampshire	149	98	86	48	44	27.9	17.0	13.9	7.1	6.4
New Jersey	2,234	1,806	1,658	1,674	1,455	44.1	32.2	26.9	24.7	20.9
New Mexico	680	469	329	288	248	91.0	53.9	33.3	28.4	24.5
New York	11,386	8,535	6,182	5,869	5,069	74.7	52.7	36.0	32.4	28.2
North Carolina	1,565	1,210	1,040	1,276	1,247	37.8	27.2	22.3	25.9	24.6
North Dakota	206	116	88	49	49	33.6	18.4	13.8	7.5	7.8
Ohio	5,124	3,269	2,503	1,729	1,548	62.9	35.2	25.2	16.9	14.7
Oklahoma	1,165	778	465	605	442	53.4	34.2	19.4	24.7	17.6
Oregon	598	495	425	361	322	37.5	28.5	23.2	18.6	16.3
Pennsylvania	4,720	4,947	3,732	2,686	2,736	44.8	45.2	32.9	23.2	23.4
Rhode Island	347	271	165	140	148	43.5	31.7	19.2	15.7	16.5
South Carolina	862	734	692	758	716	39.0	31.5	28.7	29.7	26.9
South Dakota	140	153	123	166	119	21.4	22.4	17.4	24.2	17.8
Tennessee	2,131	1,681	1,425	1,356	1,199	63.6	48.4	39.6	35.2	30.4
Texas	4,385	2,729	2,429	2,583	3,209b	52.5	29.9	24.5	24.4	29.6
Utah	153	136	66	88	65	21.0	16.2	7.0	8.9	6.4
Vermont	171	89	83	42	44	45.7	23.6	21.4	10.4	10.6
Virginia	2,960	1,519	1,833	1,754	1,521	85.1	39.7	44.7	39.7	33.5
Washington	1,223	959	653	488	507	49.7	35.0	22.2	16.4	15.8
West Virginia	1,141	755	688	518	539	57.9	40.1	38.1	28.5	29.8
Wisconsin	1,058	888	713	560	463	30.6	23.4	17.6	13.5	11.0
Wyoming	56	60	40	21	31	18.9	18.6	11.3	6.4	9.7

aIncludes all diagnosed cases, both "officially and not officially" reported.
bIn prior years data were limited to counties with organized health units.

105

Table A.3   Percent of new active pulmonary tuberculosis cases by
extent of disease[a], by state, 1967

State	Total	Minimal	Moderately Advanced	Far Advanced
United States	100.0	20.5	44.6	34.9
Conterminous United States	100.0	20.3	44.6	35.1
Alabama	100.0	15.3	46.2	38.5
Alaska	100.0	52.6	38.2	9.2
Arizona	100.0	19.9	42.8	37.3
Arkansas	100.0	16.2	33.5	50.3
California	100.0	27.0	45.5	27.5
Colorado	100.0	19.1	50.0	30.9
Connecticut	100.0	24.6	43.7	31.7
Delaware	100.0	15.4	34.1	50.5
District of Columbia	100.0	12.4	37.6	50.0
Florida	100.0	18.0	49.1	32.9
Georgia	100.0	15.0	39.2	45.8
Hawaii	100.0	40.9	48.5	10.6
Idaho	100.0	8.7	34.8	56.5
Illinois	100.0	17.0	51.0	32.0
Indiana	100.0	23.2	45.2	31.6
Iowa	100.0	6.8	35.3	57.9
Kansas	100.0	28.6	43.9	27.5
Kentucky	100.0	13.9	45.6	40.5
Louisiana	100.0	13.8	46.7	39.5
Maine	100.0	28.6	49.3	22.1
Maryland	100.0	22.4	43.9	33.7
Massachusetts	100.0	24.3	36.6	39.1
Michigan	100.0	24.3	44.1	31.6
Minnesota	100.0	29.3	50.6	20.1
Mississippi	100.0	20.3	40.0	39.7
Missouri	100.0	16.3	39.3	44.4
Montana	100.0	33.3	46.0	20.7
Nebraska	100.0	16.3	44.6	39.1
Nevada	100.0	19.0	30.2	50.8
New Hampshire	100.0	19.4	50.0	30.6
New Jersey	100.0	10.8	43.3	45.9
New Mexico	100.0	29.9	41.5	28.6
New York	100.0	21.7	46.5	31.8
North Carolina	100.0	16.3	36.2	47.5
North Dakota	100.0	36.4	39.4	24.2
Ohio	100.0	20.0	41.6	38.4
Oklahoma	100.0	11.4	54.7	33.9
Oregon	100.0	37.6	41.5	20.9
Pennsylvania	100.0	19.2	49.2	31.6
Rhode Island	100.0	18.6	41.6	39.8
South Carolina	100.0	17.0	30.5	52.5
South Dakota	100.0	25.0	34.5	40.5
Tennessee	100.0	23.8	46.1	30.1
Texas	100.0	16.9	44.5	38.6
Utah	100.0	45.3	33.3	21.4
Vermont	100.	24.2	48.5	27.3
Virginia	100.0	28.4	37.0	34.6
Washington	100.0	30.7	51.4	17.9
West Virginia	100.0	24.9	31.5	43.6
Wisconsin	100.0	18.6	51.4	30.0
Wyoming	100.0	15.4	61.5	23.1
Puerto Rico[b]	100.0	13.3	37.9	48.8

[a]Cases for which extent specified.
[b]Not included in totals.

State	Total active cases	Pulmonary						Nonpulmonary		Form not specified
		Total pulmonary	Primary	Minimal	Moderately advanced	Far advanced	Extent not specified	Unexplained pleurisy	Other	
United States	45,647	40,699	4,415	7,034	15,245	11,926	2,079	693	3,520	735
Conterminous United States	45,189	40,300	4,393	6,874	15,074	11,888	2,071	682	3,472	735
Alabama	1,379	1,322	126	165	499	416	116	14	42	1
Alaska	110	92	14	40	29	7	2	-	18	-
Arizona	436	391	52	66	142	124	7	-	44	1
Arkansas	497	444	122	50	103	155	14	14	39	-
California	4,171	3,686	349	897	1,515	915	10	74	411	-
Colorado	256	211	30	31	81	50	19	6	35	4
Connecticut	411	360	29	70	124	90	47	14	37	-
Delaware	122	104	13	14	31	46	-	-	18	-
District of Columbia	423	379	78	28	85	113	75	-	44	-
Florida	1,601	1,462	184	230	627	421	-	11	92	36
Georgia	1,223	959	125	121	315	368	30	21	75	168
Hawaii	348	307	8	120	142	31	6	11	30	-
Idaho	55	47	1	4	16	26	-	-	8	-
Illinois	2,999	2,687	58	430	1,289	809	101	-	312	-
Indiana	1,069	988	106	179	348	243	112	16	65	-
Iowa	150	140	-	9	47	77	7	-	10	-
Kansas	223	206	16	49	75	47	19	2	15	-
Kentucky	1,071	1,012	59	131	431	383	8	16	43	-
Louisiana	966	905	65	101	343	290	106	-	61	-
Maine	120	98	14	22	38	17	7	3	19	-
Maryland	1,187	1,057	97	214	418	321	7	-	130	-
Massachusetts	910	802	50	178	269	287	18	32	76	-
Michigan	1,930	1,687	276	343	622	446	0	68	141	34
Minnesota	394	329	16	89	154	61	9	7	58	-
Mississippi	616	570	52	101	199	198	20	6	40	-
Missouri	882	815	144	98	237	268	68	8	59	-
Montana	109	86	7	21	29	13	16	-	23	-
Nebraska	121	114	9	15	41	36	13	-	5	2
Nevada	147	137	74	12	19	32	-	-	10	-
New Hampshire	44	41	2	7	18	11	3	-	3	-
New Jersey	1,455	1,348	159	127	508	538	16	23	84	-
New Mexico	248	211	45	46	64	44	12	7	30	-
New York	5,069	4,427	349	722	1,548	1,058	750	185	197	260
North Carolina	1,247	1,066	150	149	332	435	-	74	107	-
North Dakota	49	37	1	12	13	8	3	-	12	-
Ohio	1,548	1,393	132	222	462	427	150	-	143	12
Oklahoma	442	405	9	42	202	125	27	8	29	-
Oregon	322	296	16	97	107	54	22	2	24	-
Pennsylvania	2,736	2,448	192	433	1,111	712	-	-	288	-
Rhode Island	148	129	9	21	47	45	7	-	19	-
South Carolina	716	592	116	81	145	250	-	-	87	37
South Dakota	119	100	15	21	29	34	1	1	18	-
Tennessee	1,199	1,111	140	226	438	286	21	-	88	-
Texas	3,209	2,873	469	383	1,007	873	141	35	196	105
Utah	65	50	4	19	14	9	4	-	15	-
Vermont	44	37	4	8	16	9	-	-	7	-
Virginia	1,521	1,453	308	325	424	396	-	-	68	-
Washington	507	414	42	113	189	66	4	18	75	-
West Virginia	539	442	49	80	101	140	72	5	23	69
Wisconsin	463	405	28	70	194	113	-	9	43	6
Wyoming	31	24	2	2	8	3	9	3	4	-
Puerto Rico[a]	1,191	1,140	189	127	360	464	-	12	39	

[a]Not included in totals.

107

Table A.5   Number of counties according to level of case rate group: average for 1962-65

Region and state	Total number of counties	New active tuberculosis case rate				
		Under 15.0	15.0 to 24.9	25.0 to 34.9	35.0 to 49.9	50.0 and over
United States	3,084	1,346	695	448	321	274
Northeast	217	124	64	19	5	5
Connecticut	8	7	1	–	–	–
Maine	16	13	3	–	–	–
Massachusetts	14	10	3	–	–	1
New Hampshire	10	9	1	–	–	–
New Jersey	21	5	9	5	2	–
New York	62	33	19	7	–	3
Pennsylvania	67	36	22	6	2	1
Rhode Island	5	2	3	–	–	–
Vermont	14	9	3	1	1	–
North Central	1,056	685	238	67	34	32
Illinois	102	45	32	14	6	5
Indiana	92	36	32	11	9	4
Iowa	99	99	–	–	–	–
Kansas	105	83	16	5	–	1
Michigan	83	35	37	5	5	1
Minnesota	87	74	10	3	–	–
Missouri	115	50	30	18	12	5
Nebraska	93	85	7	–	–	1
North Dakota	53	43	7	–	–	3
Ohio	88	44	37	7	–	–
South Dakota	67	41	13	1	2	10
Wisconsin	72	50	17	3	–	2
South	1,394	302	317	321	257	197
Alabama	67	7	12	16	18	14
Arkansas	75	1	17	28	20	9
Delaware	3	–	–	2	1	–
District of Columbia	1	–	–	–	–	1
Florida	67	12	27	17	8	3
Georgia	159	35	49	35	27	13
Kentucky	120	1	20	25	36	38
Louisiana	64	7	28	20	7	2
Maryland	24	2	8	7	5	2
Mississippi	82	7	29	30	12	4
North Carolina	100	22	22	25	22	9
Oklahoma	77	21	22	13	11	10
South Carolina	46	10	8	13	11	4
Tennessee	95	2	11	23	27	32
Texas	254	170	31	24	11	18
Virginia	105	1	15	25	34	30
West Virginia	55	4	18	18	7	8
West	417	235	76	41	25	40
Alaska	1	–	–	–	–	1
Arizona	14	1	2	2	3	6
California	58	10	16	20	7	5
Colorado	63	49	6	8	–	–
Hawaii	5	1	–	–	2	2
Idaho	44	33	8	2	–	1
Montana	56	41	8	2	1	4
Nevada	17	–	1	1	3	12
New Mexico	32	9	7	4	6	6
Oregon	36	21	12	–	2	1
Utah	29	27	1	–	–	1
Washington	39	22	13	2	1	1
Wyoming	23	21	2	–	–	–

Table A.6   Tuberculosis; number of deaths and death rate for each state:
1952, 1957, 1961, and 1965

State	Number of deaths				Death rate			
	1952	1957	1961	1965	1952	1957	1961	1965
United States	24,861	13,390	9,938	7,934	15.9	7.8	5.4	4.1
Conterminous United States	24,621	13,324	9,892	7,900	15.8	7.8	5.4	4.1
Alabama	572	318	286	260	18.5	10.0	8.6	7.5
Alaska	173	46	19	12	88.3	20.2	8.1	4.5
Arizona	358	223	131	121	42.4	20.0	9.2	7.7
Arkansas	492	253	190	109	26.4	14.1	10.5	5.6
California	1,810	906	620	596	15.4	6.4	3.8	3.2
Colorado	166	110	71	61	12.0	6.4	3.9	3.1
Connecticut	248	119	105	84	12.1	5.2	4.1	3.0
Delaware	53	46	26	20	15.6	11.0	5.7	4.0
District of Columbia	250	110	102	102	31.0	14.2	13.1	12.7
Florida	504	264	220	216	16.2	6.2	4.2	3.7
Georgia	464	261	197	150	12.8	6.8	4.9	3.4
Hawaii	67	20	27	22	13.0	3.4	4.1	3.1
Idaho	43	20	18	11	7.4	3.1	2.6	1.6
Illinois	1,575	740	502	431	17.8	7.7	5.0	4.1
Indiana	515	309	267	195	12.4	6.8	5.7	4.0
Iowa	183	79	66	43	7.0	2.9	2.4	1.6
Kansas	161	77	57	42	8.2	3.6	2.6	1.9
Kentucky	855	441	307	204	29.2	15.0	10.0	6.4
Louisiana	557	302	238	173	19.6	9.7	7.3	4.9
Maine	102	48	36	29	11.2	5.1	3.7	2.9
Maryland	642	319	259	201	25.6	11.1	8.2	5.7
Massachusetts	718	416	304	225	15.5	8.5	5.9	4.2
Michigan	787	448	334	293	11.9	5.9	4.2	3.5
Minnesota	205	108	98	68	6.7	3.3	2.8	1.9
Mississippi	418	166	116	76	19.2	7.8	5.2	3.3
Missouri	690	394	287	219	17.2	9.3	6.6	4.9
Montana	77	66	25	22	12.9	10.0	3.6	3.1
Nebraska	79	74	37	27	6.1	5.3	2.5	1.9
Nevada	28	25	17	17	15.4	9.7	5.4	3.9
New Hampshire	47	18	13	9	8.8	3.1	2.1	1.3
New Jersey	844	531	391	295	16.7	9.4	6.4	4.4
New Mexico	170	100	68	68	22.8	11.4	6.9	6.7
New York	2,639	1,552	1,165	916	17.3	9.6	6.8	5.1
North Carolina	548	222	177	160	13.2	5.0	3.8	3.2
North Dakota	53	23	8	11	8.6	3.7	1.3	1.7
Ohio	1,116	634	468	374	13.7	6.8	4.7	3.7
Oklahoma	321	162	137	110	14.7	7.1	5.7	4.5
Oregon	150	67	59	39	9.4	3.9	3.2	2.0
Pennsylvania	1,825	1,031	881	628	17.3	9.4	7.8	5.4
Rhode Island	100	53	32	30	12.5	6.2	3.7	3.4
South Carolina	360	190	132	101	16.3	8.2	5.4	4.0
South Dakota	74	31	20	26	11.3	4.5	2.8	3.8
Tennessee	883	455	289	248	26.3	13.1	8.0	6.4
Texas	1,339	793	567	436	16.0	8.7	5.7	4.1
Utah	51	21	28	13	7.0	2.5	3.0	1.3
Vermont	58	39	25	21	15.5	10.3	6.4	5.2
Virginia	663	331	184	155	19.1	8.7	4.4	3.5
Washington	260	113	83	58	10.6	4.1	2.8	2.0
West Virginia	321	166	124	89	16.3	8.8	6.9	4.9
Wisconsin	228	138	117	114	6.6	3.6	2.9	2.8
Wyoming	19	12	8	4	6.4	3.7	2.3	1.2

Table A.7   Tuberculosis deaths and age-adjusted death rates by color and sex for each state, 1959-61

State	Number of deaths					Age-adjusted death rate				
	Total	White		Nonwhite		Total	White		Nonwhite	
		Male	Female	Male	Female		Male	Female	Male	Female
United States	32,276	17,963	6,191	5,450	2,672	5.4	6.7	2.1	21.2	9.5
Conterminous United States	32,151	17,950	6,187	5,382	2,632	...	...	...	...	...
Alabama	879	305	138	278	158	9.0	8.8	3.4	23.6	12.0
Alaska	66	8	3	29	26	18.1	7.0	1.2	56.8	63.6
Arizona	493	321	77	61	34	13.3	19.0	4.6	36.6	22.6
Arkansas	566	288	92	113	73	8.9	11.3	3.1	20.9	12.8
California	2,217	1,396	493	247	81	4.2	6.0	1.9	15.4	5.2
Colorado	228	163	50	9	6	4.1	6.1	1.8	14.8	8.7
Connecticut	321	222	62	25	12	3.5	5.2	1.3	20.8	8.9
Delaware	72	33	17	17	5	5.0	5.5	2.2	20.1	6.1
District of Columbia	306	69	26	138	73	11.7	10.1	2.8	27.2	11.7
Florida	669	344	105	150	70	3.9	4.3	1.4	13.9	5.9
Georgia	630	218	96	197	119	5.5	5.5	2.0	15.6	7.6
Hawaii	59	5	1	39	14	4.1	3.2	0.6	6.6	2.9
Idaho	57	35	13	6	3	2.7	3.3	1.2	50.7	33.3
Illinois	1,795	1,034	289	332	140	5.2	6.5	1.7	25.0	9.1
Indiana	787	499	189	62	37	4.9	6.8	2.3	18.0	9.9
Iowa	212	144	56	10	2	2.0	2.7	1.1	24.0	5.3
Kansas	173	108	45	17	3	2.2	3.0	1.1	10.9	2.5
Kentucky	982	552	280	115	35	9.6	12.1	5.4	34.0	10.4
Louisiana	785	324	94	248	119	8.3	10.2	2.6	20.1	8.6
Maine	112	75	36	-	1	3.3	4.8	1.9	...	16.0
Maryland	789	351	130	208	100	8.4	9.4	2.9	31.6	14.4
Massachusetts	985	709	226	34	16	5.0	8.1	2.2	21.0	9.4
Michigan[a]	1,105	645	202	188	70	4.4	5.6	1.7	21.4	7.6
Minnesota	323	222	85	11	5	2.5	3.6	1.3	19.7	9.4
Mississippi	413	121	55	135	102	6.4	5.9	2.3	12.8	8.5
Missouri	908	575	187	103	43	5.5	7.6	2.3	18.8	7.4
Montana	94	58	11	9	16	4.0	4.7	1.0	28.4	74.2
Nebraska	94	59	19	10	6	1.9	2.3	0.9	23.7	10.9
Nevada	52	36	8	4	4	6.2	8.6	2.2	16.3	13.5
New Hampshire	54	42	11	1	-	2.2	3.7	0.8	15.8	...
New Jersey	1,201	665	222	216	98	5.7	6.9	2.2	32.2	12.8
New Mexico	225	108	74	24	19	9.7	10.2	6.9	28.0	23.3
New York	3,748	2,097	626	710	315	6.2	7.5	2.1	37.2	13.4
North Carolina	587	241	102	160	84	4.6	5.1	1.8	12.5	5.7
North Dakota	32	17	11	3	1	1.4	1.4	1.1	26.6	2.2
Ohio	1,490	864	292	247	87	4.5	5.8	1.8	24.0	7.7
Oklahoma	449	237	85	68	59	5.3	6.3	1.9	22.5	16.9
Oregon	196	136	39	14	7	3.1	4.5	1.3	27.3	16.9
Pennsylvania	2,770	1,769	439	371	191	6.9	9.6	2.2	31.8	15.1
Rhode Island	150	113	25	6	6	4.7	7.8	1.5	22.7	17.9
South Carolina	430	133	41	157	99	6.9	6.7	1.8	18.9	9.9
South Dakota	76	29	10	17	20	3.3	2.3	0.8	48.4	63.9
Tennessee	1,001	492	278	150	81	8.5	10.5	4.9	18.7	9.2
Texas	1,801	1,039	460	213	89	6.1	8.4	3.4	13.3	5.3
Utah	74	51	12	8	3	3.1	4.5	1.0	32.4	10.1
Vermont	78	68	10	-	-	4.9	9.5	1.0	...	...
Virginia	692	263	110	210	109	5.8	5.9	2.0	19.5	9.6
Washington	257	168	57	21	11	2.6	3.5	1.2	14.8	9.5
West Virginia	392	250	98	35	9	6.4	8.8	3.2	22.5	6.1
Wisconsin	370	239	99	23	9	2.5	3.3	1.3	24.6	9.2
Wyoming	31	23	5	1	2	3.0	4.3	1.0	11.9	24.3

[a]Three-year total for Michigan (1,105) understated by 2 deaths.

Table A.8   Tuberculosis deaths, by state: United States, 1959-61

State	Total	Age under 1	1-4	5-14	15-24	25-34	35-44	45-54	55-64	65-74	75-84	85 & over	Not stated
United States	32,276	110	322	141	397	1,600	3,631	5,668	7,188	7,188	4,476	1,075	21
Conterminous United States	32,151	107	319	141	397	1,595	3,615	5,652	7,173	7,612	4,454	1,068	18
Alabama	879	5	8	5	28	67	123	138	164	194	119	27	1
Alaska	66	3	3	-	-	5	8	10	5	20	7	2	3
Arizona	493	5	9	4	7	28	53	88	105	128	55	10	1
Arkansas	566	2	4	2	15	20	49	93	125	141	100	15	-
California	2,217	2	25	10	12	94	219	381	538	494	362	78	2
Colorado	228	1	1	3	1	6	9	55	54	63	27	8	-
Connecticut	321	-	2	1	3	4	29	51	79	84	56	12	-
Delaware	72	-	-	-	-	3	9	7	20	15	13	4	1
District of Columbia	306	-	2	-	4	29	58	62	71	46	25	9	-
Florida	669	3	11	2	9	33	86	125	150	147	81	22	-
Georgia	630	4	12	1	15	42	106	125	110	130	66	18	1
Hawaii	59	-	-	-	-	-	8	6	10	15	15	5	-
Idaho	57	-	1	-	-	2	6	9	14	14	10	1	-
Illinois	1,795	8	23	5	20	104	205	366	403	405	215	41	-
Indiana	787	-	3	4	15	32	78	111	157	204	136	47	-
Iowa	212	-	1	-	2	4	13	27	57	61	35	12	-
Kansas	173	-	-	1	1	3	12	36	40	43	26	11	-
Kentucky	982	2	20	7	10	62	95	142	195	231	161	57	-
Louisiana	785	5	5	2	14	46	105	166	169	160	87	24	2
Maine	112	-	2	1	-	3	10	25	24	29	16	2	-
Maryland	789	2	8	3	7	42	116	152	171	173	92	23	-
Massachusetts	985	3	1	2	8	31	95	157	238	241	164	44	1
Michigan	1,105	1	7	3	7	44	117	194	235	278	182	37	-
Minnesota	323	1	-	3	1	2	24	42	80	82	70	18	-
Mississippi	413	4	8	4	12	32	57	68	83	79	54	11	1
Missouri	908	1	3	2	4	26	82	159	214	228	151	37	1
Montana	94	-	1	2	1	2	8	11	18	34	14	3	-
Nebraska	94	1	-	1	1	2	9	21	24	18	15	2	-
Nevada	52	-	2	-	2	-	8	7	5	15	13	-	-
New Hampshire	54	-	1	2	-	1	2	6	10	18	13	1	-
New Jersey	1,201	6	14	4	14	68	167	222	252	271	157	26	-
New Mexico	225	1	5	5	6	18	26	37	46	50	25	6	-
New York	3,748	9	19	11	44	217	519	741	903	818	386	78	3
North Carolina	587	2	5	6	9	29	67	86	142	155	73	12	1
North Dakota	32	-	1	-	1	-	-	2	6	13	8	1	-
Ohio	1,490	4	15	4	6	65	162	230	337	378	234	55	-
Oklahoma	449	3	3	3	5	25	28	77	106	92	81	24	2
Oregon	196	1	-	2	2	4	18	46	45	54	23	1	-
Pennsylvania	2,770	3	4	6	24	119	268	544	666	733	327	76	-
Rhode Island	150	1	3	1	-	6	11	23	34	50	13	8	-
South Carolina	430	2	5	1	14	50	93	74	81	77	25	8	-
South Dakota	76	4	1	-	6	5	4	6	20	17	9	4	-
Tennessee	1,001	2	19	4	10	51	93	145	191	254	184	48	-
Texas	1,801	17	44	14	34	104	195	290	385	413	243	62	-
Utah	74	-	-	3	1	2	4	11	20	21	6	6	-
Vermont	78	-	-	-	-	-	6	3	17	34	14	4	-
Virginia	692	1	9	2	10	33	76	126	128	152	130	25	-
Washington	257	1	2	-	1	8	21	39	67	73	35	10	-
West Virginia	392	-	7	4	7	18	43	72	82	96	48	15	-
Wisconsin	370	-	2	1	3	9	27	49	87	96	70	25	1
Wyoming	31	-	1	-	1	-	4	5	5	10	5	-	-

111

Table A.9   Tuberculosis death rates, by state: United States, 1959-61

State	All ages	Under 1	1-4	5-14	15-24	25-34	35-44	45-54	55-64	65-74	75-84	85 & over
United States	6.0	0.9	0.7	0.1	0.6	2.3	5.0	9.2	15.4	23.2	32.2	38.6
Conterminous United States	6.0	0.9	0.7	0.1	0.6	2.3	5.0	9.2	15.4	23.1	32.1	38.4
Alabama	9.0	2.1	0.9	0.2	1.9	5.6	10.2	12.9	22.0	37.2	54.2	63.4
Alaska	9.7	14.1	3.7	...	...	4.2	8.3	17.6	18.2	178.0	172.3	232.3
Arizona	12.6	4.8	2.3	0.5	1.2	5.5	10.2	21.5	37.7	67.1	81.5	81.5
Arkansas	10.6	1.7	0.9	0.2	2.0	3.5	7.8	15.0	25.2	36.9	59.8	45.2
California	4.7	0.2	0.6	0.1	0.2	1.5	3.2	7.1	13.8	18.1	31.0	34.0
Colorado	4.3	0.8	0.2	0.3	0.1	0.9	1.3	9.9	13.3	20.8	19.1	26.1
Connecticut	4.2	...	0.3	0.1	0.3	0.4	2.6	5.5	11.7	17.2	28.5	28.4
Delaware	5.4	...	...	...	...	1.6	4.7	4.8	19.4	21.3	42.7	63.6
District of Columbia	13.4	...	1.1	...	1.2	8.8	18.1	20.7	31.1	33.1	44.7	72.8
Florida	4.5	0.9	0.9	0.1	0.5	1.8	4.4	7.5	10.8	12.6	19.3	30.4
Georgia	5.3	1.4	1.1	0.0	0.8	2.8	7.0	9.8	12.8	22.2	27.5	38.0
Hawaii	3.1	...	...	...	...	...	3.0	3.4	8.8	25.4	63.0	105.5
Idaho	2.8	...	0.5	...	...	0.9	2.4	4.1	9.3	12.4	19.3	10.3
Illinois	5.9	1.2	0.9	0.1	0.5	2.7	4.9	10.0	14.2	20.6	26.8	26.2
Indiana	5.6	...	0.2	0.1	0.8	1.8	4.3	7.3	13.3	23.8	34.2	57.0
Iowa	2.6	...	0.1	...	0.2	0.4	1.3	3.0	7.3	9.9	11.7	17.8
Kansas	2.6	...	...	0.1	0.1	0.4	1.5	5.1	6.9	9.6	11.7	22.2
Kentucky	10.8	1.0	2.4	0.4	0.7	5.7	8.5	14.5	25.3	40.9	62.1	107.7
Louisiana	8.0	1.9	0.5	0.1	1.0	3.8	8.8	16.1	22.7	33.1	43.7	57.4
Maine	3.9	...	0.8	0.2	...	0.9	2.8	7.9	9.1	14.6	16.3	8.6
Maryland	8.5	0.9	0.9	0.2	0.6	3.3	8.4	14.6	23.7	37.9	49.6	61.3
Massachusetts	6.4	0.9	0.1	0.1	0.4	1.6	4.5	8.6	15.8	21.5	33.6	41.3
Michigan	4.7	0.2	0.3	0.1	0.2	1.4	3.7	7.5	12.1	21.3	35.6	37.6
Minnesota	3.2	0.4	...	0.1	0.1	0.2	1.9	3.8	8.7	11.7	23.3	28.7
Mississippi	6.3	2.3	1.2	0.3	1.2	4.5	8.0	9.9	16.1	21.1	33.4	31.6
Missouri	7.0	0.4	0.3	0.1	0.2	1.7	5.1	10.4	16.8	23.8	33.3	38.3
Montana	4.6	...	0.5	0.5	0.4	0.8	3.1	5.0	11.5	26.4	24.4	30.0
Nebraska	2.2	1.0	...	0.1	0.2	0.4	1.8	4.5	6.0	5.7	10.3	6.4
Nevada	6.1	...	2.5	...	1.8	...	6.2	6.5	7.3	39.6	91.6	...
New Hampshire	3.0	...	0.6	0.6	...	0.5	0.8	2.9	5.8	14.0	21.7	7.0
New Jersey	6.6	1.6	0.9	0.1	0.7	2.8	6.1	9.8	14.8	23.4	35.6	31.0
New Mexico	7.9	1.2	1.6	0.7	1.4	4.5	7.3	14.1	27.4	47.7	61.8	70.6
New York	7.4	0.9	0.5	0.1	0.7	3.3	7.3	11.5	17.3	23.5	29.1	31.0
North Carolina	4.3	0.6	0.4	0.2	0.4	1.6	3.8	6.0	14.5	24.6	28.5	24.3
North Dakota	1.7	...	0.5	...	0.4	...	...	1.0	3.9	11.5	15.3	10.0
Ohio	5.1	0.6	0.5	0.1	0.2	1.7	4.1	7.1	13.8	21.5	30.2	34.9
Oklahoma	6.4	2.0	0.5	0.2	0.5	3.0	3.2	9.5	16.4	19.5	36.1	48.2
Oregon	3.7	0.9	...	0.2	0.3	0.7	2.5	7.2	9.4	14.9	14.5	3.3
Pennsylvania	8.2	0.4	0.1	0.1	0.6	2.8	5.5	13.0	20.9	32.3	35.0	41.7
Rhode Island	5.8	1.8	1.4	0.2	...	1.9	3.1	7.5	13.8	28.0	17.4	52.1
South Carolina	6.0	1.1	0.7	0.1	1.2	5.6	10.3	10.5	17.5	24.8	21.0	35.8
South Dakota	3.7	7.8	0.5	...	2.2	2.1	1.7	2.8	11.1	12.0	14.7	32.9
Tennessee	9.4	0.8	2.0	0.2	0.6	3.8	6.7	12.0	21.7	41.9	69.0	89.0
Texas	6.3	2.4	1.6	0.2	0.8	2.7	5.3	9.3	17.1	27.9	38.8	47.8
Utah	2.8	...	0.5	0.2	0.6	1.3	4.4	11.3	17.8	11.6	61.5
Vermont	6.7	...	...	...	...	...	4.3	2.3	16.1	42.0	34.3	41.8
Virginia	5.8	0.4	0.8	0.1	0.5	2.1	4.6	9.9	14.7	26.5	53.4	49.9
Washington	3.0	0.5	0.3	...	0.1	0.8	1.8	4.0	9.3	13.5	14.0	20.9
West Virginia	7.0	...	1.5	0.3	0.9	2.8	6.0	11.3	17.0	28.7	31.3	50.6
Wisconsin	3.1	...	0.2	0.0	0.2	0.6	1.8	3.7	8.0	12.0	20.4	36.8
Wyoming	3.1	...	1.0	...	0.8	...	3.1	4.6	6.5	19.0	23.8	...

112

Table A.10   Tuberculosis deaths, by residence, standard metropolitan statistical areas, 1959-61

Standard metropolitan statistical areas	Total			White			Nonwhite		
	Total	Male	Female	Total	Male	Female	Total	Male	Female
Total	21,582	15,924	5,658	15,754	11,947	3,807	5,828	3,977	1,851
Abilene, Texas	4	3	1	4	3	1	-	-	-
Akron, Ohio	44	35	9	39	33	6	5	2	3
Albany, Georgia	8	6	2	2	2	-	6	4	2
Albany-Schenectady-Troy, N. Y.	123	93	30	117	91	26	6	2	4
Albuquerque, N. Mex.	64	34	30	63	34	29	1	-	1
Allentown-Bethlehem-Easton, Pa.-N.J.	77	54	23	73	52	21	4	2	2
Altoona, Pa.	22	17	5	22	17	5	-	-	-
Amarillo, Texas	11	10	1	11	10	1	-	-	-
Ann Arbor, Mich.	15	10	5	12	7	5	3	3	-
Asheville, N.C.	43	37	6	36	30	6	7	7	-
Atlanta, Ga.	186	117	69	92	58	34	94	59	35
Atlantic City, N. J.	46	39	7	28	24	4	18	15	3
Augusta, Ga.-S.C.	47	31	16	25	19	6	22	12	10
Austin, Texas	36	23	13	30	20	10	6	3	3
Bakersfield, Calif.	43	32	11	34	24	10	9	8	1
Baltimore, Md.	573	408	165	333	251	82	240	157	83
Baton Rouge, La.	38	29	9	17	14	3	21	15	6
Bay City, Mich.	9	6	3	9	6	3	-	-	-
Beaumont-Port Arthur, Texas	59	46	13	35	32	3	24	14	10
Billings, Mont.	5	2	3	3	1	2	2	1	1
Binghamton, N. Y.	17	12	5	16	12	4	1	-	1
Birmingham, Ala.	223	158	65	83	66	17	140	92	48
Boston-Lowell-Lawrence, Mass.	653	492	161	615	465	150	38	27	11
Bridgeport-Stamford-Norwalk, Conn.	71	58	13	62	50	12	9	8	1
Brockton, Mass.	34	28	6	32	27	5	2	1	1
Brownsville-Harlingen-San Benito, Texas	51	32	19	49	30	19	2	2	-
Buffalo, N. Y.	232	179	53	197	151	46	35	28	7
Canton, Ohio	27	23	4	20	16	4	7	7	-
Cedar Rapids, Iowa	6	5	1	6	5	1	-	-	-
Champaign-Urbana, Ill.	6	3	3	6	3	3	-	-	-
Charleston, S. C.	33	25	8	15	12	3	18	13	5
Charleston, W. Va.	38	24	14	36	22	14	2	2	-
Charlotte, N. C.	26	16	10	15	10	5	11	6	5
Chattanooga, Tenn.-Ga.	123	76	47	68	43	25	55	33	22
Chicago, Ill.	1,278	985	293	859	693	166	419	292	127
Cincinnati, Ohio-Ky.	269	191	78	192	135	57	77	56	21
Cleveland, Ohio	343	270	73	231	181	50	112	89	23
Colorado Springs, Colo.	26	20	6	26	20	6	-	-	-
Columbia, S. C.	39	23	16	11	7	4	28	16	12
Columbus, Ga.-Ala.	34	15	19	13	8	5	21	7	14
Columbus, Ohio	72	55	17	51	37	14	21	18	3
Corpus Christi, Texas	53	33	20	48	28	20	5	5	-
Dallas, Texas	129	89	40	102	73	29	27	16	11
Davenport-Rock Island-Moline, Iowa-Ill.	18	14	4	16	13	3	2	1	1
Dayton, Ohio	111	90	21	75	62	13	36	28	8
Decatur, Ill.	11	8	3	11	8	3	-	-	-
Denver, Colo.	141	111	30	129	103	26	12	8	4
Des Moines, Iowa	22	15	7	18	11	7	4	4	-
Detroit, Mich.	713	541	172	505	394	111	208	147	61
Dubuque, Iowa	7	6	1	7	6	1	-	-	-

113

Table A.10   continued

Standard metropolitan statistical areas	Total			White			Nonwhite		
	Total	Male	Female	Total	Male	Female	Total	Male	Female
Duluth-Superior, Minn.-Wis.	37	27	10	36	26	10	1	1	–
Durham, N. C.	14	7	7	5	3	2	9	4	5
El Paso, Texas	86	53	33	84	52	32	2	1	1
Erie, Pa.	44	34	10	37	29	8	7	5	2
Eugene, Oregon	11	8	3	11	8	3	–	–	–
Evansville, Ind.-Ky.	30	19	11	24	18	6	6	1	5
Fall River-New Bedford, Mass.	99	75	24	96	74	22	3	1	2
Fargo-Moorhead, N. Dak.-Minn.	5	4	1	5	4	1	–	–	–
Flint, Mich.	25	16	9	16	10	6	9	6	3
Fort Lauderdale-Hollywood, Fla.	40	26	14	26	16	10	14	10	4
Fort Smith, Ark.	14	11	3	12	10	2	2	1	1
Fort Wayne, Ind.	36	26	10	30	22	8	6	4	2
Fort Worth, Texas	85	60	25	64	46	18	21	14	7
Fresno, Calif.	76	52	24	60	40	20	16	12	4
Gadsden, Ala.	34	24	10	22	14	8	12	10	2
Galveston-Texas City, Texas	26	20	6	18	13	5	8	7	1
Gary-Hammond-East Chicago, Ind.	79	58	21	49	41	8	30	17	13
Grand Rapids, Mich.	30	25	5	28	23	5	2	2	–
Great Falls, Mont.	7	4	3	6	4	2	1	–	1
Green Bay, Wisc.	10	7	3	10	7	3	–	–	–
Greensboro-High Point, N. C.	16	11	5	9	5	4	7	6	1
Greenvile, S. C.	29	19	10	15	10	5	14	9	5
Hamilton -Middletown, Ohio	24	15	9	20	12	8	4	3	1
Harrisburg, Pa.	63	48	15	55	41	14	8	7	1
Hartford-New Britain-Bristol, Conn.	119	89	30	104	79	25	15	10	5
Honolulu, Hawaii	35	24	11	1	–	1	34	24	10
Houston, Texas	254	195	59	162	127	35	92	68	24
Huntington-Ashland, W. Va.-Ky.-Ohio	64	45	19	60	44	16	4	1	3
Huntsville, Ala.	28	19	9	15	11	4	13	8	5
Indianapolis, Ind.	130	94	36	95	73	22	35	21	14
Jackson, Mich.	7	3	4	6	3	3	1	–	1
Jackson, Miss.	39	27	12	10	9	1	29	18	11
Jacksonville, Fla.	97	75	22	43	35	8	54	40	14
Jersey City, N. J.	213	166	47	176	138	38	37	28	9
Johnstown, Pa.	56	51	5	56	51	5	–	–	–
Kalamazoo, Mich.	13	8	5	13	8	5	–	–	–
Kansas City, Mo.-Kans.	208	162	46	152	121	31	56	41	15
Kenosha, Wis.	5	4	1	5	4	1	–	–	–
Knoxville, Tenn.	75	50	25	56	37	19	19	13	6
Lake Charles, La.	27	20	7	18	13	5	9	7	2
Lancaster, Pa.	28	19	9	26	18	8	2	1	1
Lansing, Mich.	15	9	6	12	7	5	3	2	1
Laredo, Texas	31	18	13	31	18	13	–	–	–
Las Vegas, Nev.	19	12	7	14	9	5	5	3	2
Lawton, Okla.	4	1	3	1	1	–	3	–	3
Lexington, Ky.	32	20	12	21	12	9	11	8	3
Lima, Ohio	18	11	7	15	9	6	3	2	1
Lincoln, Nebr.	5	3	2	5	3	2	–	–	–
Little Rock-North Little Rock, Ark.	61	39	22	43	29	14	18	10	8
Lorain-Elyria, Ohio	25	18	7	21	15	6	4	3	1

114

Table A.10   continued

Standard metropolitan statistical areas	Total			White			Nonwhite		
	Total	Male	Female	Total	Male	Female	Total	Male	Female
Los Angeles-Long Beach, Calif.	864	613	251	729	515	214	135	98	37
Louisville, Ky.-Ind.	269	206	63	187	141	46	82	65	17
Lubbock, Texas	15	11	4	13	9	4	2	2	-
Lynchburg, Va.	11	9	2	7	5	2	4	4	-
Macon, Ga.	28	13	15	11	6	5	17	7	10
Madison, Wis.	15	10	5	15	10	5	-	-	-
Manchester, N. H.	23	18	5	22	17	5	1	1	-
Memphis, Tenn.	104	74	30	49	37	12	55	37	18
Miami, Fla.	131	95	36	98	75	23	33	20	13
Midland, Texas	4	4	-	3	3	-	1	1	-
Milwaukee, Wis.	152	114	38	124	93	31	28	21	7
Minneapolis-St. Paul, Minn.	169	129	40	161	123	38	8	6	2
Mobile, Ala.	76	47	29	34	26	8	42	21	21
Monroe, La.	18	13	5	13	10	3	5	3	2
Montgomery, Ala.	28	16	12	10	6	4	18	10	8
Muncie, Ind.	22	16	6	19	14	5	3	2	1
Muskegon-Muskegon Heights, Mich.	13	9	4	8	5	3	5	4	1
Nashville, Tenn.	110	69	41	78	47	31	32	22	10
Newark, N. J.	367	282	85	219	185	34	148	97	51
New Haven-Waterbury, Conn.	84	65	19	72	58	14	12	7	5
New Orleans, La.	309	231	78	165	133	32	144	98	46
Newport News-Hampton, Va.	57	40	17	23	16	7	34	24	10
New York, N. Y.	2,856	2,153	703	1,902	1,493	409	954	660	294
Norfolk-Portsmouth, Va.	78	56	22	22	18	4	56	38	18
Odessa, Texas	6	4	2	6	4	2	-	-	-
Ogden, Utah	7	5	2	6	4	2	1	1	-
Oklahoma City, Okla.	69	51	18	54	42	12	15	9	6
Omaha, Nebr.-Iowa	46	37	9	41	33	8	5	4	1
Orlando, Fla.	35	23	12	21	14	7	14	9	5
Paterson-Clifton-Passaic, N. J.	148	93	55	127	81	46	21	12	9
Pensacola, Fla.	20	7	13	12	6	6	8	1	7
Peoria, Ill.	44	31	13	43	30	13	1	1	-
Philadelphia, Pa.-N.J.	1,175	852	323	768	592	176	407	260	147
Phoenix, Ariz.	187	143	44	170	132	38	17	11	6
Pittsburgh, Pa.	584	443	141	439	338	101	145	105	40
Pittsfield, Mass.	13	10	3	12	9	3	1	1	-
Portland, Maine	16	9	7	16	9	7	-	-	-
Portland, Oreg.-Wash.	122	100	22	106	88	18	16	12	4
Providence, R. I.	138	108	30	126	102	24	12	6	6
Provo-Orem, Utah	3	3	-	3	3	-	-	-	-
Pueblo, Colo.	10	9	1	8	8	-	2	1	1
Racine, Wis.	14	9	5	13	8	5	1	1	-
Raleigh, N. C.	20	10	10	9	3	6	11	7	4
Reading, Pa.	82	65	17	80	64	16	2	1	1
Reno, Nev.	16	14	2	15	13	2	1	1	-
Richmond, Va.	74	48	26	35	23	12	39	25	14
Roanoke, Va.	24	18	6	19	13	6	5	5	-
Rochester, N. Y.	105	74	31	97	69	28	8	5	3
Rockford, Ill.	23	15	8	22	15	7	1	-	1
Sacramento, Calif.	105	93	12	96	85	11	9	8	1

Standard metropolitan statistical areas	Total			White			Nonwhite		
	Total	Male	Female	Total	Male	Female	Total	Male	Female
Saginaw, Mich.	31	26	5	26	22	4	5	4	1
St. Joseph, Mo.	13	5	8	12	5	7	1	–	1
St. Louis, Mo.-Ill.	396	313	83	294	237	57	102	76	26
Salt Lake City, Utah	43	35	8	40	32	8	3	3	–
San Angelo, Texas	15	12	3	15	12	3	–	–	–
San Antonio, Texas	236	156	80	227	148	79	9	8	1
San Bernardino-Riverside-Ontario, Calif.	100	72	28	94	68	26	6	4	2
San Diego, Calif.	120	83	37	106	76	30	14	7	7
San Francisco-Oakland, Calif.	448	332	116	352	259	93	96	73	23
San Jose, Calif.	60	41	19	56	38	18	4	3	1
Santa Barbara, Calif.	18	11	7	17	10	7	1	1	–
Savannah, Ga.	45	31	14	9	8	1	36	23	13
Scranton, Pa.	87	76	11	87	76	11	–	–	–
Seattle, Wash.	106	83	23	92	72	20	14	11	3
Shreveport, La.	65	44	21	23	18	5	42	26	16
Sioux City, Iowa	12	9	3	11	8	3	1	1	–
Sioux Falls, S. Dak.	1	1	–	1	1	–	–	–	–
South Bend, Ind.	27	19	8	21	14	7	6	5	1
Spokane, Wash.	35	28	7	32	25	7	3	3	–
Springfield, Ill.	25	19	6	21	15	6	4	4	–
Springfield, Mo.	22	10	12	21	9	12	1	1	–
Springfield, Ohio	23	16	7	19	13	6	4	3	1
Springfield-Holyoke, Mass.	74	50	24	70	48	22	4	2	2
Steubenville-Weirton, Ohio-W. Va.	23	19	4	21	17	4	2	2	–
Stockton, Calif.	88	79	9	68	62	6	20	17	3
Syracuse, N. Y.	76	50	26	70	47	23	6	3	3
Tacoma, Wash.	28	18	10	22	16	6	6	2	4
Tampa-St. Petersburg, Fla.	122	100	22	97	81	16	25	19	6
Terre Haute, Ind.	23	19	4	21	17	4	2	2	–
Texarkana, Texas-Ark.	21	15	6	15	11	4	6	4	2
Toledo, Ohio	69	53	16	53	43	10	16	10	6
Topeka, Kans.	15	10	5	14	9	5	1	1	–
Trenton, N. J.	93	75	18	69	57	12	24	18	6
Tucson, Ariz.	146	115	31	125	101	24	21	14	7
Tulsa, Okla.	63	38	25	46	28	18	17	10	7
Tuscaloosa, Ala.	55	30	25	14	11	3	41	19	22
Tyler, Texas	8	4	4	7	4	3	1	–	1
Utica-Rome, N. Y.	32	25	7	32	25	7	–	–	–
Waco, Texas	37	25	12	29	20	9	8	5	3
Washington, D. C.-Md.-Va.	405	266	139	169	110	59	236	156	80
Waterloo, Iowa	11	7	4	8	5	3	3	2	1
West Palm Beach, Fla.	28	24	4	18	16	2	10	8	2
Wheeling, W. Va.-Ohio	40	32	8	39	32	7	1	–	1
Wichita, Kans.	29	21	8	23	15	8	6	6	–
Wichita Falls, Texas	10	10	–	9	9	–	1	1	–
Wilkes-Barre-Hazelton, Pa.	198	182	16	197	181	16	1	1	–
Wilmington, Del.-N. J.	49	37	12	31	24	7	18	13	5
Winston-Salem, N. C.	30	22	8	14	10	4	16	12	4
Worcester, Mass.	93	73	20	93	73	20	–	–	–
York, Pa.	28	17	11	26	15	11	2	2	–
Youngstown-Warren, Ohio	84	59	25	52	40	12	32	19	13

Table A.11   Age-adjusted death rates for tuberculosis: standard metropolitan statistical areas, 1959-61

Standard metropolitan statistical areas	Total			White			Nonwhite		
	Total	Male	Female	Total	Male	Female	Total	Male	Female
All areas	5.8	9.0	2.9	4.5	7.3	2.1	16.8	24.2	10.0
Abilene, Texas	1.1	1.8	0.5	1.2	1.9	0.5	...	...	...
Akron, Ohio	2.7	4.4	1.1	2.5	4.4	0.7	5.5	5.4	5.8
Albany, Ga.	4.3	7.0	2.2	2.1	5.5	...	10.2	15.2	6.2
Albany-Schenectady-Troy, N. Y.	4.9	8.1	2.2	4.7	8.0	1.9	13.4	10.8	17.8
Albuquerque, N. Mex.	10.7	12.3	9.4	10.8	12.6	9.3	7.5	...	15.7
Allentown-Bethlehem-Easton, Pa.-N. J.	4.0	6.0	2.4	3.8	5.8	2.1	35.7	37.4	34.1
Altoona, Pa.	3.9	6.4	1.8	3.9	6.4	1.8	...	...	...
Amarillo, Texas	3.0	6.1	0.5	3.1	6.3	0.6	...	...	...
Ann Arbor, Mich.	3.1	4.6	1.8	2.6	3.5	1.9	10.4	20.9	...
Asheville, N. C.	9.2	17.1	2.3	8.4	15.2	2.6	16.0	35.1	...
Atlanta, Ga.	6.4	9.2	4.3	4.0	5.8	2.6	15.4	22.3	10.1
Atlantic City, N. J.	6.6	11.5	2.5	4.0	7.6	1.2	18.8	31.4	8.1
Augusta, Ga.-S. C.	8.2	12.0	4.9	6.4	11.1	2.4	13.8	16.7	11.1
Austin, Texas	5.7	7.8	3.9	5.6	8.0	3.5	6.5	6.0	7.1
Bakersfield, Calif.	5.3	7.9	2.7	4.4	6.4	2.6	17.6	26.6	4.0
Baltimore, Md.	10.7	16.1	5.9	7.4	12.1	3.5	24.4	33.0	15.9
Baton Rouge, La.	6.8	11.6	3.0	4.9	10.1	1.5	12.2	18.9	6.5
Bay City, Mich.	2.7	4.2	1.3	2.7	4.2	1.3	...	...	...
Beaumont-Port Arthur, Texas	7.1	11.6	3.0	5.3	10.3	0.9	14.7	17.8	11.5
Billings, Mont.	2.0	1.5	2.6	1.2	0.6	1.7	102.2	96.7	106.1
Binghamton, N. Y.	2.0	3.2	1.0	2.0	3.2	0.9	13.2	...	46.2
Birmingham, Ala.	11.7	17.7	6.6	6.1	10.8	2.2	23.7	32.8	15.8
Boston-Lowell-Lawrence, Mass.	5.5	9.3	2.5	5.3	8.9	2.4	15.5	22.9	8.8
Bridgeport-Stamford-Norwalk, Conn.	3.1	5.3	1.0	2.7	4.7	1.0	10.5	19.7	2.6
Brockton, Mass.	3.6	6.3	1.3	3.4	6.2	0.9	12.9	6.9	16.5
Brownsville-Harlingen-San Benito, Texas	13.8	19.0	9.1	13.3	17.9	9.2	61.2	125.0	...
Buffalo, N. Y.	5.1	8.3	2.4	4.5	7.2	2.1	16.9	27.8	5.6
Canton, Ohio	2.2	4.0	0.6	1.6	2.7	0.6	15.6	31.1	...
Cedar Rapids, Iowa	1.3	2.3	0.4	1.3	2.3	0.4	...	...	...
Champaign-Urbana, Ill.	1.6	2.0	1.4	1.7	2.1	1.4	...	...	...
Charleston, S. C.	6.5	10.8	3.0	4.5	7.9	1.7	10.4	16.8	5.3
Charleston, W. Va.	5.0	6.6	3.6	5.2	6.6	3.9	3.4	6.8	...
Charlotte, N. C.	3.4	4.6	2.4	2.5	3.7	1.6	6.4	7.5	5.5
Chattanooga, Tenn.-Ga.	13.7	18.7	9.5	8.9	12.6	5.8	37.3	49.1	27.5
Chicago, Ill.	6.2	9.9	2.9	4.6	7.7	1.8	17.6	26.1	9.6
Cincinnati, Ohio-Ky.	7.2	11.2	4.1	5.7	8.7	3.3	20.1	31.1	10.3
Cleveland, Ohio	5.6	9.3	2.3	4.1	6.9	1.7	16.9	27.7	6.6
Colorado Springs, Colo.	6.7	11.2	3.4	6.9	11.5	3.4	...	...	...
Columbia, S. C.	5.7	7.4	4.6	2.2	3.2	1.6	15.6	19.4	12.5
Columbus, Ga.-Ala.	6.2	6.6	6.2	3.7	5.3	2.6	12.8	10.5	14.8
Columbus, Ohio	3.5	5.8	1.6	2.8	4.3	1.5	9.4	16.5	2.6
Corpus Christi, Texas	10.2	13.4	7.2	9.7	12.0	7.6	20.0	40.7	...
Dallas, Texas	4.0	6.1	2.3	3.5	5.7	1.9	6.7	8.2	5.3
Davenport-Rock Island-Moline, Iowa-Ill.	1.9	3.2	0.7	1.7	2.9	0.5	12.2	10.8	13.4
Dayton, Ohio	5.4	9.3	2.0	4.0	7.0	1.4	20.0	33.0	7.3
Decatur, Ill.	2.4	3.7	1.5	2.5	3.8	1.6	...	...	...
Denver, Colo.	4.9	8.4	2.0	4.7	8.1	1.7	12.5	17.6	8.1
Des Moines, Iowa	2.3	3.5	1.3	2.0	2.6	1.4	11.3	24.2	...
Detroit, Mich.	6.2	9.6	3.0	4.9	7.9	2.2	15.0	21.9	8.4
Dubuque, Iowa	2.4	4.8	0.6	2.4	4.8	0.6	...	...	...

117

Standard metropolitan statistical areas	Total			White			Nonwhite		
	Total	Male	Female	Total	Male	Female	Total	Male	Female
Duluth-Superior, Minn.-Wis.	3.4	4.7	2.1	3.3	4.6	2.1	21.4	30.4	...
Durham, N. C.	4.3	4.9	3.8	2.1	2.9	1.3	9.7	10.0	9.6
El Paso, Texas	12.8	17.7	8.8	12.8	17.8	8.8	11.7	16.0	8.5
Erie, Pa.	5.2	8.4	2.2	4.3	7.2	1.7	43.7	57.2	28.8
Eugene, Oreg.	2.2	3.3	1.2	2.2	3.3	1.2	...	...	...
Evansville, Ind.-Ky.	3.9	5.5	2.6	3.2	5.6	1.2	13.8	3.5	21.9
Fall River-New Bedford, Mass.	6.8	11.1	3.2	6.5	11.1	2.9	24.0	14.6	34.0
Fargo-Moorhead, N. Dak.-Minn.	1.4	2.2	0.6	1.4	2.2	0.6	...	...	...
Flint, Mich.	2.4	3.2	1.7	1.6	2.1	1.2	13.9	19.7	8.5
Fort Lauderdale-Hollywood, Fla.	3.3	4.3	2.4	2.3	2.6	1.9	13.4	20.6	7.1
Fort Smith, Ark.	5.6	9.7	1.9	5.2	9.4	1.6	10.9	14.0	7.5
Fort Wayne, Ind.	5.0	7.8	2.7	4.0	6.5	2.1	21.8	30.4	14.4
Fort Worth, Texas	5.0	7.6	2.8	4.2	6.6	2.2	12.2	17.3	7.6
Fresno, Calif.	6.9	9.4	4.3	5.8	8.0	3.6	20.6	25.5	12.1
Gadsden, Ala.	11.5	17.0	6.7	8.8	11.6	6.3	28.9	52.5	9.2
Galveston-Texas City, Texas	6.4	10.5	2.9	5.4	8.5	2.8	10.4	17.9	3.0
Gary-Hammond-East Chicago, Ind.	5.0	7.2	2.8	3.5	5.7	1.2	14.8	16.8	12.3
Grand Rapids, Mich.	2.3	4.3	0.5	2.2	4.1	0.5	7.4	14.7	...
Great Falls, Mont.	3.7	4.1	3.3	3.2	4.2	2.2	66.9	...	99.1
Green Bay, Wis.	2.6	3.7	1.6	2.6	3.8	1.6	...	...	...
Greensboro-High Point, N.C.	2.4	3.7	1.4	1.6	2.1	1.3	6.0	10.8	1.6
Greenville, S. C.	5.1	7.2	3.4	3.1	4.6	1.9	16.0	22.7	10.6
Hamilton-Middletown, Ohio	4.3	5.6	3.1	3.7	4.6	2.9	15.6	24.7	7.8
Harrisburg, Pa.	5.1	8.7	2.0	4.4	7.8	2.0	13.3	24.1	3.1
Hartford-New Britain-Bristol, Conn.	4.9	7.9	2.4	4.4	7.1	2.1	21.6	28.2	14.8
Honolulu, Hawaii	3.6	4.9	2.2	0.4	...	0.8	4.9	6.6	2.9
Houston, Texas	7.6	12.5	3.2	6.0	10.0	2.3	14.9	23.3	7.0
Huntington-Ashland, W. Va.-Ky.-Ohio	7.5	11.3	4.1	7.3	11.5	3.5	16.0	5.5	25.0
Huntsville, Ala.	9.6	14.4	5.7	7.0	11.5	3.3	23.6	28.6	19.6
Indianapolis, Ind.	5.6	8.9	2.8	4.6	8.0	1.9	12.1	15.3	9.1
Jackson, Mich.	1.4	1.3	1.6	1.4	1.4	1.4	6.9	...	13.1
Jackson, Miss.	7.8	11.9	4.3	3.1	6.3	0.6	16.5	23.2	11.0
Jacksonville, Fla.	7.7	12.9	3.3	4.4	7.9	1.5	18.9	30.5	9.1
Jersey City, N. J.	9.2	14.7	4.4	7.8	12.6	3.6	37.3	62.2	14.8
Johnstown, Pa.	5.4	10.1	0.9	5.5	10.2	0.9	...	...	...
Kalamazoo, Mich.	2.2	3.2	1.3	2.3	3.3	1.3	...	...	...
Kansas City, Mo.-Kans.	5.9	9.8	2.7	4.8	8.2	2.0	15.6	23.2	8.6
Kenosha, Wis.	1.3	2.0	0.6	1.3	2.0	0.6	...	...	...
Knoxville, Tenn.	6.7	9.6	4.1	5.4	7.8	3.5	22.1	32.9	12.5
Lake Charles, La.	8.6	12.9	4.3	7.0	10.3	3.7	14.5	22.6	6.5
Lancaster, Pa.	2.8	4.3	1.6	2.6	4.0	1.4	20.5	24.6	18.7
Lansing, Mich.	1.5	2.0	1.1	1.2	1.6	0.8	21.0	28.1	9.3
Laredo, Texas	18.3	24.3	13.3	18.3	24.4	13.3	...	...	...
Las Vegas, Nev.	5.6	7.3	3.6	4.6	5.9	3.0	20.7	27.7	9.5
Lawton, Okla.	2.0	1.4	2.9	0.7	1.5	...	12.8	...	27.0
Lexington, Ky.	7.8	10.2	5.7	6.0	7.4	5.0	17.1	25.4	9.3
Lima, Ohio	5.0	6.2	4.1	4.3	5.2	3.7	14.2	14.4	15.9
Lincoln, Nebr.	0.9	1.2	0.7	0.9	1.2	0.7	...	...	...
Little Rock-North Little Rock, Ark.	7.6	10.8	4.7	6.7	10.1	3.6	11.1	13.7	8.9
Lorain-Elyria, Ohio	4.1	5.9	2.3	3.6	5.1	2.2	15.3	21.2	8.2

Standard metropolitan statistical areas	Total			White			Nonwhite		
	Total	Male	Female	Total	Male	Female	Total	Male	Female
Los Angeles-Long Beach, Calif.	3.8	5.9	2.1	3.4	5.3	1.9	9.0	13.5	4.5
Louisville, Ky.-Ind.	11.5	19.4	5.0	8.8	15.0	3.8	30.9	51.2	12.8
Lubbock, Texas	3.7	5.6	2.0	3.3	4.8	2.1	8.2	15.4	...
Lynchburg, Va.	2.8	5.2	0.9	2.2	3.7	1.1	5.3	11.3	...
Macon, Ga.	5.8	5.8	5.6	3.2	3.6	2.6	12.1	11.8	12.5
Madison, Wis.	2.1	3.1	1.2	2.1	3.1	1.2	...	...	...
Manchester, N. H.	3.4	5.9	1.3	3.1	5.4	1.4	62.8	142.2	...
Memphis, Tenn.	5.7	9.0	2.9	4.0	7.1	1.5	9.0	12.7	5.8
Miami, Fla.	3.9	5.7	2.2	3.1	4.8	1.5	10.1	12.5	7.6
Midland, Texas	3.1	6.4	...	2.5	5.4	...	8.6	15.6	...
Milwaukee, Wis.	3.7	5.9	1.8	3.1	4.9	1.5	22.1	31.3	11.4
Minneapolis-St. Paul, Minn.	3.3	5.5	1.5	3.2	5.3	1.4	10.9	16.4	5.2
Mobile, Ala.	9.0	12.1	6.5	5.8	10.0	2.5	16.5	17.3	15.5
Monroe, La.	6.3	9.4	3.5	6.4	10.1	3.0	6.4	7.8	4.9
Montgomery, Ala.	6.0	7.9	4.8	3.4	5.0	2.4	10.5	14.1	8.1
Muncie, Ind.	5.7	9.1	2.9	5.3	8.4	2.7	18.0	23.1	12.8
Muskegon-Muskegon Heights, Mich.	3.1	4.2	2.0	2.0	2.4	1.6	17.1	25.3	7.0
Nashville, Tenn.	8.7	12.4	5.7	7.6	10.5	5.1	13.6	20.5	8.0
Newark, N. J.	6.2	10.0	2.9	3.8	7.0	1.2	23.4	33.2	15.0
New Haven-Waterbury, Conn.	3.4	5.6	1.5	3.0	5.1	1.1	15.8	20.9	11.0
New Orleans, La.	11.7	19.2	5.6	8.4	15.1	3.1	20.5	30.6	12.2
Newport News-Hampton, Va.	10.6	14.7	6.3	6.1	8.6	3.5	22.0	30.9	13.3
New York, N. Y.	7.4	11.7	3.7	5.2	8.5	2.3	25.8	39.8	14.1
Norfolk-Portsmouth, Va.	5.3	8.3	2.8	2.2	4.0	0.7	13.8	19.9	8.3
Odessa, Texas	4.1	6.6	2.1	4.3	6.9	2.2	...	...	...
Ogden, Utah	2.2	3.3	1.3	1.9	2.7	1.3	17.4	31.9	...
Oklahoma City, Okla.	4.3	6.9	2.0	3.6	6.2	1.4	12.1	14.9	9.4
Omaha, Nebr.-Iowa	3.2	5.4	1.2	3.0	5.0	1.2	7.2	11.9	2.8
Orlando, Fla.	3.2	4.5	2.3	2.1	3.0	1.5	9.8	13.0	6.7
Paterson-Clifton-Passaic, N. J.	3.6	4.7	2.8	3.2	4.2	2.4	18.3	24.3	13.2
Pensacola, Fla.	4.0	2.9	5.0	3.1	3.3	2.9	8.1	0.9	14.1
Peoria, Ill.	4.5	6.7	2.4	4.5	6.7	2.5	4.4	8.6	...
Philadelphia, Pa.-N. J.	7.9	12.2	4.4	5.7	9.5	2.5	21.7	29.4	14.7
Phoenix, Ariz.	9.9	15.4	4.6	9.4	14.9	4.1	19.4	23.8	13.4
Pittsburgh, Pa.	6.9	10.7	3.3	5.4	8.7	2.5	29.6	41.2	16.7
Pittsfield, Mass.	2.6	4.2	1.3	2.4	3.8	1.3	24.1	49.7	...
Portland, Maine	2.6	3.3	2.0	2.6	3.3	2.0	...	...	...
Portland, Oreg.-Wash.	3.9	6.7	1.3	3.5	6.1	1.1	26.9	34.7	15.9
Providence, R. I.	5.0	8.4	2.1	4.6	8.1	1.7	27.4	31.0	24.3
Provo-Orem, Utah	1.1	2.3	...	1.1	2.3	...	...	...	...
Pueblo, Colo.	2.6	4.8	0.5	2.1	4.3	...	22.2	28.8	17.7
Racine, Wis.	2.9	3.9	1.9	2.7	3.6	1.9	19.0	35.9	...
Raleigh, N. C.	4.3	4.6	3.9	2.6	1.9	3.1	9.6	13.5	6.3
Reading, Pa.	7.2	12.1	3.0	7.1	12.1	2.9	17.5	19.9	16.5
Reno, Nev.	6.0	10.0	1.9	5.8	9.6	1.9	16.1	29.4	...
Richmond, Va.	5.5	8.1	3.5	3.3	5.1	1.9	12.6	17.6	8.5
Roanoke, Va.	4.4	7.2	1.9	3.9	5.9	2.1	8.0	17.2	...
Rochester, N. Y.	4.6	7.1	2.6	4.3	6.7	2.4	16.6	24.0	9.4
Rockford, Ill.	3.5	4.7	2.4	3.4	4.8	2.1	5.4	...	10.3
Sacramento, Calif.	7.3	12.8	1.6	7.1	12.6	1.5	9.9	15.5	1.7

Standard metropolitan statistical areas	Total			White			Nonwhite		
	Total	Male	Female	Total	Male	Female	Total	Male	Female
Saginaw, Mich.	5.4	9.3	1.9	4.8	8.4	1.7	9.3	13.4	5.5
St. Joseph, Mo.	3.3	3.0	3.5	3.1	3.0	3.1	9.3	...	16.5
St. Louis, Mo.-Ill.	5.6	9.5	2.3	4.6	8.1	1.7	12.3	20.0	5.8
Salt Lake City, Utah	4.0	6.9	1.5	3.8	6.5	1.5	18.6	25.6	...
San Angelo, Texas	7.4	12.3	3.1	7.8	12.9	3.3	...	...	...
San Antonio, Texas	12.4	17.9	8.1	12.8	18.2	8.6	6.9	13.5	1.4
San Bernardino-Riverside-Ontario, Calif.	3.6	5.3	2.0	3.5	5.2	1.9	7.5	9.8	5.5
San Diego, Calif.	4.0	5.9	2.4	3.6	5.6	2.0	13.0	13.1	13.0
San Francisco-Oakland, Calif.	4.6	7.1	2.3	3.8	6.0	2.0	11.9	17.1	5.7
San Jose, Calif.	3.2	4.9	1.9	3.1	4.8	1.8	8.7	10.4	5.4
Santa Barbara, Calif.	3.2	4.3	2.0	3.0	4.1	2.0	5.9	9.1	...
Savannah, Ga.	8.4	13.1	4.7	2.5	5.2	0.5	19.8	28.8	12.7
Scranton, Pa.	8.8	16.6	2.3	8.8	16.6	2.3	...	...	...
Seattle, Wash.	2.8	4.5	1.2	2.5	4.1	1.0	9.4	12.7	3.8
Shreveport, La.	7.8	11.6	4.7	4.1	7.3	1.6	16.1	22.4	10.9
Sioux City, Iowa	3.6	5.8	1.6	3.3	5.1	1.6	22.8	40.5	...
Sioux Falls, S. Dak.	0.4	0.8	...	0.4	0.8	...	...	...	...
South Bend, Ind.	3.6	5.0	2.4	2.9	3.8	2.2	17.5	29.3	5.0
Spokane, Wash.	3.3	5.4	1.3	3.2	5.1	1.3	19.9	33.3	...
Springfield, Ill.	3.9	6.9	1.6	3.4	5.7	1.6	15.6	33.7	...
Springfield, Mo.	4.3	4.5	4.1	4.1	4.0	4.2	13.4	23.8	...
Springfield, Ohio	5.0	7.5	2.8	4.2	6.3	2.4	12.8	19.6	6.6
Springfield-Holyoke, Mass.	3.8	5.7	2.1	3.6	5.6	1.9	11.2	14.7	8.7
Steubenville-Weirton, Ohio-W. Va.	3.8	6.4	1.2	3.6	5.9	1.3	9.8	20.1	...
Stockton, Calif.	9.8	16.5	2.2	8.2	14.4	1.6	26.4	35.1	11.5
Syracuse, N. Y.	3.9	5.4	2.7	3.6	5.0	2.4	16.5	18.1	14.7
Tacoma, Wash.	2.6	3.3	2.1	2.1	3.0	1.3	21.9	14.5	35.5
Tampa-St. Petersburg, Fla.	3.7	6.1	1.6	3.1	5.3	1.2	11.0	17.3	5.0
Terre Haute, Ind.	5.5	9.4	2.1	5.3	8.9	2.2	8.6	16.9	...
Texarkana, Texas-Ark.	6.2	9.1	3.7	5.5	8.2	3.3	8.8	12.9	5.5
Toledo, Ohio	4.1	6.6	2.0	3.3	5.6	1.4	13.8	18.3	9.2
Topeka, Kans.	2.9	4.7	1.2	2.9	4.5	1.3	3.0	6.5	...
Trenton, N. J.	9.8	16.8	3.7	7.4	13.5	2.4	28.5	41.6	15.0
Tucson, Ariz.	18.2	29.7	7.6	16.5	27.8	6.4	44.4	59.4	27.3
Tulsa, Okla.	4.6	6.1	3.1	3.6	4.9	2.5	15.2	22.4	9.6
Tuscaloosa, Ala.	17.1	19.4	15.5	5.3	9.0	2.3	52.0	55.2	49.8
Tyler, Texas	2.7	3.0	2.5	3.0	3.9	2.1	2.0	...	3.6
Utica-Rome, N. Y.	2.5	4.1	1.0	2.5	4.2	1.1	...	...	...
Waco, Texas	6.4	9.4	4.1	5.8	8.8	3.5	10.4	13.6	7.9
Washington, D. C.-Md.-Va.	7.0	10.4	4.4	3.7	5.9	2.3	18.1	25.8	11.2
Waterloo, Iowa	2.9	3.7	2.3	2.1	2.6	1.7	30.3	41.9	15.6
West Palm Beach, Fla.	3.4	5.9	1.1	2.3	4.2	0.7	6.7	10.7	1.8
Wheeling, W. Va.-Ohio	5.3	8.7	2.2	5.3	8.9	1.9	7.9	...	15.8
Wichita, Kans.	3.0	4.9	1.6	2.5	3.7	1.7	13.9	27.6	...
Wichita Falls, Texas	2.5	5.5	...	2.4	5.2	...	4.5	9.2	...
Wilkes-Barre-Hazleton, Pa.	14.0	27.4	2.5	13.9	27.3	2.6	23.4	46.1	...
Wilmington, Del.-N. J.	4.3	6.7	2.0	2.9	4.9	1.2	14.7	20.8	8.1
Winston-Salem, N. C.	5.5	9.1	2.8	3.5	5.6	1.9	12.8	21.3	6.5
Worcester, Mass.	3.8	6.6	1.4	3.8	6.7	1.4	...	...	...
York, Pa.	3.3	4.4	2.3	3.1	3.9	2.4	15.7	30.8	...
Youngstown-Warren, Ohio	4.9	7.0	2.9	3.1	4.9	1.4	25.5	30.0	20.0

120

Table A.12   Crude death rates from tuberculosis: selected countries of low mortality, 1950 to 1965

Country	Average annual death rate per 100,000				Percent change			
	1962 -65	1958 -61	1954 -57	1950 -53	1958-61 to 1962-65	1954-57 to 1958-61	1950-53 to 1954-57	1950-53 to 1962-65
United States	4.6	6.2	8.9	17.7	-25.8	-30.3	-49.7	-74.0
Canada	3.8	5.1	8.6	20.2	-25.5	-40.7	-57.4	-81.2
England and Wales	5.7	8.3	13.8	28.0	-31.3	-39.9	-50.7	-79.6
Scotland	8.0	10.9	17.7	38.4	-26.6	-38.4	-53.9	-79.2
Australia	3.7	5.0	7.9	16.2	-26.0	-36.7	-51.2	-77.2
New Zealand	4.0	6.3	11.6	17.7	-36.5	-45.7	-34.5	-77.4
Union of South Africa[a]	4.9	7.2	8.3	17.1	-31.9	-13.3	-51.5	-71.3
Ireland	14.0	17.5	28.2	61.8	-20.0	-37.9	-54.4	-77.3
Netherlands	2.1	3.4	6.1	14.2	-38.2	-44.3	-57.0	-85.2
Belgium	12.3	16.9	23.8	34.2	-27.2	-29.0	-30.4	-64.0
France	16.9	22.5	30.1	49.6	-24.9	-25.2	-39.3	-65.9
Switzerland	9.6	13.7	20.2	30.0	-29.9	-32.2	-32.7	-68.0
West Germany	13.2	16.0	20.0	31.6	-17.5	-20.0	-36.7	-58.2
Denmark	2.9	4.2	5.9	11.7	-31.0	-28.8	-49.6	-75.2
Norway	4.6	6.5	11.8	22.3	-29.2	-44.9	-47.1	-79.4
Sweden	5.3	7.5	10.5	19.1	-29.3	-28.6	-45.0	-72.3
Finland	16.1	27.6	39.7	69.9	-41.7	-30.5	-43.2	-77.0
Portugal	33.6	47.2	61.6	108.2	-28.8	-23.4	-43.1	-68.9
Italy	14.2	17.9	22.2	34.1	-20.7	-19.4	-34.9	-58.4
Spain	20.8	25.9	34.7	73.8	-19.7	-25.4	-53.0	-71.8

[a]White only.

Part II / Tuberculous Infection

Lydia B. Edwards and Carroll E. Palmer

1903 — Jan. 8, 1972

Authors' Preface

For many years, the Tuberculosis Program of the United States Public Health Service has been conducting tuberculin testing surveys directed specifically at obtaining a nationwide picture of tuberculous infection in the United States. Because only those persons who have had or will have a tuberculous infection are subject to the risk of getting the disease, nationwide programs to control or eradicate tuberculosis need nationwide statistics on the population or pool of infected persons and information about the different streams of newly infected that are being added to that pool.

To obtain such statistics, it is necessary to have not only a *technique* for identifying the infected but also a *facility* for applying the technique to the population or to representative samples of it. A *technique* for identifying the infected—the tuberculin test—has been available for many years. In earlier days, this technique was thought to be very efficient. A reaction of any size to any dose of tuberculin was considered to be specific, that is, to indicate tuberculous infection. It has for some time been evident, however, that other mycobacteria infect man and cause sensitivity (cross reactions) to tuberculin.[1] Although cross reactions tend to be smaller than specific reactions, the sizes of the two overlap.

Thus, it is not possible, with the tuberculin test, to make an exact selection of those persons who are tuberculous-infected. The selection must involve a compromise; it must be based on a criterion that will define a group having the maximum of specific and the minimum of cross reactions. The criterion used in this report is induration at least 10 mm in diameter to the 0.0001 mg dose of tuberculin. We know that a small percentage of persons with tuberculous infection have reactions smaller than 10 mm and that a small percentage of those not infected with *M. tuberculosis* have cross reactions to tuberculin that are larger than 10 mm. However, for the various groups included in this report, the estimate of tuberculous infection based on the 10 mm definition is thought to be a close approximation.

To develop a *facility* for the uniform application of the tuberculin test to representative samples of the population presents very great difficulties. Although enormous numbers of tests have been given in recent years, they have been done by different persons, using different products, doses, testing methods, and population samples. Thus, it is not possible, by simply assembling the results of such tests, to construct a comprehensive picture of tuberculin sensitivity in the United States.

In 1958, an opportunity to study tuberculin sensitivity in a nation-wide sample of young men presented itself in the testing of U.S. Navy recruits. Recruits entering the Navy, at a rate of approximately 100,-000 per year, are channeled through just two training centers.* Thus, it is possible to test men from all parts of the country on a continuing basis under essentially uniform conditions. It is also possible to study changes in tuberculin sensitivity year after year in the *same* slice of the population. The recruits are of an age, 17 to 21 years, that is unusually well suited to the purpose. They are old enough to have been exposed to general community risks in addition to intrafamilial risks; they are young enough to reflect conditions of the more recent past (infections sustained only during the previous two decades); most of them are still uninfected with tuberculosis and therefore capable of reflecting small variations in the frequency of effective exposure to the disease. Though volunteers for Navy service may not be entirely representative of young males of their age group, it is difficult to conceive how a better sample involving large numbers of men could be obtained. Moreover, there is no reason to think that those entering from one part of the country are very different from those entering from another or that those entering one year are very different from those entering the next. The program has the limitation that the age span is small and that only males are in-cluded. However, for the first time, it permits studying tuberculin sensi-tivity on a nationwide basis, in adequate numbers of one age group of the population.

Part II of this monograph deals with estimates of tuberculous infec-tion, primarily in the younger age groups of the population and with some of the factors that may affect its prevalence. Most of the ma-terial to be presented is based on testing the Navy recruits. Limited material is also included for general population groups younger and older than the recruits. The difficulty of developing a facility for testing representative and numerically adequate samples of other age groups on a nationwide basis has, so far, proved insur-mountable.

The data consist of summary figures and tables, with text limited to indicating certain critical points. Detailed information on numbers tested, and so on, is given in appendix tables.

* In October 1968, the Navy opened a third training center at Orlando, Florida.

The magnitude of the tuberculin testing studies reported here makes it impossible to acknowledge properly the efforts of all of the many persons whose support we have had. There are some, however, whose contributions must be identified. Drs. R. O. Canada and John F. Chace of the U.S. Navy Medical Corps have provided immeasurable aid in setting up and supporting the Navy Recruit Program. In areas where the community and school programs were conducted, the cooperation and assistance of state and local health departments and tuberculous associations has been invaluable. The efforts and teamwork of many members of the Research Section, Tuberculosis Program, were also an essential element of the studies included in this monograph. Special thanks are extended to the exceptionally dedicated staff of nurses who were responsible for collecting the field data; to Hans Muller and later Verna Livesay, assisted by Francis Acquaviva and Carolyn Foley, who were responsible for the statistical aspects of the program; and to Forrest Cross for his infinitely painstaking work with the antigens in our laboratory.

January 1967

Lydia B. Edwards
Carroll E. Palmer

NAVY RECRUIT PROGRAM

For many years, tuberculin testing has been part of the routine examination of recruits entering the U.S. Navy. An expanded, cooperative program set up by the Navy and the Tuberculosis Program of the U.S. Public Health Service was started at the Great Lakes, Illinois, Naval Training Center in January 1958 and at the San Diego, California, Naval Training Center in April 1958. The material to be presented from this program covers the period from 1958 through 1964. All Navy recruits inducted during this period were volunteers. Prior to arrival at the training center, each had been screened at his local recruiting station and judged as meeting the fitness requirements for Navy service. Thus, men with disease or disabilities, including tuberculosis, have for the most part been eliminated from the group reporting for training.

Information obtained from recruits. Soon after arrival at the center, each recruit is asked to fill in a number of forms under the direction of Navy personnel. One of these forms is the field record card for the skin-testing program (Fig. 1). When completed, the cards are turned over to the Public Health Service staff, who make sure that a card is included for each man who has reported for training and that the information requested is complete and legible. A card with omissions or obvious errors is reviewed with the recruit when he reports for testing, and the necessary information is added or corrections made.

The information each recruit is asked to fill in (above the heavy black line on the card) includes: *Identifying data:* service number, name, date of arrival at the training center, and billet and company number. *Descriptive data:* age, date of birth, race, weight, and height. *Detailed residence history:* permanent home address and chronological listing of all places where he has lived for six months or more since birth. *History of contact with tuberculosis:* in August 1960, a question was added to the record card: "Have you ever lived in the same household with a person who had tuberculosis?" Each recruit is asked to check a box marked "Yes" or one marked "No or don't know." In 1965, a further question was added to the card: "If yes, how old were you at the time?"

Skin tests. According to the plan of the cooperative skin-testing program, each recruit is given four skin tests; tuberculin and histoplasmin are given in the upper and lower part of the left forearm, PPD-B and a fourth test (with one of a number of other mycobacterial or fungal antigens) in the right arm. All tests are given by the Mantoux method; 0.1 ml of antigen is injected intradermally into the volar surface of the forearm. Most of the injections are given by the Public Health Service nurses, some by corpsmen working under their direction. Reactions are "read" generally at 48 hours (tests given on Friday are read on Monday at about 72 hours) by the nurses, who carefully measure the widest transverse diameter of palpable induration with a ruler calibrated in millimeters. The nurses are instructed that it is neither their responsibil-

Figure 1. Field record card: Navy recruit skin-testing program

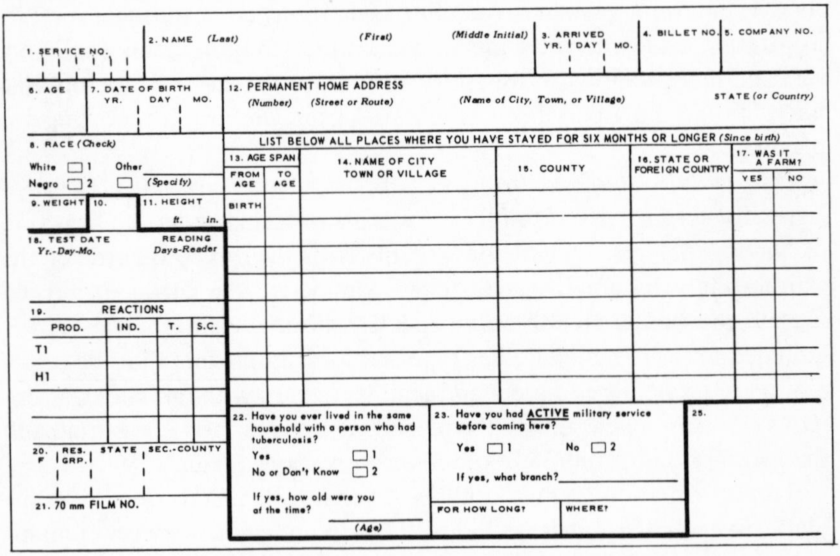
1. SERVICE NO.
2. NAME (Last) (First) (Middle Initial)
3. ARRIVED YR. DAY MO.
4. BILLET NO.
5. COMPANY NO.
6. AGE
7. DATE OF BIRTH YR. DAY MO.
12. PERMANENT HOME ADDRESS (Number) (Street or Route) (Name of City, Town, or Village) STATE (or Country)
8. RACE (Check)
White ☐ 1 Other
Negro ☐ 2 ☐ (Specify)
9. WEIGHT 10. 11. HEIGHT ft. in.
18. TEST DATE Yr.-Day-Mo. READING Days-Reader
19. REACTIONS
PROD. IND. T. S.C.
T1
H1
20. F RES. GRP. STATE SEC.-COUNTY
21. 70 mm FILM NO.
LIST BELOW ALL PLACES WHERE YOU HAVE STAYED FOR SIX MONTHS OR LONGER (Since birth)
13. AGE SPAN FROM AGE TO AGE
14. NAME OF CITY TOWN OR VILLAGE
15. COUNTY
16. STATE OR FOREIGN COUNTRY
17. WAS IT A FARM? YES NO
BIRTH
22. Have you ever lived in the same household with a person who had tuberculosis?
Yes ☐ 1
No or Don't Know ☐ 2
If yes, how old were you at the time? (Age)
23. Have you had ACTIVE military service before coming here?
Yes ☐ 1 No ☐ 2
If yes, what branch?
FOR HOW LONG? WHERE?
25.

ity nor their prerogative to interpret reactions as "positive" or "negative." The measurements of the reactions are recorded in millimeters on the record card. Special characteristics of the reactions, such as the presence of vesicles, are also noted.

Antigens. A single tuberculin, PPD-S, has been used for many years in the research studies of the Tuberculosis Program of the U.S. Public Health Service. PPD-S identifies a particular product, a very large batch prepared by Dr. Florence Seibert in 1939–40 [1] and adopted as the international standard for mammalian-type PPD tuberculin in 1952.[2] The amount of protein used in our standard test has also been the same for many years: 0.0001 mg, commonly referred to as the 5 T.U. or "intermediate strength" dose.

The histoplasmin, identified as H-42, is a culture filtrate of *Histoplasma capsulatum,* prepared in 1946 by Dr. Arden Howell, Jr., of the Public Health Service.[3] It is used in a 1/100 dilution.

PPD-B is prepared from an organism now generally referred to as *M. batteii,* according to the method developed by Seibert for preparing PPD-S.[4] It is used in the same dose (0.0001 mg) as PPD-S in terms of protein. Most of the other skin test antigens used in the Navy program are PPD's prepared from other strains of mycobacteria in our laboratory in Chamblee, Georgia, in the same way as PPD-S and PPD-B.

The PPD products are preserved in lyophilized form. Periodically, stock solutions containing 1 mg protein per ml are prepared by the addition of buffered diluent. From the stock, dilutions containing 0.0001 mg protein per 0.1 ml are then prepared as needed.[5] Both the stock and the dilutions contain 0.5 percent phenol as a preservative. In the first years of the program, fresh dilutions were made up by our laboratory every month. Later, when it became evident that under suitable storage conditions the dilutions maintained potency over a period of many months, it was decided to make them only once every four months.[6]

Equipment. One-milliliter glass tuberculin syringes (graduated in hundredths of a milliliter) with 26-gauge platinum needles are used for testing. Sterile testing "packs," including the syringes and needles required for each testing session, are supplied from the laboratory. A color coding system is used to help identify the different antigens and the syringes used for each. A piece of colored tape is attached to the label of each antigen bottle, and the syringes to be used with that antigen are identified by a rubber ring of the same color. The tuberculin bottle and syringe, for instance, are always color coded in red, histoplasmin in green, PPD-B in blue, and the color for the variable antigen changes with the product. After use, the supplies are returned to the laboratory for cleaning and sterilization (see detailed description in Appendix A).

Personnel. The nurses assigned to the recruit testing program are members of a small team of Public Health Service nurses who spend essentially all their time carrying out the skin-testing activities of the Tuberculosis Research Section. Each nurse is given several months' on-the-job training in the field and in the central office. During this period, she spends much of her time reading reactions with one of the senior nurses. Although reasonably precise performance is usually obtained within two or three months, stability of reading takes considerably longer to achieve. Therefore, throughout the duration of the program, periodic checks are made on the comparability of performance among the various readers by means of independent observations of the same reactions. Despite such efforts to develop and maintain uniformity in the testing and reading procedures, some variation seems unavoidable, partly because of turnover in personnel. Because recruits from the eastern part of the country are generally sent to Great Lakes and those from the west to San Diego, the nurses are transferred periodically from one center to the other so that reader differences are distributed as equally as possible among recruits from all parts of the country.

Data processing. After the results of the skin tests have been recorded and findings reported to the Navy, the field record cards are sent to the headquarters office of the Research Section of the Tuberculosis Program (Washington). For tabulation and analysis, the information on the field cards is transferred to punch cards and finally to magnetic tape.

Recruit population. Of the 665,162 recruits who entered training at the Navy's two centers during the years 1958–1964, a total of 632,870 or 95 percent were tested. At San Diego, where testing was done within three days after the recruits arrived, essentially all (99 percent) were tested. The percentage was lower (91 percent) at Great Lakes, where recruits were not tested until the third to the fifth week after they arrived. By that time, some were already being separated from the Navy, and others missed being tested for a wide variety of reasons.

Of the 632,870 recruits who were tested, 10,537 are excluded from the results to be presented here because of incomplete or unacceptable data: 8,461 of these entered training before **PPD-B** was adopted as a routine test in 1958; others are excluded because their reactions were read earlier or later than the accepted period of two to four days or because information on their age, race, residence, and so forth, was not complete. A small number of recruits were excluded because they did not receive all scheduled skin tests. On a few occasions, so many recruits entered training that the testing schedule permitted giving only the tuberculin test. Also, a few recruits, about 20 each year, were not tested because they were able to convince us that they had had a very severe reaction to a prior test.

Table 1 is a summary of the study population of 622,333 recruits, showing subgroups by age, race, and residence. Almost all (611,445, or

98.3 percent) reported a permanent home address in the conterminous United States.* Most of these men (587,640, or 96.1 percent) were 17 to 21 years of age, and this is the group (enclosed within the box) on which is based almost all the material to be presented. Most (94.8 percent) of these recruits were white.** A limited amount of material will be shown for the small numbers of Negroes and "others." Results for those recruits 22 years and older will be shown only in Appendix Table C. 1, in which frequency distributions of the sizes of tuberculin reactions will be given for major subgroups shown in Table 1.

Almost 11,000 recruits reported a permanent home address outside the United States and are listed under "Not Conterminous U.S." Aside

Table 1. Navy recruit population, by age, race, and residence (tested 1958–64)

Place of Residence*	Total All Ages All Races	17 – 21 Years				22+ Years All Races
		Total	White	Negro	Other	
Total All Places	622,333	594,724	559,625	26,149	8,950	27,609
Conterminous U.S.	611,445	587,640	557,355	26,129	4,156	23,805
Not Conterminous U.S.	10,888	7,084	2,270	20	4,794	3,804
Alaska	825	784	719	1	64	41
Hawaii	1,301	1,247	537	1	709	54
Philippine Islands	7,344	3,884	23	–	3,861	3,460
Other	1,418	1,069	991	18	160	249

* Based on home address at time of entry into the Navy.

from inclusion in Appendix Table C. 1, these men will be discussed only in the section of Chapter 2 on foreign residence. They will not be included in the figures in any of the other sections.

* To simplify the text (and with apologies to Alaska and Hawaii), the cumbersome "conterminous" will generally be omitted and "the United States" will be used to refer only to the first 48 states and District of Columbia. Also, because all the material to be shown for the recruits except that in Tables 1 and 8 is based on men 17 to 21 years of age, reference to age will be omitted from the text.

** Estimates based on the first seven years of the program indicate that approximately one of every 15 white males in the general population of the United States who attain the age of 17 may be expected to be tested in this program at some time between his seventeenth and twenty-second birthday. (See Appendix B.)

SURVEYS IN SPECIAL GROUPS

To supplement the results obtained in the Navy recruit program and to obtain information on tuberculin sensitivity in various age-sex groups and groups with special characteristics, the Public Health Service, in cooperation with state and local health authorities, has conducted more than 50 skin-testing programs in 17 states. The selection of study groups has been guided by the desirability of obtaining detailed information on residents of particular parts of the country, not only where reasonably large groups of persons may be tested but also where the bulk of the population may be expected to participate. These programs have included school children, college students, and persons of all ages in selected communities. The procedures followed in conducting these programs have been generally similar to those described for the Navy program with respect to the type of data collected, testing and reading methods, and data processing. The work has been done by the same small staff of nurses who work in the Navy program.

CHANGES WITH TIME

The tuberculin testing, year after year, of very large nationwide samples of young men of the same ages, affords a remarkable opportunity to measure changes with time in tuberculous infection in this country. In addition to the current program of testing Navy recruits, results are available for a limited program on recruits tested between September 1949 and August 1951. Thus it is possible to present here an estimate of changes over a 15-year period, 1949 to 1964.

Results of the 1949–51 recruit testing program are shown in Figure 2, Map A. The same tuberculin was used in the same dose as in the current program, and testing and recording procedures were similar. However, both testing and reading of reactions were done by Navy corpsmen under the supervision of a Public Health Service medical officer. Also, the 1949–1951 program was limited to recruits entering at San Diego, and too few recruits from the northern tier and eastern states were tested to furnish reliable rates. Thus, detailed results are available only for white lifetime residents of 31 states, from each of which at least 300 men were tested.[1] For these 31 states, *the average reactor rate in 1949–1951 was 6.6 percent;* no state had a rate less than 3 percent, and nine had rates of more than 8 percent.

Figure 2, Map B, shows tuberculin reactor rates for the half million white recruits tested during 1958–1964, who were lifetime residents of the United States. The numbers tested range from about 1,300 for Delaware and Nevada, to over 37,000 for New York, and nearly 52,000 for California. *The nationwide frequency of reactors for the 7-year period is 3.9 percent.* In 30 states, the rates are less than 4 percent. In 15, located chiefly in the northwest and north-central areas, the rates are less than 3 percent. Six states in the southwest and Appalachian area have rates that vary from 5 percent to a maximum of 8 percent. When an average rate is calculated for the 1958–1964 period, based only on lifetime residents of the 31 states included in the 1949–1951 program, this new rate is the same, 3.9 percent, as the rate based on all 48 states in 1958–1964.

As shown in Figure 3, the greatest decreases between earlier and later testing periods occurred in states with the highest frequency of reactors in 1949–1951 (Arizona, Kentucky, and New Mexico). The smallest decreases were in states with the lowest rates at the earlier pe-

Figure 2. Percent of Navy recruits with reactions of 10 or more mm to 0.0001 mg PPD-S: A. tested 1949–51; B. tested 1958–64 (white, ages 17–21)

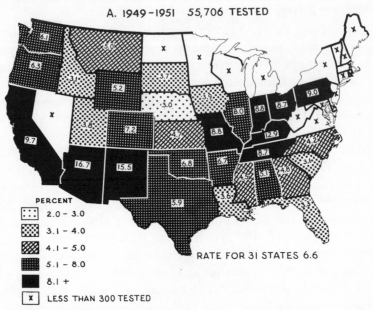

A. 1949-1951   55,706 TESTED

PERCENT
- ⋯ 2.0 – 3.0
- ▨ 3.1 – 4.0
- ▩ 4.1 – 5.0
- ▦ 5.1 – 8.0
- ■ 8.1 +
- x LESS THAN 300 TESTED

RATE FOR 31 STATES 6.6

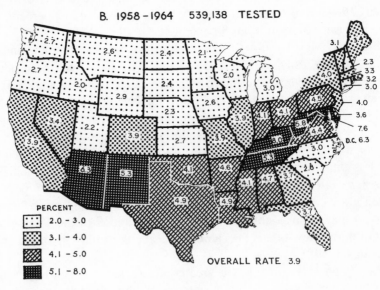

B. 1958 – 1964   539,138 TESTED

PERCENT
- ⋯ 2.0 – 3.0
- ▨ 3.1 – 4.0
- ▩ 4.1 – 5.0
- ▦ 5.1 – 8.0

OVERALL RATE 3.9

Figure 3. Correlation by state of the percent of Navy recruits with reactions of 10 or more mm to 0.0001 mg PPD-S, tested in 1949–51 and 1958–64 (white, ages 17–21)

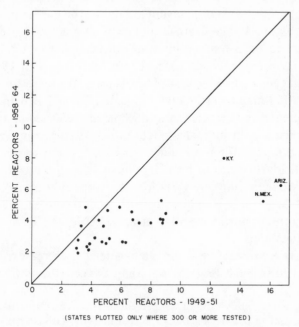

(STATES PLOTTED ONLY WHERE 300 OR MORE TESTED)

Figure 4. Percent of Navy recruits with reactions of 10 or more mm to 0.0001 mg PPD-S, for those tested during different periods in the 1958–64 program, and for comparison, those tested in 1949–51 (white, ages 17–21)

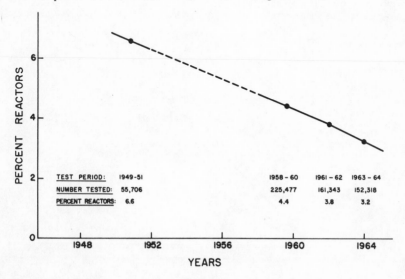

riod. The range of state rates decreased from 3 to 16.7 percent in 1949–1951 to 2 to 8 percent in 1958–1964.

The frequency of reactors in three successive groups of recruits in the current program, and the average rate for the earlier program, are plotted in Figure 4. The average frequency of reactors has dropped at what seems to be a remarkably uniform rate. It was 6.6 percent in 1949–1951; 4.4 percent in 1958–1960; 3.8 percent in 1961–1962; and 3.2 percent in 1963–1964. The observed decrease for the whole 15-year period may be estimated at one quarter of 1 percent per year.

The decreases for the country as a whole are reflected to a surprising extent by changes in individual state rates. As shown in Table 2, the drop is continuous for most states from one period to the next. For some, particularly states with small numbers tested, there are irregularities, partly due to sampling variation. It must also be appreciated that, despite all our efforts, it simply does not seem possible to maintain entirely uniform performance year after year, especially in measuring the size of reactions.

Reactor rates by state show the same pattern of decrease from 1958–1960 to 1963–1964 (Fig. 5) as seen between the early and later

Figure 5. Correlation by state of the percent of Navy recruits with reactions of 10 or more mm to 0.0001 mg PPD-S, tested in 1958–60 and 1963–64 (white, ages 17–21)

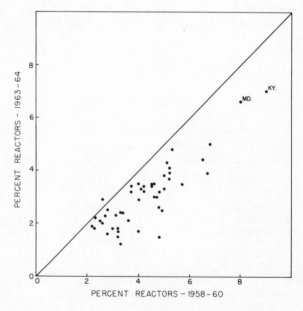

Table 2. Number of Navy recruits tested and percent with reactions of 10 or more mm to 0.0001 mg PPD-S, by test period (white, ages 17–21)

	NUMBER TESTED				PERCENT REACTORS			
	1949–51	1958–60	1961–62	1963–64	1949–51	1958–60	1961–62	1963–64
TOTAL	55,706	225,477	161,343	152,318	6.6	4.4	3.8	3.2
Alabama	1,981	3,233	2,233	1,708	5.1	5.2	4.3	4.1
Arizona	472	2,205	1,875	1,782	16.7	6.8	6.9	5.0
Arkansas	1,785	2,717	1,788	1,482	6.7	5.2	4.4	3.9
California	8,496	21,321	16,193	14,452	9.7	4.2	4.0	3.2
Colorado	1,444	3,486	2,380	2,641	7.2	4.7	3.9	3.0
Connecticut	-	3,038	2,206	2,238	-	3.6	3.2	2.1
Delaware	-	538	388	389	-	4.8	2.8	2.6
Dist. of Columbia	-	386	287	305	-	7.8	7.0	3.9
Florida	1,469	5,087	4,019	4,061	3.3	4.1	3.4	3.3
Georgia	1,961	4,157	3,013	2,578	4.8	3.7	3.9	3.4
Idaho	708	1,581	1,034	871	3.1	2.3	1.7	1.8
Illinois	879	10,377	6,600	6,897	8.0	4.5	3.5	3.5
Indiana	1,125	6,198	4,189	3,780	8.8	4.6	4.2	3.0
Iowa	2,567	4,812	3,410	3,519	3.9	2.7	2.6	2.3
Kansas	1,900	3,937	2,896	2,907	4.7	3.0	3.1	1.8
Kentucky	1,010	2,927	1,984	1,745	12.9	9.0	7.4	7.0
Louisiana	1,533	3,918	2,702	2,429	3.6	5.7	5.1	3.5
Maine	-	1,582	1,116	1,132	-	4.8	3.2	1.5
Maryland	-	2,848	2,143	2,148	-	8.0	8.1	6.6
Massachusetts	-	6,351	4,451	4,630	-	4.0	2.7	2.9
Michigan	-	10,925	7,467	6,302	-	3.4	2.9	2.4
Minnesota	-	6,162	4,882	4,926	-	2.8	1.6	1.6
Mississippi	1,337	1,786	1,109	889	4.5	4.9	4.2	2.5
Missouri	2,336	6,446	4,597	4,219	8.8	4.2	3.8	3.4
Montana	839	1,617	1,023	1,083	5.0	3.3	2.8	1.2
Nebraska	1,580	2,676	1,856	1,930	3.0	2.3	2.3	2.2
Nevada	-	455	423	461	-	4.0	2.6	3.5
New Hampshire	-	1,131	784	842	-	3.2	1.9	1.5
New Jersey	-	6,885	5,028	5,018	-	4.5	3.9	3.4
New Mexico	601	1,673	1,308	1,144	15.5	6.5	4.7	4.4
New York	-	14,807	10,888	11,509	-	4.6	3.7	3.5
North Carolina	2,645	4,121	2,769	2,673	4.2	3.3	3.0	2.4
North Dakota	-	1,137	868	715	-	2.6	2.4	2.0
Ohio	1,341	12,936	9,328	8,734	8.7	5.0	3.7	3.3
Oklahoma	2,170	3,527	2,576	2,202	6.8	4.8	3.8	3.2
Oregon	1,182	4,489	2,744	2,887	6.3	3.2	2.9	1.8
Pennsylvania	531	14,854	10,883	9,817	9.0	5.2	4.2	3.7
Rhode Island	-	885	738	758	-	3.7	2.7	3.2
South Carolina	1,308	2,400	1,597	1,466	3.1	2.8	3.1	2.5
South Dakota	401	1,220	901	919	3.7	3.2	1.9	1.7
Tennessee	1,788	3,694	2,790	2,377	8.7	5.3	5.6	4.8
Texas	6,834	11,118	9,044	8,071	5.9	5.1	5.2	4.3
Utah	976	1,362	869	779	3.8	2.5	1.7	2.1
Vermont	-	794	550	517	-	4.0	3.1	1.7
Virginia	-	2,911	2,067	1,812	-	5.0	4.1	3.8
Washington	2,180	5,725	3,582	3,481	6.1	3.1	2.6	2.3
West Virginia	-	3,175	1,853	1,376	-	6.7	5.7	3.9
Wisconsin	-	5,072	3,343	3,130	-	2.2	1.8	1.9
Wyoming	327	795	569	587	5.2	2.6	3.3	2.9

Navy programs (Fig. 3). The largest decreases tend to be in states with the highest rates in 1958–1960 and the smallest in states with the lowest rates. The *range* in reactor rates decreased from 3 to 16.7 percent in 1949–1951, to 2.2 to 9 percent in 1958–1960, and to 1.2 to 7 percent in 1963–1964.

If the downward linear trend seen in Figure 4 were to continue, a rate of approximately 1 percent would be expected by about 1972. It is not realistic, of course, to expect the trend to be linear or the observed rates to be as low as 1 percent everywhere in the country. As rates fall, with more and more states having very low frequencies of reactors, it may be expected that the curve will flatten because, with our present tuberculin testing products, the presence of cross reactions will set limits below which reactor rates will not fall. The tendency of the rates to level off in some of the southeastern states may already be reflecting the impact of this limit.

PLACE OF RESIDENCE

In order to study the influence of place of residence on the prevalence of tuberculous infection, we asked each recruit to give a complete residence history, listing all places he had lived for six months or more. Recruits who were lifetime U.S. residents were subclassified as either lifetime one-county, one-state, or not-one-state residents on the basis of this history. It was decided to use only those recruits who had lived all their lives in a single county in order to have as pure a group as possible in which to study geographic variations in tuberculin sensitivity. Many counties, however, particularly those in the south and west, have such small populations that they are represented by too few recruits to provide meaningful rates. Counties were combined, therefore, into the State Economic Areas delineated by the Bureau of Census.

State Economic Areas are geographic units intermediate in size between states and counties. They are relatively homogeneous with respect to a large number of characteristics, including industrial and commercial activities, as well as demographic, climatic, physiographic, and cultural factors. The potential usefulness of the areas for other purposes is recognized by the Bureau of the Census: "Areas of this type are well adapted for use in a wide variety of studies in which state data are neither sufficiently refined nor homogeneous, and in which the manipulations of county data present real difficulties." [2]

Figure 6 shows the frequency of tuberculin reactors, by State Economic Area, for the quarter of a million recruits who were lifetime one-county residents. Of the 506 areas into which the 3,068 counties of the United States are grouped, 37 are represented by more than 1,000 recruits, 424 by 100 to 1,000, 33 by 50 to 99, and only 12 by less than 50.

In large sections of the north-central part of the United States, rates among recruits are below 2 percent, and for most of the country in terms of land area, rates are less than 4 percent. Foci of high prevalence of tuberculous infection must exist in these areas, but the populations they represent are apparently too small to influence the rates in the recruit populations. Higher rates of 6 percent or more are concentrated in Kentucky and scattered irregularly throughout an area roughly paralleling the Appalachian Mountains, northward into Maryland and Pennsylvania, and southward into the south central states. Still higher rates, mostly above 10 percent, are found among recruits from the Mexican border areas in Texas, Arizona, and California, with much lower rates in the northern parts of these states.

Scattered throughout the country are areas where the rates among recruits are conspicuously higher than in the adjacent areas. Most of these areas represent large cities, where slightly higher rates might be expected. Some of them, however, represent rural areas. Thus, a higher rate is seen for the eastern shore of Maryland than for the western part of the state. Recruits from the coastal areas of the southeastern and south-central states, bordering on the south Atlantic and Gulf of Mexico, also generally have higher rates than those from the inland areas. The high rate in northwestern Colorado is primarily the result of tuberculin cross reactions, presumably caused by *M. balnei* infection.[3]

Although the cities represent only a small part of the nation in terms of land area, they include most of the population. Results of testing Navy recruits from 178 Standard Metropolitan Statistical Areas,* each with over 100 men tested, are given in Table 3.A, in order of increasing frequency of tuberculin reactors. In Table 3.B the same material is shown alphabetically, and in Figure 7 graphically. Results for these

---

* A Standard Metropolitan Statistical Area is a county or group of contiguous counties, metropolitan in character, containing at least one city of 50,000 or more population, or "Twin Cities" with a combined population of at least 50,000. In New England, the SMSA's are composed of cities and towns instead of counties, and the requirement for inclusion as an SMSA is a population density of 100 persons per square mile. A few counties in New England are thus divided among two or three metropolitan areas. Because it is not possible to divide the recruit material this way, such areas have been combined.

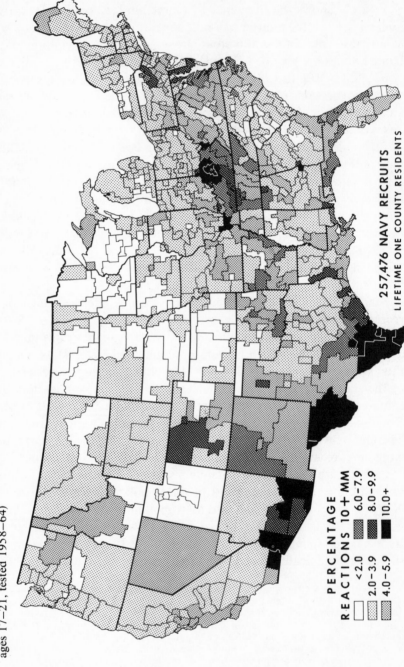

Figure 6. Percent of Navy recruits with reactions of 10 or more mm to 0.0001 mg PPD-S, by State Economic Area (white, ages 17–21, tested 1958–64)

PERCENTAGE
REACTIONS 10+ MM

<2.0   6.0-7.9
2.0-3.9   8.0-9.9
4.0-5.9   10.0+

257,476 NAVY RECRUITS
LIFETIME ONE COUNTY RESIDENTS

Table 3.A. Number of Navy recruits tested and percent with reactions of 10 or more mm to 0.0001 mg PPD-S, for lifetime residents of counties included in the specified metropolitan areas (white, ages 17–21, tested 1958–64)

Percent ≥10mm	Number tested	Metropolitan Area	Percent ≥10mm	Number tested	Metropolitan Area	Percent ≥10mm	Number tested	Metropolitan Area
0.8	118	Charleston, S. C.	2.9	205	Topeka, Kans.	4.1	246	Springfield, Ohio
0.9	106	Texarkana, Tex.-Ark.	3.0	133	Billings, Mont.	4.2	1,276	Bridgeport, Conn. area[16]
1.0	202	Dubuque, Iowa	3.0	1,528	New Haven, Conn. area[6]	4.2	332	Little Rock, Ark. area[17]
1.0	101	Durham, N. C.	3.1	869	Indianapolis, Ind.	4.2	238	Pueblo, Colo.
1.0	313	Madison, Wis.	3.1	130	Pensacola, Fla.	4.2	520	Sacramento, Calif.
1.2	347	Muskegon, Mich. area[1]	3.1	1,250	Portland, Ore.-Wash.	4.2	503	Tulsa, Okla.
1.4	296	Memphis, Tenn.	3.1	424	South Bend, Ind.	4.3	467	Chattanooga, Tenn.-Ga.
1.5	675	Grand Rapids, Mich.	3.1	455	Tampa-St. Petersburg, Fla.	4.3	463	Harrisburg, Pa.
1.5	198	Springfield, Mich.	3.2	930	Duluth-Superior, Minn.-Wis.	4.3	1,529	Kansas City, Kans.-Mo.
1.6	254	Kalamazoo, Mich.	3.2	250	Eugene, Ore.	4.3	368	Wheeling, W. Va.-Ohio
1.6	182	Ogden, Utah	3.2	563	Lancaster, Pa.	4.4	1,250	Albany, N. Y. area[18]
1.6	488	Salt Lake City, Utah	3.2	343	New London, Conn. area[7]	4.4	5,791	Philadelphia, Pa.-N. J.
1.8	169	Decatur, Ill.	3.2	347	Rockford, Ill.	4.4	2,274	San Francisco-Oakland, Calif.
1.8	273	Greensboro-High Point, N.C.	3.3	6,261	Boston, Mass. area[8]	4.5	155	Austin, Texas
1.8	169	Shreveport, La.	3.3	450	Peoria, Ill.	4.5	1,094	Denver, Colo.
1.9	411	Lansing, Mich.	3.3	399	Portland, Maine	4.5	488	San Diego, Calif.
1.9	634	Tacoma, Wash.	3.4	682	Birmingham, Ala.	4.6	5,681	Pittsburgh, Pa.
2.0	198	Asheville, N. C.	3.4	888	Gary, Ind. area[9]	4.6	216	Savannah, Ga.
2.0	460	Oklahoma City, Okla.	3.4	6,406	Los Angeles, Calif. area[10]	4.6	109	Sioux Falls, S. Dak.
2.0	450	Spokane, Wash.	3.4	438	Manchester, N. H.	4.6	263	Waterloo, Iowa
2.1	383	Binghamton, N. Y.	3.4	145	Muncie, Ind.	4.6	1,067	Youngstown-Warren, Ohio
2.1	235	Columbia, S. C.	3.4	2,356	Providence, R. I. area[11]	4.7	253	Albuquerque, N. Mex.
2.1	423	Miami, Fla.	3.4	445	Saginaw, Mich.	4.8	6,652	Chicago, Ill.
2.1	280	Springfield, Ill.	3.4	625	Wilmington, Del.-N.J.	4.9	244	Lake Charles, La.
2.1	751	Utica-Rome, N. Y.	3.5	372	Altoona, Pa.	4.9	123	Tuscaloosa, Ala.
2.1	1,639	Worcester, Mass. area[2]	3.5	648	Canton, Ohio	5.0	2,822	Buffalo, N. Y.
2.2	185	Provo-Orem, Utah	3.5	375	Lorain-Elyria, Ohio	5.0	925	Jersey City, N. J.
2.2	1,287	Springfield, Mass. area[3]	3.6	140	Champaign-Urbana, Ill.	5.0	341	Richmond, Va.
2.3	605	Flint, Mich.	3.6	2,956	Cleveland, Ohio	5.1	1,312	Houston, Texas
2.3	129	Great Falls, Mont.	3.6	331	Ft. Wayne, Ind.	5.3	190	Roanoke, Va.
2.3	221	Green Bay, Wis.	3.6	749	San Bernardino, Calif. area[12]	5.4	221	Atlantic City, N. J.
2.3	3,138	Minneapolis-St. Paul, Minn.	3.6	169	St. Joseph, Mo.	5.4	350	Evansville, Ind.-Ky.
2.3	469	Wichita, Kans.	3.6	139	Waco, Tex.	5.4	204	Galveston-Texas City, Texas
2.4	416	Bakersfield, Calif.	3.7	997	Columbus, Ohio	5.4	295	Jacksonville, Fla.
2.4	288	Bay City, Mich.	3.7	107	Monroe, La.	5.4	10,841	New York, N. Y.
2.4	292	Cedar Rapids, Iowa	3.7	1,177	Syracuse, N. Y.	5.5	1,057	Dallas, Texas
2.4	166	Fargo, N. Dak. area[4]	3.7	857	Toledo, Ohio	5.8	572	Reading, Pa.
2.4	247	Greenville, S. C.	3.8	1,045	Dayton, Ohio	5.8	139	Winston-Salem, N. C.
2.4	1,487	Hartford-New Britain, Conn.	3.8	653	Erie, Pa.	5.9	1,556	Cincinnati, Ohio-Ky.
2.4	210	Jackson, Mich.	3.8	737	Ft. Worth, Tex.	5.9	425	San Jose, Calif.
2.4	127	Macon, Ga.	3.8	313	Hamilton-Middletown, Ohio	6.0	166	Gadsden, Ala.
2.5	399	Pittsfield, Mass.	3.8	157	Lynchburg, Va.	6.1	132	Raleigh, N. C.
2.5	876	Rochester, N. Y.	3.8	1,671	Paterson, N. J. area[13]	6.4	482	Charleston, W. Va.
2.5	436	York, Pa.	3.9	232	Augusta, Ga.-S.C.	6.4	486	Nashville, Tenn.
2.6	265	Baton Rouge, La.	3.9	5,679	Detroit, Mich.	6.9	612	Scranton, Pa.
2.6	194	Charlotte, N. C.	3.9	336	Stockton, Calif.	7.6	1,006	Louisville, Ky.-Ind.
2.6	190	Racine, Wis.	4.0	354	Beaumont-Port Arthur, Tex.	7.8	908	Wilkes-Barre—Hazelton, Pa.
2.7	226	Ann Arbor, Mich.	4.0	798	Johnstown, Pa.	7.9	1,036	New Orleans, La.
2.7	820	Atlanta, Ga.	4.0	2,172	Newark, N. J.	8.2	231	Tucson, Ariz.
2.7	110	Colorado Springs, Colo.	4.0	149	Santa Barbara, Calif.	8.5	422	Huntington, W. Va. area[19]
2.7	451	Davenport, Iowa area[5]	4.0	3,280	St. Louis, Mo.-Ill.	8.7	485	Phoenix, Ariz.
2.7	221	Lima, Ohio	4.0	349	Steubenville, Ohio area[14]	9.0	356	Mobile, Ala.
2.7	222	Lincoln, Nebr.	4.0	176	Terre Haute, Ind.	9.2	206	Columbus, Ga.-Ala.
2.7	1,037	Omaha, Nebr.-Iowa	4.0	422	Trenton, N. J.	9.4	2,458	Baltimore, Md.
2.8	464	Des Moines, Iowa	4.0	742	Washington, D.C.-Md.-Va.	10.7	467	El Paso, Texas
2.8	528	Fresno, Calif.	4.0	173	Wichita Falls, Tex.	10.7	984	San Antonio, Texas
2.9	624	Knoxville, Tenn.	4.1	958	Akron, Ohio	12.4	137	Brownsville-Harlingen-San Benito, Texas
2.9	1,084	Milwaukee, Wis.	4.1	1,263	Allentown, Pa. area[15]	14.5	124	Corpus Christi, Texas
2.9	1,497	Seattle, Wash.	4.1	197	Lewiston-Auburn, Maine			
2.9	306	Sioux City, Iowa	4.1	172	Norfolk-Portsmouth, Va.			

1 Includes Muskegon Heights.
2 Includes Fitchburg-Leominster.
3 Includes Chicopee-Holyoke.
4 Includes Moorhead, Minn.
5 Includes Rock Island-Moline, Ill.
6 Includes Meriden-Waterbury.
7 Includes Groton-Norwich.
8 Includes Brockton-Lowell-Lawrence-Haverhill, Mass. (N.H.)
9 Includes Hammond-E. Chicago.
10 Includes Long Beach.
11 Includes Pawtucket-New Bedford-Fall River, R.I.-Mass.
12 Includes Riverside-Ontario.
13 Includes Clifton-Passaic.
14 Includes Weirton, W. Va.
15 Includes Bethlehem-Easton, Pa. (N. J.).
16 Includes Norwalk-Stamford.
17 Includes N. Little Rock.
18 Includes Schenectady-Troy.
19 Includes Ashland, Ky. (Ohio).

Table 3.B. Number of Navy recruits tested and percent with reactions of 10 or more mm to 0.0001 mg PPD-S, for lifetime residents of counties included in the specified metropolitan areas (white, ages 17–21, tested 1958–64)

Percent ≥10mm	Number tested	Metropolitan Area	Percent ≥10mm	Number tested	Metropolitan Area	Percent ≥10mm	Number tested	Metropolitan Area
4.1	958	Akron, Ohio	1.5	675	Grand Rapids, Mich.	2.2	185	Provo-Orem, Utah
4.4	1,250	Albany, N.Y. area [1]	2.3	129	Great Falls, Mont.	4.2	238	Pueblo, Colo.
4.7	253	Albuquerque, N. Mex.	2.3	221	Green Bay, Wis.	2.6	190	Racine, Wis.
4.1	1,263	Allentown, Pa. area [2]	1.8	273	Greensboro-High Point, N.C.	6.1	132	Raleigh, N.C.
3.5	372	Altoona, Pa.	2.4	247	Greenville, S.C.	5.8	572	Reading, Pa.
2.7	226	Ann Arbor, Mich.	3.8	313	Hamilton-Middletown, Ohio	5.0	341	Richmond, Va.
2.0	198	Asheville, N.C.	4.3	463	Harrisburg, Pa.	5.3	190	Roanoke, Va.
2.7	820	Atlanta, Ga.	2.4	1,487	Hartford-New Britain, Conn.	2.5	876	Rochester, N.Y.
5.4	221	Atlantic City, N.J.	5.1	1,312	Houston, Texas	3.2	347	Rockford, Ill.
3.9	232	Augusta, Ga.-S.C.	8.5	422	Huntington, W. Va. area [9]	4.2	520	Sacramento, Calif.
4.5	155	Austin, Texas	3.1	869	Indianapolis, Ind.	3.4	445	Saginaw, Mich.
2.4	416	Bakersfield, Calif.	2.4	210	Jackson, Mich.	1.6	488	Salt Lake City, Utah
9.4	2,458	Baltimore, Md.	5.4	295	Jacksonville, Fla.	10.7	984	San Antonio, Tex.
2.6	265	Baton Rouge, La.	5.0	925	Jersey City, N.J.	3.6	749	San Bernardino, Calif. area [17]
2.4	288	Bay City, Mich.	4.0	798	Johnstown, Pa.	4.5	488	San Diego, Calif.
4.0	354	Beaumont-Port Arthur, Texas	1.6	254	Kalamazoo, Mich.	4.4	2,274	San Francisco-Oakland, Calif.
3.0	133	Billings, Mont.	4.3	1,529	Kansas City, Kans.-Mo.	5.9	425	San Jose, Calif.
2.1	383	Binghamton, N.Y.	2.9	624	Knoxville, Tenn.	4.0	149	Santa Barbara, Calif.
3.4	682	Birmingham, Ala.	4.9	244	Lake Charles, La.	4.6	216	Savannah, Ga.
3.3	6,261	Boston, Mass. area [3]	3.2	563	Lancaster, Pa.	6.9	612	Scranton, Pa.
4.2	1,276	Bridgeport, Conn. area [4]	1.9	411	Lansing, Mich.	2.9	1,497	Seattle, Wash.
12.4	137	Brownsville, Texas area [5]	4.1	197	Lewiston-Auburn, Maine	1.8	169	Shreveport, La.
5.0	2,822	Buffalo, N.Y.	2.7	221	Lima, Ohio	2.9	306	Sioux City, Iowa
3.5	648	Canton, Ohio	2.7	222	Lincoln, Nebr.	4.6	109	Sioux Falls, S.D.
2.4	292	Cedar Rapids, Iowa	4.2	332	Little Rock, Ark. area [10]	3.1	424	South Bend, Ind.
3.6	140	Champaign-Urbana, Ill.	3.5	375	Lorain-Elyria, Ohio	2.0	450	Spokane, Wash.
0.8	118	Charleston, S.C.	3.4	6,406	Los Angeles, Calif. area [11]	2.1	280	Springfield, Ill.
6.4	482	Charleston, W. Va.	7.6	1,006	Louisville, Ky.-Ind.	1.5	198	Springfield, Mo.
2.6	194	Charlotte, N.C.	3.8	157	Lynchburg, Va.	4.1	246	Springfield, Ohio
4.3	467	Chattanooga, Tenn.-Ga.	2.4	127	Macon, Georgia	2.2	1,287	Springfield, Mass. area [18]
4.8	6,652	Chicago, Ill.	1.0	313	Madison, Wis.	3.6	169	St. Joseph, Mo.
5.9	1,556	Cincinnati, Ohio-Ky.	3.4	438	Manchester, N.H.	4.0	3,280	St. Louis, Mo.-Ill.
3.6	2,956	Cleveland, Ohio	1.4	296	Memphis, Tenn.	4.0	349	Steubenville, Ohio area [19]
2.7	110	Colorado Springs, Colo.	2.1	423	Miami, Fla.	3.9	336	Stockton, Calif.
2.1	235	Columbia, S.C.	2.9	1,084	Milwaukee, Wis.	3.7	1,177	Syracuse, N.Y.
9.2	206	Columbus, Ga.-Ala.	2.3	3,138	Mpls.-St. Paul, Minn.	1.9	634	Tacoma, Wash.
3.7	997	Columbus, Ohio	9.0	356	Mobile, Ala.	3.1	455	Tampa-St. Petersburg, Fla.
14.5	124	Corpus Christi, Texas	3.7	107	Monroe, La.	4.0	176	Terre Haute, Ind.
5.5	1,057	Dallas, Texas	3.4	145	Muncie, Ind.	0.9	106	Texarkana, Tex.-Ark.
2.7	451	Davenport, Iowa area [6]	1.2	347	Muskegon, Mich. area [12]	3.7	857	Toledo, Ohio
3.8	1,045	Dayton, Ohio	6.4	486	Nashville, Tenn.	2.9	205	Topeka, Kans.
1.8	169	Decatur, Ill.	3.0	1,528	New Haven, Conn. area [13]	4.0	422	Trenton, N.J.
4.5	1,094	Denver, Colo.	3.2	343	New London, Conn. area [14]	8.2	231	Tucson, Ariz.
2.8	464	Des Moines, Iowa	7.9	1,036	New Orleans, La.	4.2	503	Tulsa, Okla.
3.9	5,679	Detroit, Mich.	5.4	10,841	New York City, N.Y.	4.9	123	Tuscaloosa, Ala.
1.0	202	Dubuque, Iowa	4.0	2,172	Newark, N.J.	2.1	751	Utica-Rome, N.Y.
3.2	930	Duluth-Superior, Minn.-Wis.	4.1	172	Norfolk-Portsmouth, Va.	3.6	139	Waco, Tex.
1.0	101	Durham, N.C.	1.6	182	Ogden, Utah	4.0	742	Washington, D.C.-Md.-Va.
10.7	467	El Paso, Texas	2.0	460	Oklahoma City, Okla.	4.6	263	Waterloo, Iowa
3.8	653	Erie, Pa.	2.7	1,037	Omaha, Nebr.-Iowa	4.3	368	Wheeling, W.Va.-Ohio
3.2	250	Eugene, Ore.	3.8	1,671	Paterson, N.J. area [15]	2.3	469	Wichita, Kans.
5.4	350	Evansville, Ind.-Ky.	3.1	130	Pensacola, Fla.	4.0	173	Wichita Falls, Tex.
2.4	166	Fargo, N. Dak. area [7]	3.3	450	Peoria, Ill.	7.8	908	Wilkes Barre-Hazelton, Pa.
2.3	605	Flint, Mich.	4.4	5,791	Philadelphia, Pa.-N.J.	3.4	625	Wilmington, Del.-N.J.
3.6	331	Fort Wayne, Ind.	8.7	485	Phoenix, Ariz.	5.8	139	Winston-Salem, N.C.
3.8	737	Fort Worth, Texas	4.6	5,681	Pittsburgh, Pa.	2.1	1,639	Worcester-Fitchburg-Leominster, Mass.
2.8	528	Fresno, Calif.	2.5	399	Pittsfield, Mass.			
6.0	166	Gadsden, Alabama	3.3	399	Portland, Maine	2.5	436	York, Pa.
5.4	204	Galveston-Texas City, Texas	3.1	1,250	Portland, Ore.-Wash.	4.6	1,067	Youngstown-Warren, Ohio
3.4	888	Gary, Ind. area [8]	3.4	2,356	Providence, R.I. area [16]			

[1] Includes Schenectady-Troy.
[2] Includes Bethlehem-Easton, Pa. (N.J.).
[3] Includes Brockton-Lowell-Lawrence-Haverhill, Mass.(N.H.).
[4] Includes Norwalk-Stamford.
[5] Includes Harlingen-San Benito.
[6] Includes Rock Island-Moline, Ill.
[7] Includes Moorhead, Minn.
[8] Includes Hammond-E. Chicago.
[9] Includes Ashland, Ky. (Ohio).
[10] Includes N. Little Rock.
[11] Includes Long Beach.
[12] Includes Muskegon Heights.
[13] Includes Meriden-Waterbury.
[14] Includes Groton-Norwich.
[15] Includes Clifton-Passaic.
[16] Includes Pawtucket-New Bedford-Fall River, R.I.-Mass.
[17] Includes Riverside-Ontario.
[18] Includes Chicopee-Holyoke.
[19] Includes Weirton, W. Va.

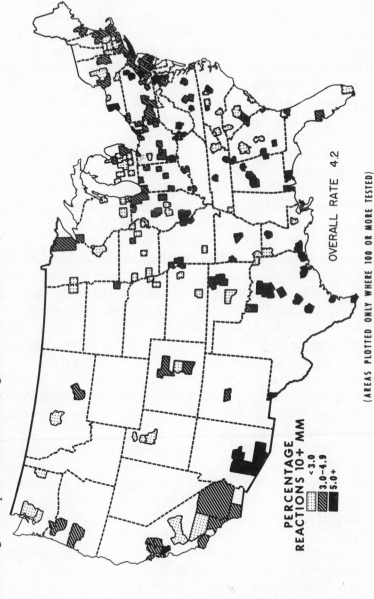

Figure 7. Percent of Navy recruits with reactions of 10 or more mm to 0.0001 mg PPD-S, for lifetime residents of counties included in large metropolitan areas (white, ages 17–21, tested 1958–64)

PERCENTAGE
REACTIONS 10+ MM

□ <3.0
▨ 3.0–4.9
■ 5.0+

OVERALL RATE 4.2

(AREAS PLOTTED ONLY WHERE 100 OR MORE TESTED)

metropolitan centers and also for the 22 with fewer than 100 recruits tested are given by county in Appendix Table C.2.

The overall rate for recruits from the large cities is 4.2 percent. According to the 1960 census, these cities account for almost two thirds of the population of the United States.[4] In a considerable number, the frequency of tuberculin reactors is surprisingly low: in 62, the rates are less than 3 percent; in 101, or more than half, rates vary from 3 to 6 percent; and only in 17 are the rates above 6 percent. Six of these 17 cities (Table 3.A) are located in Texas or Arizona near the Mexican border, where a considerable proportion of the population is of Mexican stock. The Columbus, Georgia, area was the site of two Public Health Service BCG trials; hence the high rate observed there.[5] Most other cities where rates exceed 6 percent are located along the Gulf of Mexico, and in areas bordering the Appalachian Mountains.

It should be mentioned that the metropolitan areas where recruit rates are over 6 percent account for only 4.4 percent of the population of the country, whereas those where rates are less than 3 percent account for 10.8 percent of the population. In some states, the range of rates among recruits from different metropolitan centers is small, and in others it is large. In Michigan, for instance, rates range from only 1.5 to 3.9 percent, and in Texas, they range from less than 4 percent in the north to more than 10 percent along the Mexican border.

Data given in Figure 8.A and B show the variations in frequency of reactors for recruits from the counties that make up each of the 24 largest metropolitan areas—those with populations of one million or more. These 24 areas comprise about one third of the total white population of the United States. The overall rate in these areas is 4.4 percent. In some, for instance Minneapolis–St. Paul, the rates are remarkably similar in the different counties that make up the area. In others, such as Boston, New York, Philadelphia, and San Francisco, there is considerable variation, with higher rates generally in the densely populated central counties and lower rates in the surrounding counties. However, even in the central counties, all rates are less than 10 percent.

A special tabulation was made for the 9,294 recruits tested in 1958 1963 who listed New York City as their permanent address (Table 4). All those 17 to 21 years old are included, regardless of race or residence history. The reactor rate for these recruits is 8.9 percent. For the white recruits (who constitute 94 percent of all the New York City recruits) the rate is 8.1 percent, with a higher rate for those from Manhattan

Figure 8-A. Percent of Navy recruits with reactions of 10 or more mm to 0.0001 mg PPD-S, for lifetime residents of counties included in metropolitan areas with populations of one million or more (white, ages 17–21, tested 1958–64)

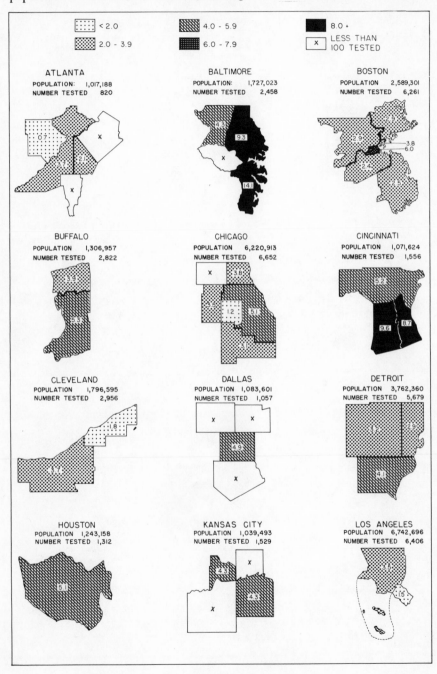

Figure 8-B. Percent of Navy recruits with reactions of 10 or more mm to 0.0001 mg PPD-S, for lifetime residents of counties included in metropolitan areas with populations of one million or more (white, ages 17–21, tested 1958–64)

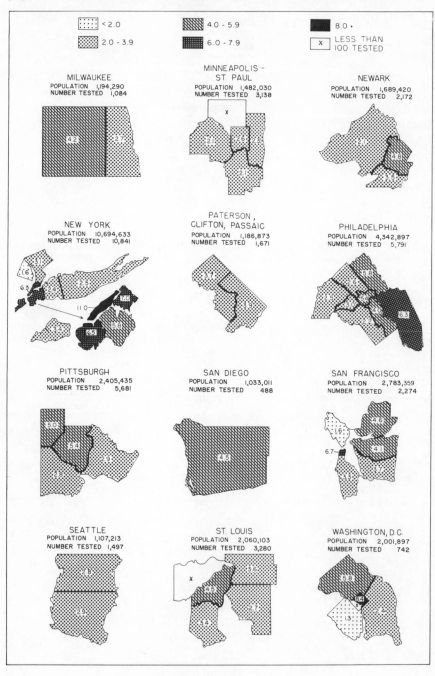

than from the other boroughs, and a very much higher rate for the group that reported that they had lived for six months or more outside the United States. (Results for the white recruits who were lifetime residents of New York City have been included as an inset in Figure 8.B.) For the 469 Negroes who were residents of New York City, the rate is 19.8 percent; for the 98 who classified themselves as "others," it is 30.6 percent.

The differences between the frequencies of tuberculin reactors among white recruits from urban and rural areas are summarized for individual states in Table 5. (See also Appendix Table C.3.) Results are

Table 4. Number of Navy recruits tested and percent with reactions of 10 or more mm to 0.0001 mg PPD-S, for residents of New York City, by race, type of residence, and borough (tested 1958–63)

Place of Residence	TOTAL All Races All Residence	WHITE				NEGRO				OTHER
		Total	Lifetime N.Y.C.	Lifetime U.S.	Some Foreign Residence	Total	Lifetime N.Y.C.	Lifetime U.S.	Some Foreign Residence	Total
					Number Tested					
Total All Places	9,294	8,727	7,066	1,110	551	469	263	150	56	98
Bronx	1,885	1,761	1,415	193	153	94	51	27	16	30
Kings	3,148	2,975	2,467	319	189	152	79	51	22	21
Queens	2,726	2,636	2,173	374	89	82	48	28	6	8
Richmond	487	475	385	78	12	11	7	4	-	1
Manhattan	1,048	880	626	146	108	130	78	40	12	38
					Percent Reactors*					
Total All Places	8.9	8.1	6.6	6.7	29.6	19.8	15.6	23.3	30.4	30.6
Bronx	9.9	8.8	7.0	4.1	31.4	21.3	15.7	(8)	(4)	(12)
Kings	8.6	7.9	6.5	6.9	27.0	18.4	12.7	23.5	(6)	(7)
Queens	6.8	6.5	5.8	6.1	24.7	17.1	(4)	(7)	(3)	(0)
Richmond	5.1	5.3	3.4	11.5	(3)	(0)	(0)	(0)	-	(0)
Manhattan	15.5	13.6	11.0	8.2	36.1	23.9	24.4	(8)	(4)	(11)

* Where less than 50 tested, the number of reactors is given in parentheses.

shown for three categories of lifetime one-county residents: lifetime residents of standard metropolitan areas; lifetime farm residents; and other nonmetropolitan residents. The nationwide rate for lifetime farm residents is lower (2.8 percent) than for the other nonmetropolitan residents (3.6 percent), and both are lower than the rate for lifetime residents of metropolitan counties (4.2 percent). This same pattern of differences prevails in most of the states, although there is some variation, particularly in the rates for the relatively few farm residents.

Another finding about the recruits in these categories is illustrated in Figure 9. It can be seen that, for each state, the rates in one group corre-

Table 5. Number of Navy recruits tested and percent with reactions of 10 or more mm to 0.0001 mg PPD-S, for lifetime one-county residents of metropolitan areas, farms, and other non-metropolitan areas, by state (white, ages 17–21, tested 1958–64)

	NUMBER TESTED				PERCENT REACTORS*			
	Total	Metro-politan	Non-Metropolitan Farm	Non-Metropolitan Other	Total	Metro-politan	Non-Metropolitan Farm	Non-Metropolitan Other
TOTAL	257,476	151,637	27,312	78,527	3.8	4.2	2.8	3.6
Alabama	3,454	1,543	767	1,144	4.5	5.5	3.4	4.0
Arizona	1,115	716	31	368	8.2	8.5	(1)	7.9
Arkansas	2,387	442	886	1,059	4.9	4.3	5.0	5.2
California	14,706	12,291	460	1,955	3.7	3.7	3.7	3.8
Colorado	2,634	1,442	355	837	4.3	4.3	2.3	5.0
Connecticut	4,797	4,634	20	143	3.1	3.2	(1)	1.4
Delaware	701	468	52	181	3.3	3.4	(2)	2.8
Dist. of Columbia	166	166	-	-	8.4	8.4	-	-
Florida	2,846	1,525	294	1,027	4.1	3.1	3.7	5.7
Georgia	4,089	1,592	933	1,564	3.4	4.0	2.5	3.3
Idaho	1,069	-	315	754	2.0	-	2.2	1.9
Illinois	13,273	9,138	804	3,331	3.9	4.3	2.9	3.3
Indiana	7,119	3,335	794	2,990	3.7	3.5	2.1	4.4
Iowa	5,999	1,998	1,203	2,798	2.3	2.8	1.2	2.5
Kansas	3,838	1,143	722	1,973	2.4	3.1	1.8	2.2
Kentucky	3,526	1,290	906	1,330	8.1	8.5	8.5	7.4
Louisiana	4,334	1,821	803	1,710	5.1	5.9	4.5	4.5
Maine	2,278	596	215	1,467	3.3	3.5	0.9	3.6
Maryland	3,978	2,828	147	1,003	7.7	8.6	5.4	5.5
Massachusetts	10,494	10,189	18	287	3.0	3.1	(0)	1.7
Michigan	13,461	9,140	899	3,422	3.1	3.2	2.4	2.8
Minnesota	8,464	3,989	1,635	2,840	1.9	2.4	1.3	1.4
Mississippi	1,602	64	696	842	3.8	(3)	3.9	3.7
Missouri	7,120	3,850	1,178	2,092	3.8	4.2	3.0	3.4
Montana	1,329	262	264	803	2.3	2.7	0.8	2.6
Nebraska	2,950	996	688	1,266	2.2	2.9	1.6	1.9
Nevada	182	141	2	39	3.3	2.8	(0)	(2)
New Hampshire	1,487	648	86	753	2.4	3.5	(0)	1.6
New Jersey	8,811	6,989	92	1,730	3.8	4.1	(2)	2.9
New Mexico	1,126	253	160	713	5.9	4.7	4.4	6.6
New York	23,574	18,100	727	4,747	4.2	4.8	1.9	2.3
North Carolina	5,105	1,037	1,293	2,775	2.8	3.0	1.9	3.1
North Dakota	1,406	97	531	778	1.1	(4)	0.8	1.0
Ohio	17,125	11,457	957	4,711	3.7	3.9	1.8	3.4
Oklahoma	3,013	1,025	631	1,357	3.8	3.0	3.6	4.4
Oregon	2,693	1,324	361	1,008	2.9	3.3	1.9	2.8
Pennsylvania	24,534	16,691	887	6,956	4.5	4.7	1.6	4.4
Rhode Island	1,543	1,543	-	-	2.8	2.8	-	-
South Carolina	2,842	676	649	1,517	2.4	1.8	2.8	2.4
South Dakota	1,247	109	431	707	2.1	4.6	1.6	2.0
Tennessee	4,467	1,792	1,116	1,559	5.1	4.0	4.3	6.9
Texas	9,910	6,457	1,018	2,435	6.1	6.6	3.5	6.2
Utah	1,285	855	140	290	1.5	1.8	0.7	1.0
Vermont	1,090	-	156	934	3.6	-	2.6	3.7
Virginia	3,098	1,133	601	1,364	4.3	4.3	3.5	4.7
Washington	4,397	2,757	449	1,191	2.4	2.4	1.6	2.7
West Virginia	3,795	1,056	657	2,082	5.4	6.9	4.3	4.9
Wisconsin	6,399	2,039	1,154	3,206	2.0	2.6	1.6	1.8
Wyoming	618	-	129	489	3.4	-	5.4	2.9

* Where less than 100 tested, the number of reactors is given in parentheses.

late rather well with the rates in the other two. The significance of this correlation is probably not that the association among the three categories is so strong and the differences among them so small, but rather, that in the United States today the frequency of reactors in the metropolitan areas is so low. The conditions that are traditionally believed to increase the frequency and spread of tuberculosis—poverty, crowding, and more intimate contact with greater numbers of people, not only within but also outside the home—must obviously be more common in the large urban centers of the nation. Moreover, the foreign-born and first-generation Americans tend to congregate in such areas,

Figure 9. Correlation by state of the percent of Navy recruits with reactions of 10 or more mm to 0.0001 mg PPD-S, for: A. lifetime residents of metropolitan and non-metropolitan counties; B. non-metropolitan residents, according to lifetime farm and other residence (white, ages 17–21, tested 1958–64)

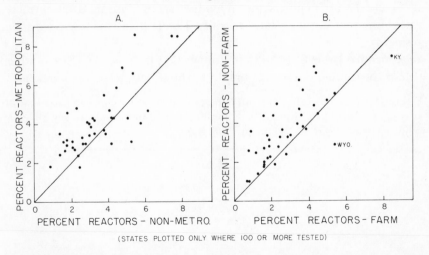

(STATES PLOTTED ONLY WHERE 100 OR MORE TESTED)

bringing with them high rates of tuberculosis. Yet, despite these conditions, the observed frequency of tuberculin reactors is low.

Several factors probably contribute to these low rates. One is the migration in recent years of so many young people, and their children, from rural areas (with even lower infection rates) into the large cities. Although the number of recruits who had spent their lifetimes on farms is small, just under 30,000, the 2.8 percent frequency of reactors would hardly have been credible a few decades ago. Another factor is the continuing migration of the population, again particularly the younger age groups, from the centers of the cities to the suburban fringes. Finally, the concentration in the cities of the antituberculosis efforts of the past has no doubt been a major factor in the decrease in tuberculous infection.

MOBILITY OF RESIDENCE

When tuberculosis control measures are being planned for a constantly migrating population such as lives in the United States today, it would seem pertinent to ask: "How much tuberculous infection is endemic to an area; how much is being brought in from the outside?" To attempt to answer this question, we separated recruits from each state into two groups: those who had spent all their lives in that state, and those who had at some time lived elsewhere. For the country as a whole, the frequency of tuberculin reactors among 372,289 one-state residents was 3.8 percent as compared with 4.6 percent for the 185,066 not-one-state group. Differences of about the same magnitude are seen in Figure 10 for many of the individual states. In only a few are the rates for the not-one-state recruits lower than for the one-state residents.

Appendix Table C.4 shows that migration from one state to another *within* the United States has only a slight effect on the rates (see also

Figure 10. Correlation by state of the percent of Navy recruits with reactions of 10 or more mm to 0.0001 mg PPD-S, for lifetime one-state residents, and all other residents (white, ages 17–21, tested 1958–64)

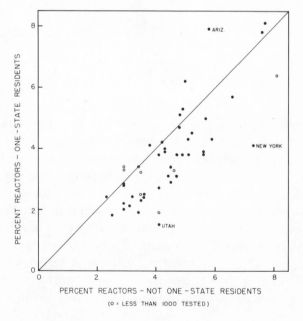

Appendix Table C.5). Men who had moved about in the United States but had never been out of the country had, on the average, almost the same rates as those who had lived continuously in a single state—4.0 percent as compared with 3.8 percent. It thus appears that almost all the differences between rates for lifetime and not-lifetime residents of a state are due to the very high frequency of reactors among those who had been born in, or had lived in, foreign countries.

New York state furnishes a striking example of the impact of foreign residence. The frequency of reactors for lifetime New York residents is 4.1 percent, as compared with 3.3 percent for those who at some time had lived outside the state but never outside the United States; for the remainder, those with some foreign residence but whose permanent address is now New York, the rate is 21.5 percent. The effect of combining the two groups of not-one-state New York residents, one with a rate of 3.3 percent and the other a rate of 21.5 percent, is an average of 7.3 percent. Although the number of recruits with a history of foreign residence is small, the very high frequency of reactors among them is sufficient to conspicuously affect the rate for the state as a whole (4.7 percent).

The frequency of reactors in Utah also is conspicuously higher for not-one-state (4.1 percent) than for one-state residents (1.5 percent). But here the difference is a function not of a high rate for the former, but rather of an exceptionally low rate for the latter—actually lower than for any other state.

This extremely low rate can illustrate how another factor, one that has nothing to do with the prevalence of tuberculous infection, can influence observed frequencies of tuberculin reactors, and how important it is, or soon will be, to take account of place of residence, and former residence, in studies of the statistics of tuberculin reactors. Compared with residents of other areas in the country, residents of the northwestern states are relatively free of tuberculin cross reactions.[6] The result is a lower observed frequency of tuberculin reactors. Rates for those who move to the northwest will tend to be inflated by cross reactions because of infections acquired in other areas, particularly the southeastern part of the country. We can see, for example, how migration of long-time residents of Georgia into Utah would tend to raise the overall frequency of reactors for Utah residents, whereas migration in the opposite direction, from Utah to Georgia, would reduce the overall reactor rate for Georgia residents.

At the present time, migration of the population within the United

States may not be responsible for very prominent problems in tuberculosis control work. As tuberculous infection and disease decrease, however, it would seem inevitable that place of residence and former residences will become crucial elements.

RACE

One of the items on the Navy field record card (Figure 1) relates to race. Each recruit is asked to check either a box marked "White," "Negro," or "Other-specify." Of the 587,000 recruits who were U.S. residents, about 26,000 checked "Negro," and 4,000, "Other." The lat-

Figure 11. Percent of Navy recruits with reactions of 10 or more mm to 0.0001 mg PPD-S, by region (U.S. Bureau of the Census), by race (ages 17–21, tested 1958–64)

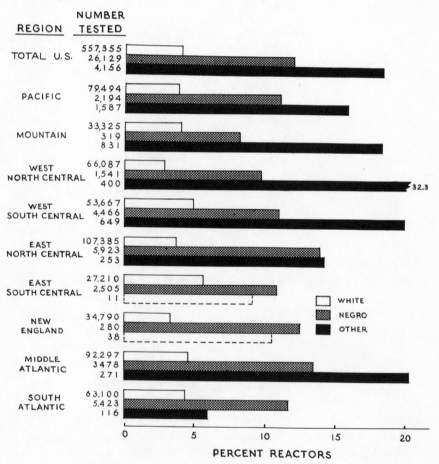

REGION	NUMBER TESTED
TOTAL U.S.	557,355 / 26,129 / 4,156
PACIFIC	79,494 / 2,194 / 1,587
MOUNTAIN	33,325 / 319 / 831
WEST NORTH CENTRAL	66,087 / 1,541 / 400
WEST SOUTH CENTRAL	53,667 / 4,466 / 649
EAST NORTH CENTRAL	107,385 / 5,923 / 253
EAST SOUTH CENTRAL	27,210 / 2,505 / 11
NEW ENGLAND	34,790 / 280 / 38
MIDDLE ATLANTIC	92,297 / 3,478 / 271
SOUTH ATLANTIC	63,100 / 5,423 / 116

ter group specified their race as Spanish, Malayan, Indian, Mexican, and so on, and although some of these terms refer to national origin rather than race, no attempt is made to correct or change them. The recruit's classification of himself is accepted.

The overall frequency of tuberculin reactors is much higher for Negro recruits (12 percent) and "Others" (18.4 percent) than for white recruits (4.1 percent). Similar racial differences prevail for all major subdivisions of the country (Fig. 11). Everywhere the frequency of re-actors is lowest for the whites, with the Negro rates generally inter-mediate between the other two. (See also Appendix Table C.5.)

For the Negroes, further details of geographic variations in rates are given in Figure 12. Rates are shown for individual states if 100 or more Negroes were tested but are based on combined figures for contiguous states with smaller numbers tested. The lowest frequencies of reactors —less than 9 percent—are found in the northwest and north-central areas. Throughout the rest of the country, the rates generally range from slightly more than 9 percent to just under 13 percent. A few states have higher rates, from 13 to 18 percent (Florida, New York, Connect-icut, Maryland, Delaware, and Illinois).

Figure 12. Percent of Negro Navy recruits with reactions of 10 or more mm to 0.0001 mg PPD-S (ages 17–21, tested 1958–64)

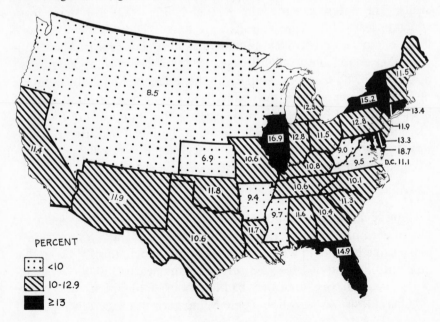

Figure 13. Correlation by state of the percent of Navy recruits with reactions of 10 or more mm to 0.0001 mg PPD-S, for whites and Negroes (ages 17–21, tested 1958–64)

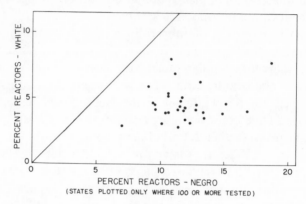

Rates are usually higher for Negro recruits who had moved into a state than for those who had lived in that state all their lives. However, for Illinois and Maryland, the states with the highest rates among the Negroes, the frequency is about the same for lifetime and non-lifetime residents. (See Appendix Table C.6.)

Comparison of Figures 12 and 2-B will show that, geographically, the frequencies of reactors are quite different for white and Negro recruits. The differences are summarized in Figure 13 for states from which at least 100 Negro recruits were tested. There is a conspicuous lack of association between the state rates for the two races. The conditions that contribute to high reactor rates for one race apparently do not apply, or do not apply equally, to the other. Although the numbers of Negroes are not large, the comparison has unusual validity because both whites and Negroes from all parts of the country were tested by the same staff, with the same products, at the same time. Errors of observation or unavoidable variations in technique should have been distributed uniformly over all groups.

CONTACT WITH TUBERCULOSIS

Beginning in August 1960, each recruit was asked to check on the record card his answer to the following question: "Have you ever lived in the same household with a person who had tuberculosis?" From that time until the end of 1964, 2.8 percent of the nearly 350,000 white recruits checked "yes," that they had had household contact with a case of tuberculosis. As shown in Table 6, the percent of recruits reporting

Table 6. Number of Navy recruits tested, percent with household contact with tuberculosis, and percent of recruits with reactions of 10 or more mm to 0.0001 mg PPD-S, for contacts and non-contacts by state (ages 17–21, tested 1960–64)

| | TOTAL TESTED | TB CONTACTS | | REACTORS AMONG | | | |
| | | | | TB Contacts | | Non-contacts | |
		Number	Percent	Number	Percent	Number	Percent
			WHITE, AGES 17 TO 21 YEARS, LIFETIME U.S. RESIDENTS				
TOTAL	352,876	9,820	2.8	2,253	22.9	10,521	3.1
Alabama	4,451	137	3.1	40	29.2	156	3.6
Arizona	4,052	197	4.9	66	33.5	182	4.7
Arkansas	3,735	139	3.7	34	24.5	129	3.6
California	34,692	1,209	3.5	242	20.0	1,051	3.1
Colorado	5,652	175	3.1	35	20.0	166	3.0
Connecticut	4,984	134	2.7	37	27.6	100	2.1
Delaware	866	25	2.9	6	24.0	18	2.1
Dist. of Columbia	652	22	3.4	7	31.8	32	5.1
Florida	8,992	202	2.2	45	22.3	268	3.0
Georgia	6,384	157	2.5	33	21.0	205	3.3
Idaho	2,140	62	2.9	10	16.1	27	1.3
Illinois	15,313	431	2.8	96	22.3	450	3.0
Indiana	8,936	271	3.0	52	19.2	280	3.2
Iowa	7,734	166	2.1	35	21.1	152	2.0
Kansas	6,496	166	2.6	26	15.7	136	2.1
Kentucky	4,231	197	4.7	64	32.5	257	6.4
Louisiana	5,821	143	2.5	26	18.2	248	4.4
Maine	2,489	75	3.0	22	29.3	46	1.9
Maryland	4,757	130	2.7	41	31.5	320	6.9
Massachusetts	10,158	248	2.4	69	27.8	227	2.3
Michigan	15,619	416	2.7	81	19.5	342	2.2
Minnesota	10,890	274	2.5	43	15.7	152	1.4
Mississippi	2,302	59	2.6	12	20.3	81	3.6
Missouri	9,883	342	3.5	72	21.1	295	3.1
Montana	2,365	64	2.7	3	4.7	49	2.1
Nebraska	4,194	83	2.0	17	20.5	78	1.9
Nevada	956	33	3.5	5	15.2	25	2.7
New Hampshire	1,842	44	2.4	9	20.5	24	1.3
New Jersey	11,427	241	2.1	68	28.2	356	3.2
New Mexico	2,701	90	3.3	20	22.2	107	4.1
New York	25,190	550	2.2	158	28.7	778	3.2
North Carolina	6,072	151	2.5	36	23.8	135	2.3
North Dakota	1,813	46	2.5	9	19.6	31	1.8
Ohio	20,383	565	2.8	124	21.9	615	3.1
Oklahoma	5,368	166	3.1	35	21.1	168	3.2
Oregon	6,387	272	4.3	50	18.4	116	1.9
Pennsylvania	23,225	460	2.0	148	32.2	817	3.6
Rhode Island	1,689	52	3.1	15	28.8	36	2.2
South Carolina	3,492	58	1.7	14	24.1	85	2.5
South Dakota	2,043	38	1.9	4	10.5	34	1.7
Tennessee	5,728	236	4.1	62	26.3	248	4.5
Texas	19,013	538	2.8	126	23.4	820	4.4
Utah	1,858	25	1.3	5	20.0	35	1.9
Vermont	1,196	23	1.9	4	17.4	29	2.5
Virginia	4,372	127	2.9	34	26.8	148	3.5
Washington	8,028	280	3.5	48	17.1	165	2.1
West Virginia	3,776	104	2.8	35	33.7	154	4.2
Wisconsin	7,225	167	2.3	24	14.4	116	1.6
Wyoming	1,304	30	2.3	6	20.0	32	2.5
			NEGRO, AGES 17 TO 21 YEARS, LIFETIME U.S. RESIDENTS				
TOTAL	17,384	537	3.1	191	35.6	1,747	10.4

contact varied by state from less than 2 percent to nearly 5 percent. In general, the percentage increased with the prevalence of tuberculosis in the state, as measured by the new-case rate (Fig. 14).*

Despite what must be regarded as a crude, and probably not very accurate way of obtaining information on exposure to tuberculosis, the answers to the contact question separate the men into two groups with sharply contrasting frequencies of tuberculin reactors. Among the 340,000 recruits who checked "No or Don't Know," only 3.1 percent reacted to tuberculin; among the nearly 10,000 who checked that they had had contact, the rate was seven times greater, 22.9 percent. (See also Appendix Table C. 7.)

Among the relatively large numbers of noncontacts from each state, the frequency of reactors ranges from less than 2 percent to almost 7 percent. As shown in Figure 15.A, the reactor rates for these groups correlate rather closely with the new tuberculosis case rates by state, although the findings for Maryland and Kentucky deviate conspicuously from the trend established by the other states.

Figure 14. Correlation by state of the percent of Navy recruits with history of contact with tuberculosis, and new tuberculosis case rates (white recruits, ages 17–21, tested 1960–64; new case rates—white population, 1959–61)

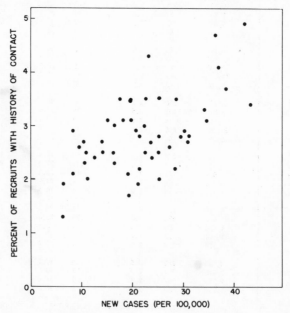

* New tuberculosis case rates were obtained through the courtesy of Mr. Anthony Lowell.

The frequency of reactors among the contacts also varies considerably by state, ranging from about 15 percent to more than 30 percent (Figure 15.B). Because the number of contacts in many states is rather small, these rates cannot be regarded with the same confidence as those for the noncontacts. However, there again appears to be some association between frequency of reactors and new-case rates. (Note that the reactor scale for contacts is five times smaller than that for noncontacts.) Because, in addition to the risk of becoming infected by someone in his own household, a contact is also exposed to the community risk, some correlation might be expected. The association remains, however, even when the rates for noncontacts are subtracted from those for contacts and the resultant rates correlated with the new-case rates.

Many factors no doubt influence the frequency of reactors among contacts: the accuracy of diagnosis of the disease in the "index" case;

Figure 15. Correlations by state of the percent of Navy recruits with reactions of 10 or more mm to 0.0001 mg PPD-S, with new tuberculosis case rates for: A. recruits with no history of contact with tuberculosis; B. recruits with history of contact with tuberculosis (white recruits, ages 17–21, tested 1960–64; new case rates—white population, 1959–61)

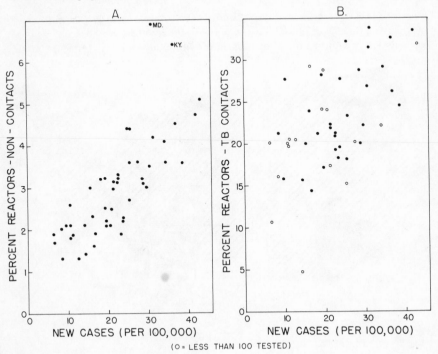

how early the disease was discovered and how adequately treated; the relationship of the recruit to the person having tuberculosis; the age of the recruit when contact occurred, and so on. It is not unreasonable to believe, also, that the conditions thought to foster a high tuberculosis morbidity rate in a community (poverty, crowding, and so on) would facilitate the spread of infection within the household.

The affirmative responses to the contact question identify among the white recruits a group which is very small (2.8 percent) but which none-theless accounts for a sizable proportion (18 percent) of all tuberculin reactors. The map in Figure 16 shows the varying percentage of all re-actors found in the contacts—from 10 to 30 percent. The states with the highest percentages are scattered throughout the country; those with the lowest are concentrated in the south-central and southeastern areas. These lower rates no doubt reflect inclusion of an unusually high proportion of cross reactions in the reactor group.

Too few Negroes (about 17,000) have been tested since the contact question was introduced to show details by state, so results for all Negro recruits are given in Table 6. Certain summary statistics for white and Negro recruits are also given in Table 7. New tuberculosis case rates

Figure 16. Navy recruits with reactions of 10 or more mm to 0.0001 mg PPD-S, who have a history of household contact with tuberculosis, as a percentage of all recruits with reactions of 10 or more mm (white, ages 17–21, tested 1960–64)

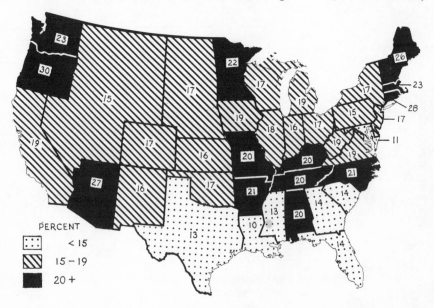

are not available for the Negro population for 1959–1961, but the rate for the nonwhite population, composed chiefly of Negroes, is a little more than three times as high as that for the white population. The frequency of reactors among all recruits, and among recruits with no history of household contact, is also a little more than three times higher for Negroes than for whites.

Among recruits who have a history of contact with tuberculosis, the frequency of reactors is half again as high for Negroes as for whites, 35.6 percent as compared with 22.9 percent. As has been shown for the white contacts, the frequency of reactors tends to increase with the new-case rate. Actually, the overall rate for Negroes is only a little higher than the rates for white contacts from states with the highest new case rates for tuberculosis.

Table 7. Summary statistics on history of household contact with tuberculosis, and frequency of tuberculin reactions of 10 or more mm to 0.0001 mg PPD-S, for white and Negro recruits and for white student nurses (recruits, ages 17–21, tested 1960–64) (student nurses, ages 17–24, tested 1943–49)

	Navy Recruits 1960–64		Student Nurses 1943–49
	White	Negro	White
Percent with household contact	2.8	3.1	2.8
Percent reactors among:			
Total of group tested	3.6	11.1	10.9
No history of household contact	3.1	10.4	10.1
History of household contact	22.9	35.6	37.0
Percent of all reactors in the group that report contact	17.6	9.9	9.4
New tuberculosis case rate (U.S. Population, 1959–61)	24/100,000	82/100,000*	

* Nonwhite rate

Because tuberculosis is much more prevalent among Negroes than whites, it might be expected that the percentage of Negro recruits reporting contact with the disease might also be much higher. This, however, is not the case. The percentage of recruits reporting household contact is almost the same in the two races: 2.8 percent for the white recruits, and 3.1 percent for the Negro. The high frequency of reactors among all Negroes, combined with the low percentage of Negroes giving a history of contact, even though more than a third of them are tuberculin reactors, results in a low proportion of all Negro reactors being found among the contacts. Instead of 18 percent as for the white, less than 10 percent of all Negro reactors are found among recruits reporting contact.

Between 1943 and 1949, a study of tuberculosis among young women entering nurses' training was carried out by the U.S. Public Health Service, the National Tuberculosis Association, and 76 schools in ten metropolitan areas spread over the country from Philadelphia to San Francisco and from Minneapolis to New Orleans.[7] The study provided a nationwide, fairly representative poopulation of about 22,000 white women, 17 to 24 years of age during the middle 1940's. All student nurses were tuberculin tested by a single Public Health Service team which went from school to school. The same tuberculin (PPD-S), in the same dose (0.0001 mg), and a generally similar working plan were used as in the Navy Program. On entry to training, each student was asked to fill out a detailed questionnaire regarding previous contact with someone who had tuberculosis. Results from this study are included in Table 7. New tuberculosis case rates were not generally available before 1953, but from the national statistics on tuberculosis morbidity and mortality it seems likely that the prevalence of tuberculosis in the white population about 1945 may not have been very different from that for the Negro population in 1959–1961. The percentage of the nurses with a history of household contact, and the frequency of reactors among the total group of student nurses, contacts and noncontacts, is surprisingly similar for these young white women of twenty years ago and the Negro recruits tested in 1960–1964.

The contrast between the findings among student nurses and Negro recruits on the one hand, and white recruits on the other, might suggest that as the prevalence of tuberculosis falls, the infected in the population become increasingly concentrated in the immediate environment of persons with tuberculous disease. However, a correlation of the percent of all reactors found among recruits reporting contact and the new tuberculosis case rates by state fails to show the negative relationship that might be expected.

For a long time, the tuberculin test has been used to find active cases of tuberculosis among reactors or their contacts. However, as emphasis changes from finding the cases of "today" to preventing the cases of "tomorrow," tuberculin testing of young people may become the most effective way to find household groups in whom tuberculous infection is concentrated and to whom chemoprophylaxis may be offered.

FOREIGN RESIDENCE

Two categories of recruits reported residence outside the United States.* More than 17,000 listed a *permanent home address within the United States* but indicated that they had lived outside the country for periods of six months or more. Approximately 11,000 recruits gave a *permanent home address outside the United States.* Figure 17 shows the frequency of reactors for the first group, those whose home was in the United States, according to whether they had been born outside the country or had been born in the United States and subsequently lived abroad. Rates are shown separately for whites and nonwhites. For comparison, rates for lifetime residents of the United States are also shown. For both whites and nonwhites, the frequency of tuberculin re-actors among foreign-born is very much higher than among lifetime U.S. residents. Among whites born in the United States who later lived in a foreign area, the rate is only a little higher than for the lifetime U.S. group. Among nonwhite recruits, the rate for the U.S.-born with some foreign residence, is intermediate between the other two groups.

As shown in Figure 18, the frequencies of reactors for recruits born in the Pacific Islands or North America (Canada and Alaska) are not very different than those for men who were born in the United States and later lived in these areas. For recruits born in Europe, South America, and the remaining areas listed, the rates are very high (24 to 31 percent); rates for the U.S.-born who lived in these areas are much lower (all below 7.4 percent).

Among the foreign-born recruits, the high frequency of reactors is not unexpected. Tuberculosis is much more prevalent in most other areas of the world than in the United States, and birth and early resi-dence in a high-rate area are not the end of higher risk of exposure to the disease. For many foreign-born recruits, part of the risk must have immigrated with them in infected family members. Moreover, national groups tend to form closely knit colonies in the new world, sharing their cultural heritages and their tubercle bacilli.

Finally, it must be emphasized that BCG vaccination against tuber-culosis has been carried out extensively in many of the countries in

* In this section, as in the others, "The United States" refers to the conterminous United States. Foreign residence means residence in any area outside the conterminous United States.

Figure 17. Percent of Navy recruits, U.S. residents, with reactions of 10 or more mm to 0.0001 mg PPD-S, by color, place of birth, and residence (ages 17–21, tested 1958–64)

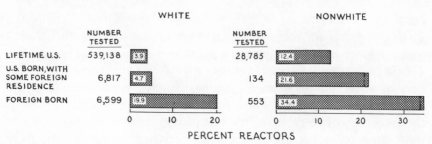

which these recruits were born and some of them must have been vaccinated. Because no way has been found to distinguish tuberculin sensitivity produced by BCG from that produced by virulent tubercle bacilli, or by both, it is impossible to determine how much of the high frequency of reactors is the result of naturally acquired tuberculous infection.

The comparatively low rate in U.S.-born recruits who have lived outside the United States is somewhat unexpected. In part it may be related to the inclination of persons (including Americans) living in

Figure 18. Percent of Navy recruits, U.S. residents, with reactions of 10 or more mm to 0.0001 mg PPD-S, for foreign-born, and for U.S.-born with some foreign residence, by place of foreign residence (white, ages 17–21, tested 1958–64)

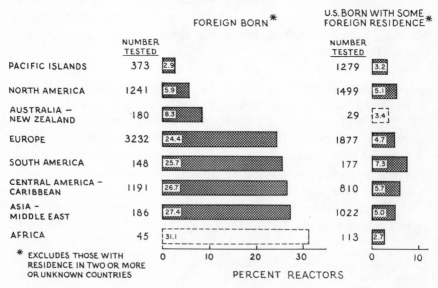

countries other than their own to associate principally with groups of the same national origin. Moreover, the greater the known risk of becoming infected with tuberculosis, the greater the effort these persons probably make to protect themselves and their children from infectious environments. U.S. citizens going abroad are not advised to be vaccinated with BCG even though it may be popular in the countries where they expect to live. The absence of BCG-induced reactions may thus also account in part for the low frequency of reactors among U.S.-born recruits who have lived outside the country.

The effect of BCG can also be seen among the nearly 11,000 recruits who reported a *permanent home address outside the United States*. As seen in Table 8, the average frequency of reactors for these recruits is

Table 8. Number tested and percent of Navy recruits, not conterminous U.S. residents, with reactions of 10 or more mm to 0.0001 mg PPD-S, by age, color, and place of residence.

Place of Residence*	Total All Ages All Races	17 – 21 Years			22+ Years All Races
		Total	White	Nonwhite	
	NUMBER TESTED				
Not Conterminous U.S.	10,888	7,084	2,270	4,814	3,804
Alaska	825	784	719	65	41
Hawaii	1,301	1,247	537	710	54
Philippine Islands	7,344	3,884	23	3,861	3,460
Other	1,418	1,069	991	178	249
	PERCENT REACTORS**				
Not Conterminous U.S.	54.0	44.9	12.6	60.1	70.9
Alaska	20.8	19.6	14.5	(50)	(18)
Hawaii	8.4	8.0	5.6	9.9	(9)
Philippine Islands	72.3	70.2	(10)	70.4	74.7
Other	20.0	18.6	14.4	31.5	34.1

* Based on home address at time of entry into the Navy.
** Where less than 100 tested, the number of reactors is given in parentheses.

more than 50 percent (see also Appendix Table C. 1). Rates are particularly high for the more than 7,000 Filipinos; over 72 percent had reactions at least 10 mm in diameter. Since 1951, BCG has been widely used in the Philippines as a tuberculosis control measure. By the end of 1964, seven million persons, almost all in the younger age groups, had been vaccinated.[8] An attempt was made in the Navy program to determine which recruits had been BCG-vaccinated, but the task proved to be so difficult and results so dubious that the effort had to be abandoned. Our experience is no different from that of many other investigators around the world. Wherever BCG vaccination has been used, it is virtually impossible later, by means of the tuberculin test, to appraise accurately the amount of tuberculous infection in the population or to identify the infected individuals.

To supplement the material from the Navy recruit program, the Tuberculosis Program of the U.S. Public Health Service has conducted extensive skin-testing surveys in schools, universities, and general population groups in various parts of the country. Results are available for 58,000 school children in six states (Georgia, Maryland, Massachusetts, Minnesota, North Carolina, and North Dakota), nearly 15,000 college students in six states (Alabama, Georgia, Kentucky, North Dakota, Wisconsin, and Utah), and four community-wide or adult-age surveys. (See Appendix Table C. 8.) One purpose of the studies was to obtain information on the frequency of tuberculin reactors among females and in groups younger and older than the recruits. Another was to provide material for evaluating the representativeness of the results observed among the recruits and to determine how well such results correspond with those collected in a different way, by on-the-spot testing of young people of comparable ages in different parts of the United States.

SURVEYS IN SCHOOLCHILDREN AND COLLEGE STUDENTS
The results of testing 48,000 white children, ranging from preschool youngsters to high school seniors, are given in Figures 19 and 20. On entry to school, less than 0.5 percent of the children are tuberculin reactors. With increasing age there is an increase in the frequency of reactors. The *differences* among rates in the various groups also increase. The highest rates are seen in children living in the southeastern states, where tuberculin cross reactions undoubtedly inflate the rates. The frequency of reactors varies little by sex, although after ten years of age, the boys tend to have slightly higher rates than the girls.

One of the significant findings from these surveys is not that differences exist among groups but rather how low, and how consistently low, the frequency of tuberculin reactors has been during the past decade among white children from widely separated areas of the country. An estimate of the frequency of reactors for children of elementary school age, roughly an average for 6 to 14 year olds, is only a little more than 1 percent; for high school students, an average for 14 to 18 year olds, it is about 2.5 percent. It must be realized that these estimates are based on material that is now 4 to 10 years old and that more recent rates are no doubt even lower.

Results of testing 14,000 white college students, principally freshmen, with an average age of about 19 years, are also shown in Figures 19 and 20. Because the number of foreign students (generally with high tuberculin reactor rates) varies so widely among the participating universities, it seemed best to base the rates only on students who had always lived in the United States. To do otherwise would be to give undue weight to an artificial variable—the frequency and country of origin of the foreign students. Some variation is seen in the frequency of reactors for students from the different institutions (from 2 to 5 percent), and again we observe the effects of cross reactions in students from the southeast. For the students included in this testing program, the rates are considerably lower for college women than for college men. However, again the striking findings are that the frequency of tuberculin reactors is low among young adults and that the differences among groups from different parts of the country are small.

The number of Negroes included in the community programs is small: only 10,000 Negro children living in Georgia, North Carolina, and Maryland (Fig. 19). The frequency of tuberculin reactors is much higher among these children on entry to school than among the whites, on the average, almost four times as high; and the increase in frequency with age is much more precipitous. For the small number of Negro college students (limited to Georgia colleges), the frequency of reactors is much higher than among the whites. Except for the young children, the frequency of reactors is appreciably higher in males than females.

As a point of reference, summary rates for 17 to 21 year old recruits are plotted on both Figures 19 and 20. The rates for white recruits are somewhat higher than for all college students but almost identical with the rate for white college men. This finding adds to our confidence that the Navy recruits must represent fairly well their age group in the population with respect to the frequency of tuberculin reactors. Whatever factors may influence young men's decisions to join the Navy or enter college, for the country as a whole they do not conspicuously affect the frequency of tuberculin reactors. The tuberculin reactor rate among white recruits, moreover, fits reasonably well with the age curves of the frequency of reactors among other groups we have tested in the community surveys.

COMMUNITY-WIDE SURVEYS

Figure 21 summarizes results for three community-wide surveys: Pamlico County, North Carolina;[1] the Crookston and Fosston areas of

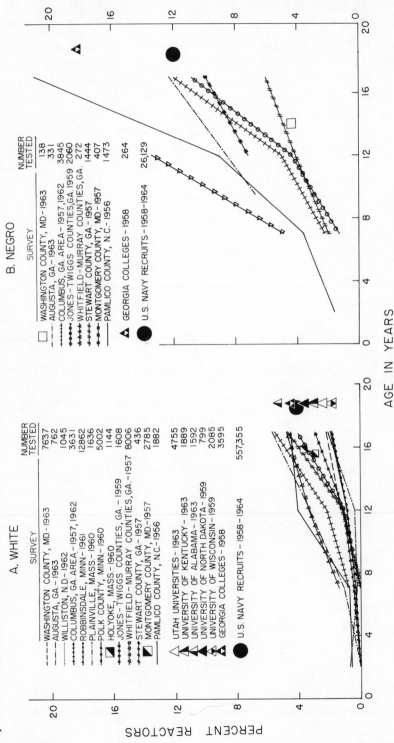

Figure 19. Percent of school children and college students with reactions of 10 or more mm to 0.0001 mg PPD-S, in specified places throughout the United States, by race and age (tested 1956–64)

A. WHITE

SURVEY	NUMBER TESTED
WASHINGTON COUNTY, MD.-1963	7637
AUGUSTA, GA.-1963	762
WILLISTON, N.D.-1962	1045
COLUMBUS, GA. AREA-1957,1962	3631
ROBBINSDALE, MINN.-1961	12862
PLAINVILLE, MASS.-1960	1636
POLK COUNTY, MINN.-1960	5002
HOLYOKE, MASS.-1960	1144
JONES-TWIGGS COUNTIES, GA.-1959	1608
WHITFIELD-MURRAY COUNTIES, GA.-1957	8006
STEWART COUNTY, GA.-1957	436
MONTGOMERY COUNTY, MD.-1957	2785
PAMLICO COUNTY, N.C.-1956	1882
UTAH UNIVERSITIES-1963	4755
UNIVERSITY OF KENTUCKY-1963	1889
UNIVERSITY OF ALABAMA-1963	1592
UNIVERSITY OF NORTH DAKOTA-1959	799
UNIVERSITY OF WISCONSIN-1959	2085
GEORGIA COLLEGES-1958	3595
U.S. NAVY RECRUITS-1958-1964	557,355

B. NEGRO

SURVEY	NUMBER TESTED
WASHINGTON COUNTY, MD.-1963	138
AUGUSTA, GA.-1963	331
COLUMBUS, GA. AREA-1957,1962	3845
JONES-TWIGGS COUNTIES, GA.-1959	2060
WHITFIELD-MURRAY COUNTIES, GA.-1957	272
STEWART COUNTY, GA.-1957	1444
MONTGOMERY COUNTY, MD.-1957	407
PAMLICO COUNTY, N.C.-1956	1473
GEORGIA COLLEGES-1958	264
U.S. NAVY RECRUITS-1958-1964	26,129

PERCENT REACTORS

AGE IN YEARS

Polk County, Minnesota; and Plainville, Massachusetts. Another survey was conducted among the employees of an industrial plant in Austin, Minnesota. Results are given only for whites, because, except in Pamlico, there were very few nonwhites in the surveyed populations. The similarity of the rates among the children of these communities is in sharp contrast with the divergence of rates among the adults. Among the children, reactor rates are everywhere low, though lowest in Plainville and highest in Pamlico. (As noted earlier, rates in the southeast, to some extent, reflect the high prevalence of cross reactions.) Among the adults, the curves fan out after age 25; the Plainville curve rises rapidly, the curve for the Pamlico residents only slowly, and the Minnesota curves are intermediate between the other two.

It is not unlikely that the curves shown in Figure 21 represent a framework into which age curves of reactors for many of the white communities of the country would fit. Available evidence indicates that low rates of tuberculin reactors may be expected among the white children and very young adults of most areas today. The rates among the older adults may be expected to vary much more widely, reflecting the

Figure 20. Percent of school children with reactions of 10 or more mm to 0.0001 mg PPD-S, by age and sex, and for comparison, percent reactors among college students and Navy recruits (white children and college students, tested 1956–63; white recruits, tested 1958–64)

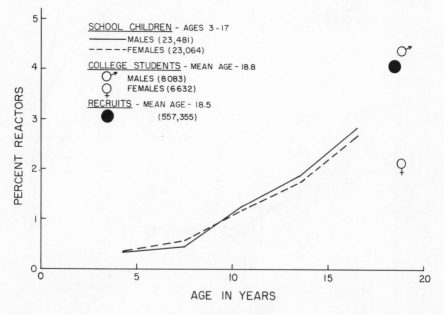

tuberculous infections accumulated through lifetimes extending back into the latter part of the nineteenth century. A major factor influencing the differences between the younger and older segments of the population is the precipitous fall in the incidence of tuberculous disease during the past 25 to 30 years. Another factor is the dramatic decrease in the frequncy of bovine tuberculosis, which was highly prevalent in some parts of the United States up to the early 1920's. In this country, as has been shown recently to be the case in Denmark,[2] tuberculosis of cattle no doubt increased enormously the frequency of tuberculin reactors in certain areas among the individuals who now constitute the older age groups of the populations.

Figure 21. Percent of community residents with reactions of 10 or more mm to 0.0001 mg PPD-S, by age (white, tested 1956–60)

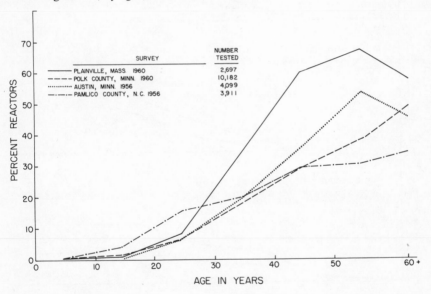

Finally, this century has witnessed a tremendous movement of people into and within the United States. Streams of immigrants have entered the United States, most of them coming from countries where tuberculosis was and is much more prevalent than in this country. Moreover, the immigrants from many of these countries tended to concentrate in certain areas. Within the United States there have been major population shifts from the more densely populated east toward the west, from farms to cities, from city centers to suburbs. Thus, the

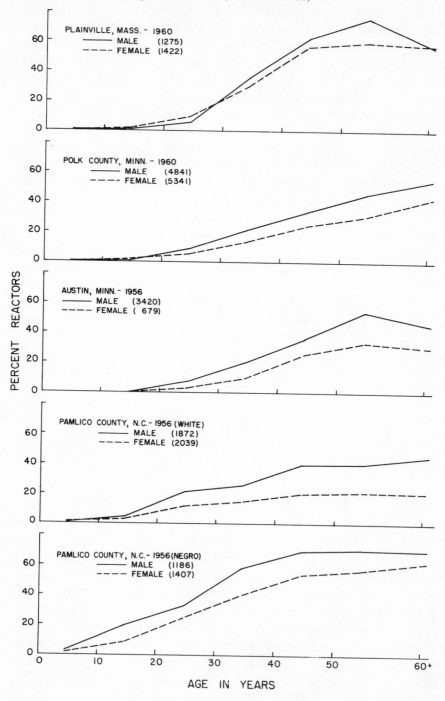

Figure 22. Percent of community residents with reactions of 10 or more mm to 0.0001 mg PPD-S, by age, sex and race (tested 1956–60)

reactor rate in each community will necessarily depend not only on the past experience with tuberculosis in that community but also on where the people who make up its population came from. Of interest is the parallel between reactor rates for the older residents of the communities shown in Figure 21 and the frequency of foreign born in the counties in which these communities are included. Plainville is a small town in the highly urbanized area between Boston and Providence. According to the 1960 Census,[3] 10 percent of the residents of Norfolk County, Massachusetts (which includes Plainville), are foreign born, in contrast to only 0.2 percent of the residents of Pamlico County, North Carolina, with intermediate rates for Polk and Mower Counties in Minnesota. The reactor rates for the adults of these communities parallel also the degree of urbanization of the counties—Norfolk County is 86 percent urban, Mower County, 58 percent, Polk County, 43 percent, and Pamlico County is entirely rural. However, one of the critical points illustrated in Figure 21 is that wide differences in tuberculin reactor rates among the adults are not necessarily reflected in the reactor rates of the young children. The rates among children and even young adults reflect only the recent past. Rates may be low because tuberculous disease has been infrequent in the community during the lifetime of the children or because effective tuberculosis control procedures achieved early diagnosis of infectious cases and stopped the spread of infection by isolation—in the past by hospitalization and recently by the use of highly effective drugs.

For all groups of adults, the frequency of tuberculin reactors is higher for males than females (Fig. 22). The difference is generally very small up to young adult life but tends to increase progressively in the older age groups. The differences are least in Plainville, where reactor rates are highest, and greatest in Pamlico, where they are lowest. Tuberculosis morbidity and mortality are higher among males than females, and a contributing factor no doubt is that more males than females are infected. However, the sex differences in the frequency of reactors are not sufficient to account for the differences in morbidity and mortality.

The significance of former residence can be illustrated by the material from Polk County, Minnesota, where a residence history was obtained from each participant. The frequencies of reactors are lowest among persons who had spent their entire lives in Minnesota (Fig. 23). Rates are somewhat higher for those who had lived at some time outside the state but never outside the United States. Still higher rates appear among men who reported overseas military service in the First or Second World Wars or in the Korean War. Although based on small numbers, the highest rates are found among persons born outside the United States.

Tuberculosis control programs carried on for many years in this country no doubt deserve much of the credit for the very low tuberculin reactor rates among the children and for the very low tuberculosis death and new-case rates in the general population. However, as long as there are persons in the population who have had a tuberculous in-

Figure 23. Percent of Polk County, Minnesota residents with reactions of 10 or more mm to 0.0001 mg PPD-S, by age, residence, and sex (tested 1960)

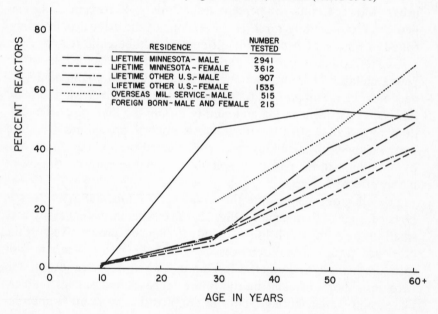

fection, even though it may have occurred many years ago, new cases of the disease will continue to occur.[4] The wide divergence of reactor rates among the adults in different communities and in different subgroups within the same community suggests that the time is approaching when tuberculin testing of the older age group should become a feasible way of identifying older individuals at risk of developing manifest disease. The very low rate at which new infection occurs among the uninfected today means that once tuberculin testing is done, the identity of most of the infected is established for a long time to come, provided careful records are kept. Procedures to prevent the appearance of endogenous disease (chemoprophylaxis) can then be undertaken as facilities permit.[5]

Since 1956, the Tuberculosis Program of the U.S. Public Health Service has conducted tuberculin skin-testing surveys involving more than a half million Navy recruits and nearly 75,000 schoolchildren, college students, and adults in various communities throughout the United States. The results of these tests have been summarized here in terms of percent "reactors" in order to obtain a nationwide picture of tuberculous infection.

The most striking finding has been the low rate of tuberculin reactors found among almost all the young people tested during the past ten years. At an average age of about 19 years, only 4 percent of the white recruits tested during 1958–1964 reacted to tuberculin with an induration 10 or more mm in diameter. About the same frequency of reactors was found among young white men of the same age tested in colleges and other community groups. Slightly lower rates were found among college women, and still lower rates among children. Approximately 1 percent of the white children of elementary school age and 2.5 percent of the high school students were reactors.

These rates represent the results of testing done an average of 5 years ago and are higher than might be expected today. The frequency of reactors among successive cohorts of the Navy recruits has been steadily decreasing at a rate of about a quarter of 1 percent per year. The best estimate that can be made of the prevalence of tuberculous infection today among the white recruits is close to 3 percent. This rate reflects all the tuberculous infections that have accumulated during the lifetimes of these young men. Because the incidence of tuberculosis has declined steadily during this period, the rate of new infections with tubercle bacilli may now be substantially less than one per thousand per year.

The results from the Navy Recruit Program have been summarized in Figure 24 to show variations in the frequency of reactors by place of residence (for white recruits only) and by certain other characteristics of the recruits. The frequency of tuberculin reactors shows some relation to place of residence in a geographic sense. In the upper left hand section of the figure, states have been grouped into quartiles according to frequency of reactors. The average rate for the states with the lowest frequencies is 2.5 percent (the lowest rate state is Idaho, at 2.1 percent), and the average rate for the states (and the District of Columbia) with

Figure 24. Percent of Navy recruits with reactions of 10 or more mm to 0.0001 mg PPD-S by place of residence (for white recruits only), and by color, place of birth, and contact with tuberculosis (for all recruits) (ages 17–21, tested 1958–64)

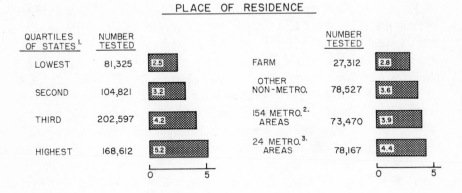

PLACE OF RESIDENCE

QUARTILES OF STATES[1.]	NUMBER TESTED			NUMBER TESTED	
LOWEST	81,325	2.5	FARM	27,312	2.8
SECOND	104,821	3.2	OTHER NON-METRO.	78,527	3.6
THIRD	202,597	4.2	154 METRO.[2.] AREAS	73,470	3.9
HIGHEST	168,612	5.2	24 METRO.[3.] AREAS	78,167	4.4

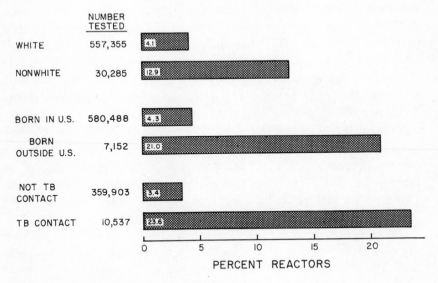

OTHER CHARACTERISTICS

	NUMBER TESTED	
WHITE	557,355	4.1
NONWHITE	30,285	12.9
BORN IN U.S.	580,488	4.3
BORN OUTSIDE U.S.	7,152	21.0
NOT TB CONTACT	359,903	3.4
TB CONTACT	10,537	23.6

PERCENT REACTORS

1. QUARTILE POSITION DETERMINED BY FREQUENCY OF REACTORS
2. EACH WITH LESS THAN ONE MILLION POPULATION.
3. EACH WITH MORE THAN ONE MILLION POPULATION.

the highest frequencies is 5.2 percent (the highest rate state is Kentucky, at 8.0 percent). The frequency of reactors is also associated with the degree of urbanization; 2.8 percent of farm residents react to tuberculin, in contrast to 4.4 percent of the residents of very large metropolitan areas.

These differences in frequency of reactors according to where the recruits lived are dwarfed by the tremendous differences found according to certain other characteristics of the individual, as shown in the lower section of the figure. The frequency of tuberculin reactors is three times as high for nonwhite as for white recruits. Foreign-born recruits have rates five times higher than those for recruits born within the conterminous United States. Recruits with a history of household contact with a case of tuberculosis have rates nearly seven times higher than those for recruits who reported no such contact.

All these high-rate subgroups account for only a small percentage of the recruit population, but they contribute a large percentage of all reactors. The nonwhite recruits, for example, represent only 5 percent of the recruit population, but contribute 15 percent of the tuberculin reactors. Only 1 percent of the recruits were born outside the conterminous United States, but they account for 6 percent of the reactors. Approximately 3 percent of the recruits reported household contact with a case of tuberculosis, but this small group includes 18 percent of all the tuberculin reactors.

The recruit population may thus be separated into two groups with respect to the concentration of tuberculous infection: a low-rate group, composed of native-born white recruits without history of contact with tuberculosis; and a high-rate group, composed of all nonwhites, tuberculosis contacts, and recruits born abroad. The low-rate group with a tuberculin reactor rate of 3.3 percent would include 91 percent of all of the recruits and 67 percent of the tuberculin reactors. The high-rate group with a rate of 16.7 percent would include only 9 percent of the recruit population but 33 percent of the reactors.

There is little reason to think that results among the Navy recruits are very different from those for their age group in the general population. Thus, the search for the infected among the younger age groups would be expected to be most profitable if concentrated on nonwhites, on contacts, and on foreign born.

In several community-wide surveys, uniformly low frequencies of reactors were found among the children, but wide differences in rates were found among the adults. Moreover, there were large differences in rates among adults in the same community, according to mobility of residence. As in the recruits, the highest rates were found among the foreign born. The rates for adult males were consistently higher than for adult females.

Although these surveys show that older people can no longer be regarded as universally infected with tuberculosis (less than half of those 40 years and older were tuberculin reactors), they illustrate the concentration of the reactors in the older age group. Rough estimates based on these studies suggest that less than 4 percent of the infected are under 20 years of age and nearly 75 percent are 40 years and older. If tuberculosis is to be eradicated, it is not sufficient to concentrate on finding the cases of "today." Methods must be developed, and chemoprophylaxis seems a promising approach, to prevent the infections of the past from developing into "tomorrow's" cases. Skin-testing surveys, especially among older age groups, will serve to define the size and characteristics of the infected pool and to identify the individuals to be treated.

Appendix A / Cleaning and Sterilization of Supplies Used for Tuberculin Testing

A. For all glassware which is used in the preparation or administration of skin test dilutions of tuberculin (that is, pipettes, flasks, beakers, syringes, and vials):

(1) Wash glassware in warm water to remove debris (remove all metal parts, syringe clips and adapters) and soak in detergent solution for 30 minutes to 1 hour. (Solution is 1 tablespoon of strong alkaline detergent or tri sodium phosphate per gallon of warm water.)

(2) Remove glassware and rinse under running tap water to remove detergent.

(3) Place in sulphuric acid–dichromate acid cleaning solution for a minimum of 12 hours.

(4) Remove from acid (use rubber gloves and stainless steel tongs) and rinse under tap water until all visible traces of acid are removed. (Protective goggles and rubber apron are recommended in case of splashing.)

(5) Flush with tapwater for four hours in suitable container (pipette container or container in which water is introduced at the bottom and flows up, around, and through). This is to remove any dichromate which may be adsorbed on the ground surfaces of the syringes. (Dichromate is very toxic to BCG, and in case the tuberculin syringes are used for this vaccine, it is very important that no residual dichromate remains.)

(6) Rinse in distilled water.

(7) Place glassware in fresh distilled water for 3 separate changes, allowing it to remain in each change at least 30 minutes.

(8) Remove, drain, and dry in dust-free atmosphere. (Cover with towels or dry in hood or oven.)

(9) Wrap or assemble as required.

(10) Sterilize by high pressure steam 30 minutes, 15 lbs or dry heat as indicated.

B. For needles and metal parts (that is, syringe adapters and clips):

(1) Boil needles and metal parts for 30 minutes (in stainless steel sponge bowl) in a solution of detergent (1 teaspoon of strong alkaline detergent per pint of water).

(2) Flush needles under tap water. (Do not pour hot solution off of

the needles; if this is done a film of detergent is very rapidly formed on the hot metal.)

(3) Rinse metal parts in running tap water 15 to 20 minutes.

(4) Rinse in distilled water.

(5) Cover needles with distilled water and bring to boil; boil for 10 minutes; flush with distilled water and drain.

(6) Flush individual needles, using new clean syringe, with water and acetone or ether. Tube and sterilize by high pressure steam 30 minutes, 15 to 18 lbs. (fast exhaust and dry).

Appendix B / Data on Age-Representativeness of White Navy Recruit Population

Table B.1. U.S. Navy recruits, by age at time of test (white, tested 1958–64)

	TOTAL	AGE AT TEST				
		17	18	19	20	21
NUMBER	557,355	233,513	187,304	82,733	34,717	19,088
PERCENT	100.0	41.90	33.61	14.84	6.23	3.42

Table B.2. Percentage of all white males, aged 17–21 during 1958–64, who were skin-tested as Navy recruits

WHITE MALES, 1960 CENSUS		WHITE NAVY RECRUITS TESTED							YEAR OF TEST
		NUMBER	PERCENT OF ALL WHITE MALES AVAILABLE						
				AGE AT TEST					
AGE	NUMBER		TOTAL	17	18	19	20	21	
23	905,462	1,111	0.12					0.12	1958
22	930,934	4,064	0.44				0.28	0.16	1959
21	950,807	13,152	1.38			0.83	0.39	0.16	1960
20	928,590	38,846	4.18		2.29	1.18	0.44	0.27	1961
19	967,340	76,331	7.89	2.80	2.93	1.27	0.53	0.36	1962
18	1,094,690	90,080	8.23	3.46	2.80	1.21	0.53	0.23	1963
17	1,284,386	100,985	7.86	3.45	2.34	1.15	0.42	0.50	1964
16	1,273,781	81,735	6.42	2.51	2.30	0.98	0.63		
15	1,254,176	66,960	5.34	2.42	2.04	0.88			
14	1,223,528	51,805	4.23	2.42	1.81				
13	1,582,755	32,286	2.04	2.04					
Total (weighted average)			6.83	2.69	2.33	1.07	0.47	0.27	

Table C.1. Distributions by sizes of reactions to 0.0001 mg PPD-S for all Navy recruits tested 1958–64

	TOTAL	INDURATION TO PPD-S (IN GROUPS OF 2 MILLIMETERS)															
		0	2	4	6	8	10	12	14	16	18	20	22	24	26	28	≥30
CONTERMINOUS U S		AGES 17 TO 21 YEARS ALL RACES (587,640)															
ALABAMA	8139	7183	120	144	125	127	92	96	70	63	68	27	11	6	2	2	3
ARIZONA	6480	5682	94	125	83	51	70	71	71	63	61	44	32	18	9	3	3
ARKANSAS	6680	5949	116	126	80	68	51	54	78	54	42	31	22	2	6		1
CALIFORNIA	58857	53755	696	754	479	380	414	419	427	385	385	309	220	133	57	29	15
COLORADO	9100	8356	97	133	67	65	56	58	55	54	56	45	32	16	4	3	3
CONNECTICUT	7856	7345	76	65	43	43	44	52	44	41	43	30	18	5	2	2	3
DELAWARE	1489	1366	17	11	15	11	13	15	11	10	8	3	5	1	2		1
DIST.OF COLUMBIA	1552	1357	24	13	10	20	16	18	23	19	20	11	11	6	4		
FLORIDA	14490	12689	262	375	284	261	196	129	101	75	63	27	17	6	4	1	
GEORGIA	11084	9823	197	253	198	132	118	108	74	57	55	31	26	7	2	2	1
IDAHO	3621	3420	39	47	16	17	11	16	15	10	9	7	8	3	1	2	
ILLINOIS	26715	24307	315	268	227	202	223	226	238	206	204	144	73	42	22	9	9
INDIANA	14955	13773	191	128	96	89	94	103	99	102	112	77	48	29	8	4	2
IOWA	11989	11274	119	131	70	68	68	57	55	42	39	22	26	8	5	1	4
KANSAS	10406	9674	102	156	82	78	57	60	50	51	33	34	18	8	1	2	
KENTUCKY	7299	6436	83	59	62	62	80	116	113	104	90	40	26	20	3	3	2
LOUISIANA	10739	8969	226	375	276	256	180	144	104	83	51	37	20	12	4	1	1
MAINE	3956	3727	32	25	26	11	21	19	17	25	14	12	16	8	3		
MARYLAND	7954	6757	108	119	142	155	137	129	119	111	72	48	33	12	5	4	3
MASSACHUSETTS	15999	14980	174	118	84	81	81	76	82	88	101	50	37	27	9	7	4
MICHIGAN	26517	24831	291	199	114	119	122	131	143	132	166	124	66	48	12	12	7
MINNESOTA	16386	15567	178	118	68	79	71	52	38	41	61	51	24	18	12	6	2
MISSISSIPPI	4316	3757	81	113	89	74	63	43	37	23	14	13	6	2			1
MISSOURI	16439	15124	177	190	131	108	113	126	132	114	91	59	36	24	9	3	2
MONTANA	3930	3659	34	53	22	21	25	23	17	19	17	15	11	6	5	3	
NEBRASKA	6742	6311	74	98	40	33	32	29	18	28	27	19	12	10	5	3	3
NEVADA	1490	1371	20	19	14	7	8	15	6	13	5	9	2		1		
NEW HAMPSHIRE	2865	2743	24	8	11	8	9	11	10	9	9	11	7	1	1	2	1
NEW JERSEY	18325	16746	193	208	171	127	135	139	142	125	114	88	66	41	21	4	5
NEW MEXICO	4639	4146	58	67	50	35	35	38	42	48	44	36	20	14	3	2	1
NEW YORK	40058	36734	429	334	267	261	295	385	324	310	280	205	136	58	24	10	6
NORTH CAROLINA	10882	9829	161	216	155	119	81	81	68	54	55	30	14	12	3	2	2
NORTH DAKOTA	2807	2653	30	12	13	12	7	10	13	15	13	6	7	10	3	3	
OHIO	33506	30892	365	276	202	202	235	242	289	250	226	147	95	54	15	6	10
OKLAHOMA	9362	8449	118	146	107	76	71	85	80	80	66	38	25	13	5	2	1
OREGON	10581	9962	115	109	52	32	35	37	42	54	49	48	20	14	4	1	7
PENNSYLVANIA	37663	34437	419	368	294	276	274	334	302	300	271	161	120	60	24	17	6
RHODE ISLAND	2497	2334	21	21	17	18	15	9	13	14	15	9	2	5	2	1	1
SOUTH CAROLINA	6239	5534	115	158	131	77	66	40	38	26	33	10	5	5		1	
SOUTH DAKOTA	3259	3031	27	33	15	8	14	19	19	28	18	16	16	6	3	4	2
TENNESSEE	9972	8991	122	148	54	84	83	116	106	89	81	40	35	15	4	3	1
TEXAS	32001	27891	558	760	570	410	394	343	310	247	201	141	85	57	19	12	3
UTAH	3159	2958	34	38	25	22	26	13	11	8	9	8	3	2		2	
VERMONT	1935	1828	26	8	7	4	7	5	7	11	10	9	12				1
VIRGINIA	8280	7463	112	122	70	78	85	86	81	59	54	43	15	10		2	
WASHINGTON	13837	13009	142	130	73	48	58	70	69	64	57	41	32	22	14	6	2
WEST VIRGINIA	6669	6013	101	58	41	59	49	78	68	75	49	42	24	3	6	2	1
WISCONSIN	11868	11282	125	82	66	34	35	47	42	44	40	33	20	8	3	3	4
WYOMING	2056	1919	14	27	18	10	7	15	9	12	10	6	5	4			
NOT CONTERMINOUS U S		AGES 17 TO 21 YEARS ALL RACES (2,295)															
ALASKA	784	575	10	15	13	17	13	17	26	22	26	13	15	11	6	4	1
HAWAII	1247	1013	37	36	28	33	23	19	14	13	14	6	4	5	1	1	
PUERTO RICO/V.I.	121	78		3	2	2	5	9	6	5	3	4	3	1			
U.S. POSSESSIONS	143	77	4	14	5	6	4	6	6	6	3	4	4	1	2	1	
FOREIGN COUNTRIES		AGES 17 TO 21 YEARS ALL RACES (4,789)															
PHILIPPINE IS.	3884	456	50	156	223	271	445	443	488	403	344	295	141	98	42	23	6
OTHER COUNTRIES	905	717	9	13	21	19	26	12	21	14	20	17	9	3	1	3	
TOTAL ALL AREAS		AGES 22 YEARS OR MORE ALL RACES (27,609)															
CONTERMINOUS U S	23805	20514	210	362	336	336	344	355	344	249	295	202	125	71	31	20	11
PHILIPPINE IS.	3460	304	26	101	206	238	366	438	470	384	382	229	162	88	37	14	15
OTHER	344	197	1	9	11	14	14	23	22	14	11	9	8	7	2	1	1

Table C.2. Number of Navy recruits tested and percent with reactions of 10 or more mm to 0.0001 mg PPD-S, for lifetime residents of counties included in metropolitan areas (white, ages 17–21, tested 1958–64)

Area	County	State	Number Tested	Reactions (10+) Number	Percent
Abilene	Jones	Tex.	19	0	
	Taylor	Tex.	78	2	
Total			97	2	
Akron	Summit	Ohio	958	39	4.1
Albany	Dougherty	Ga.	26	2	
Albany–	Albany	N.Y.	452	29	6.4
Schenectady–	Rensselaer	N.Y.	335	15	4.5
Troy	Saratoga	N.Y.	198	5	2.5
	Schenectady	N.Y.	265	6	2.3
Total			1,250	55	4.4
Albuquerque	Bernalillo	N.Mex.	253	12	4.7
Allentown–	Warren	N.J.	121	0	
Bethlehem–	Lehigh	Pa.	565	18	3.2
Easton	Northampton	Pa.	577	34	5.9
Total			1,263	52	4.1
Altoona	Blair	Pa.	372	13	3.5
Amarillo	Potter	Tex.	94	7	
	Randall	Tex.	4	2	
Total			98	9	
Ann Arbor	Washtenaw	Mich.	226	6	2.7
Asheville	Buncombe	N.C.	198	4	2.0
Atlanta	Clayton	Ga.	27	0	
	Cobb	Ga.	137	1	0.7
	De Kalb	Ga.	140	3	2.1
	Fulton	Ga.	486	18	3.7
	Gwinnett	Ga.	30	0	
Total			820	22	2.7
Atlantic City	Atlantic	N.J.	221	12	5.4
Augusta	Richmond	Ga.	156	9	5.8
	Aiken	S.C.	76	0	
Total			232	9	3.9
Austin	Travis	Tex.	155	7	4.5
Bakersfield	Kern	Calif.	416	10	2.4
Baltimore	Anne Arundel	Md.	170	24	14.1
	Baltimore	Md.	2,118	198	9.3
	Carroll	Md.	138	6	4.3
	Howard	Md.	32	3	
Total			2,458	231	9.4
Baton Rouge	East Baton	La.	265	7	2.6
Bay City	Bay	Mich.	288	7	2.4
Beaumont–	Jefferson	Tex.	319	13	4.1
Port Arthur	Orange	Tex.	35	1	
Total			354	14	4.0
Billings	Yellowstone	Mont.	133	4	3.0
Binghamton	Broome	N.Y.	383	8	2.1
Birmingham	Jefferson	Ala.	682	23	3.4
Boston-Brockton–	Essex	Mass.	1,552	45	2.9
Lowell-Lawrence–	Middlesex	Mass.	2,182	64	2.9
Haverhill	Norfolk	Mass.	828	20	2.4
	Plymouth	Mass.	482	12	2.5
	Suffolk	Mass.	1,007	60	6.0
	Rockingham	N.H.	210	8	3.8
Total			6,261	209	3.3
Bridgeport-Norwalk- Stamford	Fairfield	Conn.	1,276	54	4.2
Brownsville– Harlingen– San Benito	Cameron	Tex.	137	17	12.4
Buffalo	Erie	N.Y.	2,199	116	5.3
	Niagara	N.Y.	623	24	3.9
Total			2,822	140	5.0
Canton	Stark	Ohio	648	23	3.5
Cedar Rapids	Linn	Iowa	292	7	2.4
Champaign-Urbana	Champaign	Ill.	140	5	3.6
Charleston	Charleston	S.C.	118	1	0.8
Charleston	Kanawha	W.Va.	482	31	6.4
Charlotte	Mecklenburg	N.C.	194	5	2.6
Chattanooga	Walker	Ga.	81	2	
	Hamilton	Tenn.	386	18	4.7
Total			467	20	4.3
Chicago	Cook	Ill.	5,708	291	5.1
	DuPage	Ill.	165	2	1.2
	Kane	Ill.	310	11	3.5
	Lake	Ill.	132	5	3.8
	McHenry	Ill.	82	1	
	Will	Ill.	255	8	3.1
Total			6,652	318	4.8
Cincinnati	Campbell	Ky.	115	10	8.7
	Kenton	Ky.	156	15	9.6
	Hamilton	Ohio	1,285	67	5.2
Total			1,556	92	5.9
Cleveland	Cuyahoga	Ohio	2,785	102	3.7
	Lake	Ohio	171	3	1.8
Total			2,956	105	3.6
Colorado Springs	El Paso	Colo.	110	3	2.7
Columbia	Lexington	S.C.	81		
	Richland	S.C.	154	5	3.2
Total			235	5	2.1
Columbus	Russell	Ala.	40	4	
	Chattahoochee	Ga.	1	1	
	Muscogee	Ga.	165	14	8.5
Total			206	19	9.2
Columbus	Franklin	Ohio	997	37	3.7
Corpus Christi	Nueces	Tex.	124	18	14.5
Dallas	Collin	Tex.	52	8	
	Dallas	Tex.	921	45	4.9
	Denton	Tex.	35	1	
	Ellis	Tex.	49	4	
Total			1,057	58	5.5
Davenport-Rock	Rock Island	Ill.	243	5	2.1
Island-Moline	Scott	Iowa	208	7	3.4
Total			451	12	2.7
Dayton	Greene	Ohio	118	4	3.4
	Miami	Ohio	154	4	2.6
	Montgomery	Ohio	773	32	4.1
Total			1,045	40	3.8
Decatur	Macon	Ill.	169	3	1.8
Denver	Adams	Colo.	81	4	
	Arapahoe	Colo.	70	3	
	Boulder	Colo.	82	7	
	Denver	Colo.	758	34	4.5
	Jefferson	Colo.	103	1	1.0
Total			1,094	49	4.5
Des Moines	Polk	Iowa	464	13	2.8
Detroit	Macomb	Mich.	412	12	2.9
	Oakland	Mich.	899	29	3.2
	Wayne	Mich.	4,368	180	4.1
Total			5,679	221	3.9

Area	County	State	Number Tested	Reactions (10+) Number	Percent
Dubuque	Dubuque	Iowa	202	2	1.0
Duluth-Superior	St. Louis	Minn.	782	23	2.9
	Douglas	Wis.	148	7	4.7
Total			930	30	3.2
Durham	Durham	N.C.	101	1	1.0
El Paso	El Paso	Tex.	467	50	10.7
Erie	Erie	Pa.	653	25	3.8
Eugene	Lane	Oreg.	250	8	3.2
Evansville	Vandenburgh	Ind.	326	17	5.2
	Henderson	Ky.	24	2	
Total			350	19	5.4
Fargo-Moorhead	Clay	Minn.	69	0	
	Cass	N. Dak.	97	4	
Total			166	4	2.4
Flint	Genesee	Mich.	605	14	2.3
Fort Lauderdale-Hollywood	Broward	Fla.	49	0	
Fort Smith	Sebastian	Ark.	74	5	
Fort Wayne	Allen	Ind.	331	12	3.6
Fort Worth	Johnson	Tex.	35	0	
	Tarrant	Tex.	702	28	4.0
Total			737	28	3.8
Fresno	Fresno	Calif.	528	15	2.8
Gadsden	Etowah	Ala.	166	10	6.0
Galveston-Texas City	Galveston	Tex.	204	11	5.4
Gary-Hammond-East Chicago	Lake	Ind.	803	30	3.7
	Porter	Ind.	85	0	
Total			888	30	3.4
Grand Rapids	Kent	Mich.	675	10	1.5
Great Falls	Cascade	Mont.	129	3	2.3
Green Bay	Brown	Wis.	221	5	2.3
Greensboro-High Pt.	Guilford	N.C.	273	5	1.8
Greenville	Greenville	S.C.	247	6	2.4
Hamilton-Middletwn	Butler	Ohio	313	12	3.8
Harrisburg	Cumberland	Pa.	157	4	2.5
	Dauphin	Pa.	306	16	5.2
Total			463	20	4.3
Hartford-New Britain	Hartford	Conn.	1,285	33	2.6
	Middlesex	Conn.	118	3	2.5
	Tolland	Conn.	84	0	
Total			1,487	36	2.4
Houston	Harris	Tex.	1,312	67	5.1
Huntington-Ashland	Boyd	Ky.	76	7	
	Lawrence	Ohio	90	3	
	Cabell	W. Va.	188	20	10.6
	Wayne	W. Va.	68	6	
Total			422	36	8.5
Huntsville	Madison	Ala.	77	7	
Indianapolis	Marion	Ind.	869	27	3.1
Jackson	Jackson	Mich.	210	5	2.4
Jackson	Hinds	Miss.	64	3	
Jacksonville	Duval	Fla.	295	16	5.4

Area	County	State	Number Tested	Reactions (10+) Number	Percent
Jersey City	Hudson	N.J.	925	46	5.0
Johnstown	Cambria	Pa.	643	25	3.9
	Somerset	Pa.	155	7	4.5
Total			798	32	4.0
Kalamazoo	Kalamazoo	Mich.	254	4	1.6
Kansas City	Johnson	Kans.	72	2	
	Wyandotte	Kans.	397	17	4.3
	Clay	Mo.	84	4	
	Jackson	Mo.	976	42	4.3
Total			1,529	65	4.3
Kenosha	Kenosha	Wis.	83	2	
Knoxville	Anderson	Tenn.	91	2	
	Blount	Tenn.	109	4	3.7
	Knox	Tenn.	424	12	2.8
Total			624	18	2.9
Lake Charles	Calcasieu	La.	244	12	4.9
Lancaster	Lancaster	Pa.	563	18	3.2
Lansing	Clinton	Mich.	67	4	
	Eaton	Mich.	87	4	
	Ingham	Mich.	257	0	0.0
Total			411	8	1.9
Laredo	Webb	Tex.	56	12	
Las Vegas	Clark	Nev.	82	2	
Lawton	Comanche	Okla.	62	1	
Lewiston-Auburn	Androscoggin	Maine	197	8	4.1
Lexington	Fayette	Ky.	89	7	
Lima	Allen	Ohio	221	6	2.7
Lincoln	Lancaster	Nebr.	222	6	2.7
Little Rock-North Little Rock	Pulaski	Ark.	332	14	4.2
Lorain-Elyria	Lorain	Ohio	375	13	3.5
Los Angeles-Long Beach	Los Angeles	Calif.	6,147	215	3.5
	Orange	Calif.	259	4	1.5
Total			6,406	219	3.4
Louisville	Clark	Ind.	95	5	
	Floyd	Ind.	81	2	
	Jefferson	Ky.	830	69	8.3
Total			1,006	76	7.6
Lubbock	Lubbock	Tex.	83	2	
Lynchburg	Amherst	Va.	12	0	
	Campbell	Va.	145	6	4.1
Total			157	6	3.8
Macon	Bibb	Ga.	112	3	2.7
	Houston	Ga.	15	0	
Total			127	3	2.4
Madison	Dane	Wis.	313	3	1.0
Manchester	Hillsborough	N.H.	438	15	3.4
Memphis	Shelby	Tenn.	296	4	1.4
Miami	Dade	Fla.	423	9	2.1
Midland	Midland	Tex.	25	0	
Milwaukee	Waukesha	Wis.	118	5	4.2
	Milwaukee	Wis.	966	26	2.7
Total			1,084	31	2.9

Area	County	State	Number Tested	Reactions (10+) Number	Percent
Minneapolis–	Anoka	Minn.	97	2	
St. Paul	Dakota	Minn.	140	3	2.1
	Hennepin	Minn.	1,752	37	2.1
	Ramsey	Minn.	1,018	26	2.6
	Washington	Minn.	131	3	2.3
Total			3,138	71	2.3
Mobile	Mobile	Ala.	356	32	9.0
Monroe	Ouachita	La.	107	4	3.7
Montgomery	Montgomery	Ala.	99	3	
Muncie	Delaware	Ind.	145	5	3.4
Muskegon–	Muskegon	Mich.	347	4	1.2
Muskegon Hgts					
Nashville	Davidson	Tenn.	486	31	6.4
New Haven–	Litchfield	Conn.	259	6	2.3
Meriden-Waterbury	New Haven	Conn.	1,269	40	3.2
Total			1,528	46	3.0
New London–	New London	Conn.	343	11	3.2
Groton-Norwich					
New Orleans	Jefferson	La.	213	12	5.6
	Orleans	La.	808	67	8.3
	St. Bernard	La.	15	3	
Total			1,036	82	7.9
New York City	Nassau	N.Y.	917	22	2.4
	New York City	N.Y.	8,207	519	6.3
	Rockland	N.Y.	190	3	1.6
	Suffolk	N.Y.	600	15	2.5
	Westchester	N.Y.	927	29	3.1
Total			10,841	588	5.4
Newark	Essex	N.J.	1,220	58	4.8
	Morris	N.J.	332	7	2.1
	Union	N.J.	620	22	3.5
Total			2,172	87	4.0
Newport News–	Elizabeth	Va.	27	2	
Hampton	Warwick	Va.	27	3	
	York	Va.	13	1	
Total			67	6	
Norfolk-Portsmouth	Norfolk	Va.	166	7	4.2
	Princess Anne	Va.	6	0	
Total			172	7	4.1
Odessa	Ector	Tex.	35	1	
Ogden	Weber	Utah	182	3	1.6
Oklahoma City	Canadian	Okla.	49	0	
	Cleveland	Okla.	16	0	
	Oklahoma	Okla.	395	9	2.3
Total			460	9	2.0
Omaha	Pottawattamie	Iowa	263	5	1.9
	Douglas	Nebr.	741	22	3.0
	Sarpy	Nebr.	33	1	
Total			1,037	28	2.7
Orlando	Orange	Fla.	75	2	
	Seminole	Fla.	11	1	
Total			86	3	
Paterson-Clifton-	Bergen	N.J.	939	37	3.9
Passaic	Passaic	N.J.	732	27	3.7
Total			1,671	64	3.8
Pensacola	Escambia	Fla.	105	3	2.9
	Santa Rosa	Fla.	25	1	
Total			130	4	3.1
Peoria	Peoria	Ill.	319	11	3.4
	Tazewell	Ill.	131	4	3.1
Total			450	15	3.3
Philadelphia	Burlington	N.J.	315	20	6.3
	Camden	N.J.	754	30	4.0
	Gloucester	N.J.	231	5	2.2
	Bucks	Pa.	329	19	5.8
	Chester	Pa.	317	8	2.5
	Delaware	Pa.	745	22	3.0
	Montgomery	Pa.	620	16	2.6
	Philadelphia	Pa.	2,480	133	5.4
Total			5,791	253	4.4
Phoenix	Maricopa	Ariz.	485	42	8.7
Pittsburgh	Allegheny	Pa.	3,565	192	5.4
	Beaver	Pa.	535	27	5.0
	Washington	Pa.	675	19	2.8
	Westmoreland	Pa.	906	26	2.9
Total			5,681	264	4.6
Pittsfield	Berkshire	Mass.	399	10	2.5
Portland	Cumberland	Maine	399	13	3.3
Portland	Clackamas	Oreg.	176	6	3.4
	Multnomah	Oreg.	741	27	3.6
	Washington	Oreg.	157	3	1.9
	Clark	Wash.	176	3	1.7
Total			1,250	39	3.1
Providence–	Bristol	Mass.	813	37	4.6
Pawtucket–	Bristol	R.I.	80	0	
New Bedford	Kent	R.I.	208	0	
	Newport	R.I.	66	1	
	Providence	R.I.	1,110	42	3.8
	Washington	R.I.	79	0	
Total			2,356	80	3.4
Provo-Orem	Utah	Utah	185	4	2.2
Pueblo	Pueblo	Colo.	238	10	4.2
Racine	Racine	Wis.	190	5	2.6
Raleigh	Wake	N.C.	132	8	6.1
Reading	Berks	Pa.	572	33	5.8
Reno	Washoe	Nev.	59	2	
Richmond	Chesterfield	Va.	87	3	
	Henrico	Va.	254	14	5.5
Total			341	17	5.0
Roanoke	Roanoke	Va.	190	10	5.3
Rochester	Monroe	N.Y.	876	22	2.5
Rockford	Winnebago	Ill.	347	11	3.2
Sacramento	Sacramento	Calif.	520	22	4.2
Saginaw	Saginaw	Mich.	445	15	3.4
Salt Lake City	Salt Lake	Utah	488	8	1.6
San Angelo	Tom Green	Tex.	66	4	
San Antonio	Bexar	Tex.	984	105	10.7
San Bernardino–	Riverside	Calif.	219	11	5.0
Riverside	San Bernardino	Calif.	530	16	3.0
Total			749	27	3.6
San Diego	San Diego	Calif.	488	22	4.5
San Francisco–	Alameda	Calif.	848	31	3.7
Oakland	Contra Costa	Calif.	370	15	4.1
	Marin	Calif.	122	2	1.6
	San Francisco	Calif.	611	41	6.7
	San Mateo	Calif.	215	7	3.3
	Solano	Calif.	108	5	4.6
Total			2,274	101	4.4

Area	County	State	Number Tested	Reactions (10+) Number	Percent
San Jose	Santa Clara	Calif.	425	25	5.9
Santa Barbara	Santa Barbara	Calif.	149	6	4.0
Savannah	Chatham	Ga.	216	10	4.6
Scranton	Lackawanna	Pa.	612	42	6.9
Seattle	King	Wash.	1,250	36	2.9
	Snohomish	Wash.	247	7	2.8
Total			1,497	43	2.9
Shreveport	Bossier	La.	22	1	
	Caddo	La.	147	2	1.4
Total			169	3	1.8
Sioux City	Woodbury	Iowa	306	9	2.9
Sioux Falls	Minnehaha	S. Dak.	109	5	4.6
South Bend	St. Joseph	Ind.	424	13	3.1
Spokane	Spokane	Wash.	450	9	2.0
Springfield	Sangamon	Ill.	280	6	2.1
Springfield	Greene	Mo.	198	3	1.5
Springfield	Clark	Ohio	246	10	4.1
Springfield-	Hampden	Mass.	1,091	25	2.3
Chicopee-Holyoke	Hampshire	Mass.	196	3	1.5
Total			1,287	28	2.2
St. Joseph	Buchanan	Mo.	169	6	3.6
St. Louis	Madison	Ill.	449	16	3.6
	St. Clair	Ill.	408	11	2.7
	Jefferson	Mo.	116	4	3.4
	St. Charles	Mo.	68	1	
	St. Louis	Mo.	2,239	100	4.5
Total			3,280	132	4.0
Steubenville-	Jefferson	Ohio	240	11	4.6
Weirton	Brooke	W. Va.	47	2	
	Hancock	W. Va.	62	1	
Total			349	14	4.0
Stockton	San Joaquin	Calif.	336	13	3.9
Syracuse	Madison	N.Y.	146	4	2.7
	Onondaga	N.Y.	834	34	4.1
	Oswego	N.Y.	197	6	3.0
Total			1,177	44	3.7
Tacoma	Pierce	Wash.	634	12	1.9
Tampa-	Hillsborough	Fla.	340	11	3.2
St. Petersburg	Pinellas	Fla.	115	3	2.6
Total			455	14	3.1
Terre Haute	Vigo	Ind.	176	7	4.0
Texarkana	Miller	Ark.	36	0	
	Bowie	Tex.	70	1	
Total			106	1	0.9
Toledo	Lucas	Ohio	857	32	3.7
Topeka	Shawnee	Kans.	205	6	2.9
Trenton	Mercer	N.J.	422	17	4.0
Tucson	Pima	Ariz.	231	19	8.2
Tulsa	Creek	Okla.	63	4	
	Osage	Okla.	54	2	
	Tulsa	Okla.	386	15	3.9
Total			503	21	4.2
Tuscaloosa	Tuscaloosa	Ala.	123	6	4.9

Area	County	State	Number Tested	Reactions (10+) Number	Percent
Tyler	Smith	Tex.	84	5	
Utica-Rome	Herkimer	N.Y.	117	1	0.9
	Oneida	N.Y.	634	15	2.4
Total			751	16	2.1
Waco	McLennan	Tex.	139	5	3.6
Washington, D.C.	Washington	D.C.	166	14	8.4
	Montgomery	Md.	120	7	5.8
	Prince Georges	Md.	250	6	2.4
	Arlington	Va.	54	1	
	Fairfax	Va.	152	2	1.3
Total			742	30	4.0
Waterloo	Black Hawk	Iowa	263	12	4.6
West Palm Beach	Palm Beach	Fla.	87	1	
Wheeling	Belmont	Ohio	159	3	1.9
	Marshall	W. Va.	90	6	
	Ohio	W. Va.	119	7	5.9
Total			368	16	4.3
Wichita	Sedgwick	Kans.	469	11	2.3
Wichita Falls	Archer	Tex.	7	0	
	Wichita	Tex.	166	7	4.2
Total			173	7	4.0
Wilkes Barre-	Luzerne	Pa.	908	71	7.8
Hazleton					
Wilmington	New Castle	Del.	468	16	3.4
	Salem	N.J.	157	5	3.2
Total			625	21	3.4
Winston-Salem	Forsyth	N.C.	139	8	5.8
Worcester-Fitchburg-	Worcester	Mass.	1,639	35	2.1
Leomister					
York	York	Pa.	436	11	2.5
Youngstown-Warren	Mahoning	Ohio	601	35	5.8
	Trumbull	Ohio	466	14	3.0
Total			1,067	49	4.6

Table C.3. Distributions by sizes of reactions to 0.0001 mg PPD-S among Navy recruits by state, for metropolitan, farm, and other non-metropolitan residents (white, ages 17–21, tested 1958–64)

	TOTAL	INDURATION TO PPD - S (IN GROUPS OF 2 MILLIMETERS)															
		0	2	4	6	8	10	12	14	16	18	20	22	24	26	28	≥30
ALABAMA																	
METROPOLITAN	1543	1375	16	31	15	21	19	20	16	7	16	5	1	1			
NON METRO. FARM	767	694	8	12	16	11	8	4	3	5	4			1	1		
NON METRO. OTHER	1144	1035	17	15	19	12	10	9	9	6	5	2	2		1		2
ARIZONA																	
METROPOLITAN	716	600	15	18	13	9	11	12	9	6	6	7	5	3	1		1
NON METRO. FARM	31	29								1							
NON METRO. OTHER	368	323	2	6	6	2	3	5	6	6	2	2	2		2	1	
ARKANSAS																	
METROPOLITAN	442	397	6	10	6	4	2	4	4	2	5	1		1			
NON METRO. FARM	886	795	16	18	6	7	10	8	12	6	3	3	2				
NON METRO. OTHER	1059	939	18	20	16	11	7	7	16	8	8	4	3	1	1		
CALIFORNIA																	
METROPOLITAN	12291	11388	144	140	100	59	64	80	66	61	59	56	45	16	6	5	2
NON METRO. FARM	460	432	4	5	2		2	3	2	2	1	1	1	2	1	2	
NON METRO. OTHER	1955	1817	23	20	14	7	12	15	8	14	11	7	3	2	2		
COLORADO																	
METROPOLITAN	1442	1335	15	18	4	8	6	11	6	6	10	6	12	3	1	1	
NON METRO. FARM	355	337	4	4	4	2	2	1	2	1	2						
NON METRO. OTHER	837	764	7	9	8	7	3	8	8	6	7	4	3	3			
CONNECTICUT																	
METROPOLITAN	4634	4365	49	40	19	14	24	27	24	19	21	17	7	4	1	1	2
NON METRO. FARM	20	19								1							
NON METRO. OTHER	143	138	3				1			1							
DELAWARE																	
METROPOLITAN	468	438	6	1	3	4	3	4	3		2	1	2	1			
NON METRO. FARM	52	45	2		2	1						1	1				
NON METRO. OTHER	181	170		2	4		1	1		2	1						
DIST. OF COL.																	
METROPOLITAN	166	141	4		3	4	2	2	5	1	2	1			1		
NON METRO. FARM																	
NON METRO. OTHER																	
FLORIDA																	
METROPOLITAN	1525	1331	27	51	40	29	21	8	5	8	3	2					
NON METRO. FARM	294	241	11	13	12	6	6	2	1	2							
NON METRO. OTHER	1027	858	15	35	28	32	28	8	9	6	4	2	2				
GEORGIA																	
METROPOLITAN	1592	1453	20	24	19	13	21	16	8	7	4	3	3	1			
NON METRO. FARM	933	816	20	32	20	22	1	4	6	6	1	2	3				
NON METRO. OTHER	1564	1400	34	39	21	18	14	14	9	5	7	2		1			
IDAHO																	
METROPOLITAN																	
NON METRO. FARM	315	301	4	1	1	1	1	2			1		2	1			
NON METRO. OTHER	754	728	3	5	3	1		3	2	1	2	3	2	1			
ILLINOIS																	
METROPOLITAN	9138	8389	115	97	71	76	74	66	73	54	56	34	14	10	5	1	3
NON METRO. FARM	804	764	8	7	1	1	9	5	1	4	1	1	1	1			
NON METRO. OTHER	3331	3134	25	19	24	18	21	14	15	20	15	9	11	4	1	1	
INDIANA																	
METROPOLITAN	3335	3091	48	28	29	21	26	18	17	15	21	13	2	4	1		1
NON METRO. FARM	794	758	6	4	4	5	2	3	3	2	2	2	1	1			1
NON METRO. OTHER	2990	2783	31	24	12	9	18	21	21	15	16	13	15	10	1	1	

	TOTAL	INDURATION TO PPD-S (IN GROUPS OF 2 MILLIMETERS)															
		0	2	4	6	8	10	12	14	16	18	20	22	24	26	28	≥30
IOWA																	
METROPOLITAN	1998	1847	22	33	17	24	15	14	8	5	5	3	1	1	2		1
NON METRO. FARM	1203	1170	7	8	1	3	4	5		1	3		1				
NON METRO. OTHER	2798	2641	30	28	19	10	10	10	15	14	9	6	3	2			1
KANSAS																	
METROPOLITAN	1143	1039	17	32	5	14	7	5	8	5	3	6	1	1			
NON METRO. FARM	722	686	6	7	5	5	4	4	1				2	2			
NON METRO. OTHER	1973	1868	20	18	14	10	9	11	4	10	2	4	2			1	
KENTUCKY																	
METROPOLITAN	1290	1129	7	13	18	13	13	25	16	20	17	8	3	5	2	1	
NON METRO. FARM	906	792	16	7	6	8	13	13	16	14	12	4	1	2		1	1
NON METRO. OTHER	1330	1187	14	11	9	11	12	21	19	20	13	3	6	2		1	1
LOUISIANA																	
METROPOLITAN	1821	1536	31	59	48	39	29	34	14	13	5	8	4	1			
NON METRO. FARM	803	660	20	37	23	27	11	12	5	5	1		1	1			
NON METRO. OTHER	1710	1439	45	71	42	36	25	19	10	10	5	3	3	2			
MAINE																	
METROPOLITAN	596	559	5	4	5	2	3	2	3	3	2	4	2	1	1		
NON METRO. FARM	215	207	2	2	1	1	1			1							
NON METRO. OTHER	1467	1376	15	8	9	6	8	9	7	10	4	3	8	3	1		
MARYLAND																	
METROPOLITAN	2828	2367	36	52	62	67	54	48	45	46	23	17	8	3			
NON METRO. FARM	147	134	2		3		1	1	1	2	2	1					
NON METRO. OTHER	1003	901	13	9	11	14	6	13	13	8	5	5	3	1			1
MASSACHUSETTS																	
METROPOLITAN	10189	9612	103	71	42	50	37	46	37	61	54	25	26	15	4	5	1
NON METRO. FARM	18	15		1	1	1											
NON METRO. OTHER	287	279		2		1			1			1	1	1		1	
MICHIGAN																	
METROPOLITAN	9140	8631	78	65	34	38	39	44	50	44	44	34	17	11	5	2	4
NON METRO. FARM	899	855	14	5	1	2	3	3	3	2	3		3	3	1		1
NON METRO. OTHER	3422	3244	37	22	9	13	9	3	14	12	26	17	8	6	1		1
MINNESOTA																	
METROPOLITAN	3989	3787	45	32	17	14	20	14	4	8	17	14	7	6	1	2	1
NON METRO. FARM	1635	1573	20	10	3	7	1	2	2	1	6	6	3	1			
NON METRO. OTHER	2840	2730	33	20	7	9	9	5	5	4	8	5	2	1	1	1	
MISSISSIPPI																	
METROPOLITAN	64	59	1		1		2							1			
NON METRO. FARM	696	608	18	21	12	10	9	6	5	1	4	1					1
NON METRO. OTHER	842	752	11	20	18	10	8	8	3	6	1	4		1			
MISSOURI																	
METROPOLITAN	3850	3542	40	51	37	20	23	27	25	20	26	14	12	6	2	3	2
NON METRO. FARM	1178	1107	12	10	6	8	5	9	7	5	4	3	2				
NON METRO. OTHER	2092	1968	16	10	9	17	13	14	14	11	9	6	2	2	1		
MONTANA																	
METROPOLITAN	262	245	2	3	2	3	1	2	3						1		
NON METRO. FARM	264	255	2	3	2								1		1		
NON METRO. OTHER	803	759	9	8	4	2	3	1	2	3	5	4	3				
NEBRASKA																	
METROPOLITAN	996	926	9	21	7	4	6	6	3	2	4	3	1			1	2	1
NON METRO. FARM	688	660	8	5	2	2	4	3	1	1			2				
NON METRO. OTHER	1266	1197	17	13	8	7		3	4	6	2	5	1	3			

189

	TOTAL	INDURATION TO PPD-S (IN GROUPS OF 2 MILLIMETERS)															
		0	2	4	6	8	10	12	14	16	18	20	22	24	26	28	≥30
NEVADA																	
METROPOLITAN	141	132	3		1	1		3		1							
NON METRO. FARM	2	2															
NON METRO. OTHER	39	37						1				1					
NEW HAMPSHIRE																	
METROPOLITAN	648	613	7		4	1	3	1	3	2	4	6	3	1			
NON METRO. FARM	86	85				1											
NON METRO. OTHER	753	727	6	4	3	1	3	5		1		1	1			1	
NEW JERSEY																	
METROPOLITAN	6989	6437	73	84	61	48	47	46	54	39	34	26	20	13	4	1	2
NON METRO. FARM	92	88	2						2								
NON METRO. OTHER	1730	1624	15	15	16	10	12	6	9	6	6	4	4	1	1	1	
NEW MEXICO																	
METROPOLITAN	253	231	7	1	1	1	3	1	4	1		3					
NON METRO. FARM	160	145	4	2	2				1	4	1	1					
NON METRO. OTHER	713	643	5	8	6	4	7	5	11	5	6	3	5	4		1	
NEW YORK																	
METROPOLITAN	18100	16649	210	152	119	97	130	165	140	138	130	80	51	29	6	4	
NON METRO. FARM	727	705	6	1	1		1	1	3	3	2	3	1				
NON METRO. OTHER	4747	4524	44	32	19	18	11	21	17	17	16	15	10	1	1		1
NORTH CAROLINA																	
METROPOLITAN	1037	951	17	18	13	7	3	8	6	7	2	2	1	1		1	
NON METRO. FARM	1293	1164	27	36	26	16	4	5	4	3	4	2	1				1
NON METRO. OTHER	2775	2558	31	46	25	29	20	16	18	14	11	5		1			1
NORTH DAKOTA																	
METROPOLITAN	97	90		1		2			1	2		1					
NON METRO. FARM	531	518	6		1	2				1		1	1	1			
NON METRO. OTHER	778	747	11	4	4	4				1	4	1	1			1	
OHIO																	
METROPOLITAN	11457	10681	110	88	60	68	86	71	82	71	66	35	24	8	4	1	2
NON METRO. FARM	957	919	12	5	3	1	4	3		2	2	5	1				
NON METRO. OTHER	4711	4417	59	27	24	23	21	21	36	22	22	15	14	6	3	1	
OKLAHOMA																	
METROPOLITAN	1025	946	10	16	13	9	5	9	1	7	6	2		1			
NON METRO. FARM	631	577	11	7	8	5	5	3	1	6	4	1	2		1		
NON METRO. OTHER	1357	1233	18	19	18	9	13	9	14	8	6	5	3	2			
OREGON																	
METROPOLITAN	1324	1251	15	7	4	3	8	9	4	4	5	7	2	4	1		
NON METRO. FARM	361	346	4	3	1				1	1	1	2		1			1
NON METRO. OTHER	1008	963	5	5	6	1	5	1	7	7	4	2	2				
PENNSYLVANIA																	
METROPOLITAN	16691	15314	174	165	130	129	132	132	131	132	110	54	53	16	9	7	3
NON METRO. FARM	887	851	9	5	7	1	2	3		2	2	2	1	2			
NON METRO. OTHER	6956	6435	79	47	51	40	33	63	49	45	41	38	18	9	4	3	
RHODE ISLAND																	
METROPOLITAN	1543	1454	14	13	9	10	9	5	5	8	9	3	1	1	1		1
NON METRO. FARM																	
NON METRO. OTHER																	
SOUTH CAROLINA																	
METROPOLITAN	676	616	8	20	12	8	4	2	3	2	1						
NON METRO. FARM	649	568	10	28	13	12	9	4	1	1	1	1		1			
NON METRO. OTHER	1517	1369	32	24	41	14	13	6	9	1	7			1			

	TOTAL	INDURATION TO PPD - S (IN GROUPS OF 2 MILLIMETERS)															
		0	2	4	6	8	10	12	14	16	18	20	22	24	26	28	≥30
SOUTH DAKOTA																	
METROPOLITAN	109	101	1	2			2	1	1				1				
NON METRO. FARM	431	414	4	5		1	1	1		3			2				
NON METRO. OTHER	707	679	6	3	4	1	7	2	1		2	1					1
TENNESSEE																	
METROPOLITAN	1792	1661	16	21	11	12	13	12	13	13	11	4	2	1		1	1
NON METRO. FARM	1116	1024	10	15	5	14	4	14	7	6	9	2	4	2			
NON METRO. OTHER	1559	1387	20	24	6	14	16	19	17	17	15	10	9	2	2	1	
TEXAS																	
METROPOLITAN	6457	5582	124	143	100	85	86	90	54	67	48	37	15	13	8	4	1
NON METRO. FARM	1018	916	16	13	22	15	11	12	3	3	3	1	3				
NON METRO. OTHER	2435	2115	39	73	33	25	26	31	27	18	16	15	9	5	2		1
UTAH																	
METROPOLITAN	855	812	9	8	7	4	5	5	2		2		1				
NON METRO. FARM	140	136	3									1					
NON METRO. OTHER	290	283		3	1		1				1	1					
VERMONT																	
METROPOLITAN																	
NON METRO. FARM	156	145	7					1	1	1	1						
NON METRO. OTHER	934	883	9	3	1	3	3	4	3	6	3	4	11				1
VIRGINIA																	
METROPOLITAN	1133	1030	12	21	14	7	15	9	6	9	5	4	1				
NON METRO. FARM	601	560	5	5	7	3	2	7	3	2	5	2					
NON METRO. OTHER	1364	1250	20	16	7	7	10	16	10	9	5	6	4	4			
WASHINGTON																	
METROPOLITAN	2757	2625	23	20	14	8	8	7	15	9	9	5	5	3	3	2	1
NON METRO. FARM	449	430	4	6	2			2		1	2			2			
NON METRO. OTHER	1191	1129	9	12	6	3	4	1	7	2	5	5	5	1	2		
WEST VIRGINIA																	
METROPOLITAN	1056	946	12	10	5	10	3	14	20	14	10	9	1		1	1	
NON METRO. FARM	657	603	10	8	1	7	5	7	3	8	2	1	1	1			
NON METRO. OTHER	2082	1898	32	17	13	19	10	24	13	18	12	11	10	1	3	1	
WISCONSIN																	
METROPOLITAN	2039	1941	14	13	11	7	6	11	3	8	13	6	1	3	1	1	
NON METRO. FARM	1154	1112	14	6	2	2	2	4	6	1	2		1	1			1
NON METRO. OTHER	3206	3061	38	23	14	13	11	9	7	8	12	6	3		1		
WYOMING																	
METROPOLITAN																	
NON METRO. FARM	129	117	2	3				2		2	3						
NON METRO. OTHER	489	463	2	7	2	1	2	1	2	4	1	2	1	1			

Table C.4. Number of Navy recruits tested, and percent with reactions of 10 or more mm to 0.0001 mg PPD-S, by type of residence, by state (white, ages 17–21, tested 1958–64)

	NUMBER TESTED						PERCENT REACTORS*					
	Grand Total	Lifetime U.S.				Some Foreign Residence**	Grand Total	Lifetime U.S.				Some Foreign Residence**
		Total	Lifetime One-State		Not 1-State			Total	Lifetime One-State		Not 1-State	
			1-County	Other					1-County	Other		
Total	557,355	372,289	257,476	114,813	166,849	18,217	4.1	3.8	3.8	3.7	4.0	10.6
Alabama	7,430	5,047	3,454	1,593	2,127	256	4.8	4.3	4.6	3.8	5.5	9.4
Arizona	6,168	1,563	1,115	448	4,299	306	6.3	7.9	8.2	7.1	5.7	6.9
Arkansas	6,168	3,515	2,387	1,128	2,472	181	4.7	4.7	4.9	4.1	4.6	7.7
California	55,360	27,100	14,706	12,394	24,866	3,394	4.2	3.8	3.8	3.8	4.0	10.0
Colorado	8,835	4,308	2,634	1,674	4,199	328	4.1	3.9	4.3	3.2	4.0	7.6
Connecticut	7,737	5,530	4,797	733	1,952	255	3.5	3.1	3.1	2.7	3.0	15.3
Delaware	1,370	778	701	77	537	55	3.9	3.3	3.3	(3)	3.9	(6)
Dist. of Columbia	1,041	771	166	605	207	63	6.8	6.4	8.4	5.8	6.3	(9)
Florida	13,963	4,498	2,846	1,652	8,669	796	3.9	4.1	4.1	4.1	3.4	7.7
Georgia	10,126	7,015	4,089	2,926	2,733	378	3.8	3.4	3.4	3.5	4.3	6.3
Idaho	3,594	1,745	1,069	676	1,741	108	2.2	1.8	2.0	1.5	2.2	7.4
Illinois	24,328	17,767	13,273	4,494	6,107	454	4.1	3.8	4.0	3.3	4.3	13.4
Indiana	14,406	10,152	7,119	3,033	4,015	239	4.2	3.8	3.7	4.1	4.6	12.6
Iowa	11,889	8,824	5,999	2,825	2,917	148	2.7	2.4	2.3	2.4	3.2	10.8
Kansas	9,970	6,052	3,838	2,214	3,688	230	2.8	2.3	2.4	2.3	3.2	8.3
Kentucky	6,798	4,807	3,526	1,281	1,849	142	8.0	8.1	8.1	8.1	7.7	7.7
Louisiana	9,291	6,660	4,334	2,326	2,389	242	5.0	5.1	5.1	5.1	4.5	7.0
Maine	3,949	2,974	2,278	696	856	119	3.4	3.4	3.3	3.7	3.2	5.0
Maryland	7,409	4,870	3,978	892	2,269	270	7.7	7.8	7.7	8.1	7.1	11.1
Massachusetts	15,854	12,750	10,494	2,256	2,682	422	3.4	3.1	3.0	3.7	4.0	9.2
Michigan	25,357	19,857	13,461	6,396	4,837	663	3.2	2.9	3.1	2.5	3.4	12.4
Minnesota	16,198	12,342	8,464	3,878	3,628	228	2.2	2.0	1.9	2.3	2.3	11.0
Mississippi	3,909	2,504	1,602	902	1,280	125	4.2	4.2	3.8	4.8	4.1	5.6
Missouri	15,543	10,479	7,120	3,359	4,783	281	3.9	3.8	3.8	4.0	3.9	7.8
Montana	3,833	2,206	1,329	877	1,517	110	2.8	2.4	2.3	2.7	2.8	9.1
Nebraska	6,608	4,464	2,950	1,514	1,998	146	2.4	2.1	2.2	1.9	2.7	8.9
Nevada	1,421	243	182	61	1,096	82	3.3	2.5	3.3	(0)	3.6	(2)
New Hampshire	2,859	1,746	1,487	259	1,011	102	2.5	2.2	2.4	1.5	2.5	6.9
New Jersey	17,481	12,200	8,811	3,389	4,731	550	4.4	3.9	3.8	4.1	4.2	17.6
New Mexico	4,326	1,686	1,126	560	2,439	201	5.5	6.2	5.9	7.0	4.7	8.5
New York	38,722	31,824	23,574	8,250	5,380	1,518	4.7	4.1	4.2	3.8	3.3	21.5
North Carolina	9,824	7,344	5,105	2,239	2,219	261	3.1	2.7	2.8	2.6	3.8	6.5
North Dakota	2,770	2,033	1,406	627	687	50	2.5	1.9	1.1	3.7	3.6	(5)
Ohio	31,588	23,443	17,125	6,318	7,555	590	4.3	3.8	3.7	4.1	5.2	10.8
Oklahoma	8,628	4,888	3,013	1,875	3,417	323	4.1	4.0	3.8	4.3	4.3	4.6
Oregon	10,491	4,846	2,693	2,153	5,274	371	2.8	2.8	2.9	2.6	2.7	5.9
Pennsylvania	36,094	30,549	24,534	6,015	5,005	540	4.6	4.5	4.5	4.8	4.1	15.4
Rhode Island	2,460	1,839	1,543	296	542	79	3.3	3.2	2.8	5.4	3.3	(4)
South Carolina	5,669	4,063	2,842	1,221	1,400	206	2.8	2.8	2.4	3.7	3.0	2.4
South Dakota	3,109	1,935	1,247	688	1,105	69	2.4	2.4	2.1	3.1	2.3	(2)
Tennessee	9,073	6,020	4,467	1,553	2,841	212	5.3	5.0	5.1	5.0	5.7	4.7
Texas	29,580	19,268	9,910	9,358	8,965	1,347	5.2	5.3	6.2	4.4	4.1	10.3
Utah	3,120	1,818	1,285	533	1,192	110	2.6	1.5	1.5	1.7	3.1	14.5
Vermont	1,931	1,307	1,090	217	554	70	3.2	3.3	3.6	1.8	2.7	(3)
Virginia	7,186	4,457	3,098	1,359	2,333	396	4.6	4.3	4.3	4.3	4.5	8.3
Washington	13,643	7,140	4,397	2,743	5,648	855	3.0	2.5	2.4	2.5	3.1	6.7
West Virginia	6,512	5,001	3,795	1,206	1,403	108	5.9	5.7	5.4	6.6	6.3	10.2
Wisconsin	11,706	9,187	6,399	2,788	2,358	161	2.3	1.9	2.0	1.8	2.4	18.0
Wyoming	2,028	874	618	256	1,077	77	3.1	3.4	3.4	3.5	2.5	(6)

* Where less than 100 tested, the number of reactors is given in parentheses.
** Includes recruits with prior military service.

Table C.5. Distributions by sizes of reactions to 0.0001 mg PPD-S for Navy recruits by state, race, and type of residence (ages 17–21, tested 1958–64)

	TOTAL	INDURATION TO PPD-S (IN GROUPS OF 2 MILLIMETERS)															
		0	2	4	6	8	10	12	14	16	18	20	22	24	26	28	≥30
ALABAMA																	
WHITE: ONE STATE	5047	4532	78	82	67	71	51	50	34	30	33	10	4	2	1		2
OTHER U S	2127	1875	30	42	28	35	21	26	19	15	17	11	5	2		1	
FOREIGN	256	211	5	6	6	4	5	4	4	4	5	2					
NEGRO	705	562	6	14	24	17	15	16	13	14	13	4	2	2	1	1	1
OTHER NONWHITE	4	3	1														
ARIZONA																	
WHITE: ONE STATE	1563	1336	23	35	29	17	19	21	22	18	12	12	9	3	4	2	1
OTHER U S	4299	3840	60	79	46	28	39	44	42	35	37	25	15	6	2		1
FOREIGN	306	264	5	5	7	4	4	3	3	3	3	1	3		1		
NEGRO	122	96	3	5		2	3		3	3	2	3		1	1		
OTHER NONWHITE	190	146	3	1	1		5	3	1	4	7	3	5	8	1	1	1
ARKANSAS																	
WHITE: ONE STATE	3515	3159	57	66	38	31	29	27	46	22	20	11	6	2	1		
OTHER U S	2472	2200	51	47	33	28	12	23	22	20	12	12	9		3		
FOREIGN	181	158	2	3	3	1	2	1	2	1	5		2				1
NEGRO	508	431	6	10	5	8	8	3	8	10	4	8	5		2		
OTHER NONWHITE	4	1			1					1	1						
CALIFORNIA																	
WHITE: ONE STATE	27100	25162	298	306	196	121	144	160	147	149	150	104	85	36	22	14	6
OTHER U S	24866	22907	307	319	201	148	165	156	172	133	121	91	70	46	23	3	4
FOREIGN	3394	2897	35	51	26	47	47	50	58	42	44	46	22	18	5	3	3
NEGRO	2075	1697	24	48	37	33	35	30	31	30	37	26	27	11	4	3	2
OTHER NONWHITE	1422	1092	32	30	19	31	23	23	19	31	33	42	16	22	3	6	
COLORADO																	
WHITE: ONE STATE	4308	3985	38	60	26	33	22	29	23	22	24	19	17	7	1	1	1
OTHER U S	4199	3858	52	60	34	25	29	23	26	23	25	24	11	4	2	1	2
FOREIGN	328	282	4	9	6	2	2	5	3	4	4	1	2	3	1		
NEGRO	88	75	2	4	1	3		1	2								
OTHER NONWHITE	177	156	1			2	3		1	5	3	1	2	2		1	
CONNECTICUT																	
WHITE: ONE STATE	5530	5217	57	46	23	17	29	31	25	26	25	19	7	4	1	1	2
OTHER U S	1952	1833	15	15	10	21	8	11	11	7	8	4	6		1	1	1
FOREIGN	255	201	2	2	8	3	4	9	6	4	7	4	4	1			
NEGRO	112	90	1	2	2	2	3	1	2	3	2	3	1				
OTHER NONWHITE	7	4	1								1	1					
DELAWARE																	
WHITE: ONE STATE	778	723	9	4	10	6	5	6	3	2	5	1	3	1			
OTHER U S	537	498	8	3	3	4	4	7	3	4		1	1				1
FOREIGN	55	45		2	2		2		2	1				1			
NEGRO	113	95		2		1	2	2	3	2	3	1	1		1		
OTHER NONWHITE	6	5									1						
DIST.OF COL.																	
WHITE: ONE STATE	771	690	12	4	6	10	8	10	11	7	5	4	3		1		
OTHER U S	207	183	3	1	2	5			3	5	4			1			
FOREIGN	63	52	1	1		1	2	1	2			1	1		1		
NEGRO	506	429	8	7	1	5	7	5	8	5	11	6	7	5	2		
OTHER NONWHITE	5	3	1					1									
FLORIDA																	
WHITE: ONE STATE	4498	3811	95	160	136	112	78	38	26	22	11	5	3	1			
OTHER U S	8669	7823	149	178	116	106	75	62	55	33	40	17	8	4	2	1	
FOREIGN	796	685	11	15	12	12	18	8	9	11	7	3	3	1	1		
NEGRO	517	361	7	22	20	30	25	21	11	9	5	2	3		1		
OTHER NONWHITE	10	9				1											
GEORGIA																	
WHITE: ONE STATE	7015	6274	129	165	119	87	68	57	41	30	19	13	8	4	1		
OTHER U S	2733	2440	47	60	42	27	22	24	20	14	23	6	8				
FOREIGN	378	334	8	3	8	1	5	8	2	4	1	2	2				
NEGRO	951	769	12	25	29	17	23	19	11	9	12	10	8	3	1	2	1
OTHER NONWHITE	7	6	1														

	TOTAL	INDURATION TO PPD-S (IN GROUPS OF 2 MILLIMETERS)															
		0	2	4	6	8	10	12	14	16	18	20	22	24	26	28	≥30
IDAHO																	
WHITE: ONE STATE	1745	1677	13	12	6	6	2	6	5	3	4	4	4	2	1		
OTHER U S	1741	1625	25	33	10	9	9	8	7	4	5	1	3	1		1	
FOREIGN	108	96	1	1		2		1	2	3				1			1
NEGRO	2	1		1													
OTHER NONWHITE	25	21						1	1				2				
ILLINOIS																	
WHITE: ONE STATE	17767	16470	207	163	129	127	125	105	118	103	97	59	29	20	9	3	3
OTHER U S	6107	5625	70	59	52	41	37	53	40	43	37	31	10	3	4	1	1
FOREIGN	454	366	7	8	7	5	9	18	9	4	7	5	5	2		1	1
NEGRO	2329	1799	30	38	39	29	51	49	69	54	63	48	27	17	9	4	3
OTHER NONWHITE	58	47	1				1	1	2	2		1	2				1
INDIANA																	
WHITE: ONE STATE	10152	9459	117	77	58	51	58	61	62	52	63	44	24	17	5	2	2
OTHER U S	4015	3673	67	34	32	23	24	29	26	33	31	20	16	3	2	2	
FOREIGN	239	196	2	2	1	8	3	2	5	7	5	4	3	1			
NEGRO	537	436	5	15	5	7	9	10	6	10	13	9	4	7	1		
OTHER NONWHITE	12	9						1					1	1			
IOWA																	
WHITE: ONE STATE	8824	8348	79	96	50	43	43	39	35	29	30	12	10	5	2		3
OTHER U S	2917	2717	37	32	17	21	21	13	17	11	7	8	10	2	3	1	
FOREIGN	148	124	2	2	2	2	3	4	2		1	1	3	1			1
NEGRO	80	73	1	1	1	2							2				
OTHER NONWHITE	20	12					1	1	1	2	1	1	1				
KANSAS																	
WHITE: ONE STATE	6052	5673	66	93	36	42	29	35	21	22	8	17	5	4			1
OTHER U S	3688	3439	29	52	25	25	18	18	23	23	16	10	7	2			1
FOREIGN	230	200	2	3	4	2	4	3	1	2	3	2	3	1			
NEGRO	389	327	4	7	15	9	4	4	5	3	4	4	3				
OTHER NONWHITE	47	35	1	1	2		2			1	2	1		1	1		
KENTUCKY																	
WHITE: ONE STATE	4807	4236	54	41	44	43	55	87	62	72	60	24	12	10	2	3	2
OTHER U S	1849	1639	26	11	16	14	20	20	38	18	21	10	9	6	1		
FOREIGN	142	127	1		1	2	1	2	4	2	1		1				
NEGRO	501	434	2	7	1	3	4	7	9	12	8	6	4	4			
LOUISIANA																	
WHITE: ONE STATE	6660	5606	151	240	170	154	107	86	52	42	21	15	10	5		1	
OTHER U S	2389	2055	54	84	46	42	33	23	13	11	9	10	5	1	2		1
FOREIGN	242	204	2	5	8	6	1	4	3	6		2		1			
NEGRO	1431	1093	19	45	52	54	38	29	36	23	21	9	5	5	2		
OTHER NONWHITE	17	11		1			1	2		1		1					
MAINE																	
WHITE: ONE STATE	2974	2799	27	20	17	9	14	13	12	21	11	8	12	8	3		
OTHER U S	856	811	5	4	8	1	7	4	3	3	3	4	3				
FOREIGN	119	111		1	1			2	2	1			1				
NEGRO	5	5															
OTHER NONWHITE	2	1				1											
MARYLAND																	
WHITE: ONE STATE	4870	4147	72	75	94	103	80	81	73	65	35	25	14	4	1	1	
OTHER U S	2269	1975	30	28	36	38	42	31	20	24	25	7	5	4	2	2	
FOREIGN	270	222	3	7	3	5	6	5	9	3	2	3	2				
NEGRO	540	409	3	9	9	9	9	12	17	19	10	13	12	3	2	1	3
OTHER NONWHITE	5	4												1			
MASSACHUSETTS																	
WHITE: ONE STATE	12750	12018	127	90	51	65	56	53	50	69	70	37	29	21	6	5	3
OTHER U S	2682	2478	39	20	22	15	19	15	26	10	17	10	5	2	3		1
FOREIGN	422	364	5	6	7	1	5	2	5	6	12	2	3	3		1	
NEGRO	126	103	2	2	4		1	6	1	2	2	1		1		1	
OTHER NONWHITE	19	17	1							1							

	TOTAL	INDURATION TO PPD-S (IN GROUPS OF 2 MILLIMETERS)															
		0	2	4	6	8	10	12	14	16	18	20	22	24	26	28	≥30
MICHIGAN																	
WHITE: ONE STATE	19857	18790	218	137	63	76	66	85	89	79	103	68	41	25	7	4	6
OTHER U S	4837	4532	55	35	29	22	32	22	28	11	23	29	6	10	1	1	1
FOREIGN	663	550	8	10	5	8	13	9	10	14	14	6	6	5	2	3	
NEGRO	1078	891	10	16	16	12	11	13	16	27	24	18	12	7	2	3	
OTHER NONWHITE	82	68		1	1	1		2		1	2	3	1	1		1	
MINNESOTA																	
WHITE: ONE STATE	12342	11785	140	90	44	38	49	32	24	19	43	37	17	16	4	3	1
OTHER U S	3628	3436	35	22	19	31	16	15	9	12	13	8	5			5	2
FOREIGN	228	189	2	3	4	5	4	3	4	4	4	3		1	1		1
NEGRO	89	75	1	2		1	2	2		1		1	2		1	1	
OTHER NONWHITE	99	82		1	1	4			1	5	1	2		1	1		
MISSISSIPPI																	
WHITE: ONE STATE	2504	2205	48	69	44	34	28	23	16	14	11	7	3	1			1
OTHER U S	1280	1123	24	29	29	23	19	10	12	6	1	3	1				
FOREIGN	125	107	1	2	3	5	2	2	1		1		1				
NEGRO	403	318	8	13	13	12	14	8	8	3	1	3	2				
OTHER NONWHITE	4	4															
MISSOURI																	
WHITE: ONE STATE	10479	9731	107	104	67	67	64	70	78	66	55	32	19	9	5	3	2
OTHER U S	4783	4405	54	58	47	32	28	36	39	28	23	15	11	5	2		
FOREIGN	281	245	5	3	3	3	3	2	5	1	5	4	1	1			
NEGRO	877	729	13	22	14	6	18	18	9	19	7	7	4	9	2		
OTHER NONWHITE	19	14		1					1		1	1	1				
MONTANA																	
WHITE: ONE STATE	2206	2088	19	24	15	6	8	9	6	8	9	6	5	2	1		
OTHER U S	1517	1419	14	27	6	9	10	7	6	7	2	4	3		2	1	
FOREIGN	110	96	1			3	3	1	1	2	2	1					
NEGRO	5	5															
OTHER NONWHITE	92	51		2	1	3	4	6	4	2	4	4	3	4	2	2	
NEBRASKA																	
WHITE: ONE STATE	4464	4216	52	62	25	16	18	15	10	14	9	10	5	5	3	2	2
OTHER U S	1998	1869	19	31	11	15	8	9	7	10	11	6	1	1			
FOREIGN	146	128	2	1	1	1	1	2		2	2	2	1	1	1	1	
NEGRO	99	75	1	3	3	1	4	2	1	1	2		4	1			1
OTHER NONWHITE	35	23		1			1	1		1	3	1	1	2	1		
NEVADA																	
WHITE: ONE STATE	243	232	3		1	1		4		1		1					
OTHER U S	1096	1015	14	14	9	5	7	9	3	11	2	5	1		1		
FOREIGN	82	77		1	2			1				1					
NEGRO	50	38	3	4	1	1		1	1		1						
OTHER NONWHITE	19	9			1		1		2	1	2	3					
NEW HAMPSHIRE																	
WHITE: ONE STATE	1746	1677	14	5	8	3	7	6	3	5	4	7	4	1		1	1
OTHER U S	1011	970	9	3	2	2	2	3	7	3	4	2	2		1	1	
FOREIGN	102	90	1		1	3		2			1	1	2	1			
NEGRO	4	4															
OTHER NONWHITE	2	2															
NEW JERSEY																	
WHITE: ONE STATE	12200	11281	125	134	105	77	78	75	80	68	57	43	45	16	10	3	3
OTHER U S	4731	4357	55	43	43	34	29	33	33	32	26	19	8	12	4	1	2
FOREIGN	550	416	5	11	11	10	17	17	15	9	16	10	4	6	3		
NEGRO	822	681	7	19	12	5	10	14	13	16	12	14	8	7	4		
OTHER NONWHITE	22	11	1	1		1	1		1		3	2	1				
NEW MEXICO																	
WHITE: ONE STATE	1686	1513	29	18	13	8	13	12	21	14	12	18	8	6		1	
OTHER U S	2439	2215	23	38	28	20	17	19	11	21	22	10	4	7	3		1
FOREIGN	201	172	2	4	3	3	1	2	4	3	3	2	2				
NEGRO	46	38		2	1	1	1			2	1						
OTHER NONWHITE	267	208	4	5	5	3	3	5	6	8	6	6	6	1		1	

	TOTAL	INDURATION TO PPD-S (IN GROUPS OF 2 MILLIMETERS)															
		0	2	4	6	8	10	12	14	16	18	20	22	24	26	28	≥30
NEW YORK																	
WHITE: ONE STATE	31824	29594	339	242	185	152	189	252	220	199	182	131	83	37	12	5	2
OTHER U S	5380	5029	61	38	34	38	29	48	32	25	16	14	10	2	3		1
FOREIGN	1518	1080	19	28	24	40	50	55	42	52	48	35	26	12	5	1	1
NEGRO	1119	871	9	21	20	28	22	23	26	28	26	21	11	6	1	4	2
OTHER NONWHITE	217	160	1	5	4	3	5	7	4	6	8	4	6	1	3		
NORTH CAROLINA																	
WHITE: ONE STATE	7344	6726	114	137	95	73	40	40	37	29	28	15	4	3		1	2
OTHER U S	2219	2028	26	36	28	17	13	20	12	16	12	3	5	1	2		
FOREIGN	261	231	2	6	3	2	7	4	1		1	2		2			
NEGRO	988	790	17	33	24	24	21	17	18	8	14	9	5	6	1	1	
OTHER NONWHITE	70	54	2	4	5	3				1		1					
NORTH DAKOTA																	
WHITE: ONE STATE	2033	1943	23	9	10	9	2	6	6	9	5	4	3	2	1	1	
OTHER U S	687	650	6	2	2	2	2	3	4	3	6		1	4	2		
FOREIGN	50	42	1	1		1	1			1	1	1				1	
OTHER NONWHITE	37	18			1		2	1	3	2	1	1	3	4		1	
OHIO																	
WHITE: ONE STATE	23443	21908	256	159	115	120	160	132	159	144	125	80	47	24	8	2	4
OTHER U S	7555	6906	74	79	52	49	52	72	77	61	48	34	27	16	3	1	4
FOREIGN	590	481	7	10	13	15	8	13	10	12	11	6	3	1			
NEGRO	1885	1572	28	28	22	18	15	24	40	31	41	27	17	13	4	3	2
OTHER NONWHITE	33	25						1	3	2	1		1				
OKLAHOMA																	
WHITE: ONE STATE	4888	4478	54	70	55	36	36	35	33	34	28	12	9	5	3		
OTHER U S	3417	3100	54	54	38	25	25	28	28	27	14	12	6	4	1	1	
FOREIGN	323	291	2	6	4	5	2	3	2	2	2	2					
NEGRO	458	371	5	10	8	10	3	12	12	9	8	5	4			1	
OTHER NONWHITE	276	209	3	6	2		5	7	5	8	14	7	4	4	1		1
OREGON																	
WHITE: ONE STATE	4846	4601	47	38	19	7	16	16	20	25	18	18	8	8	1		4
OTHER U S	5274	4954	60	64	29	25	16	17	15	22	25	26	9	6	3	1	2
FOREIGN	371	336	6	4	3		3	3	5	3	3	3	2				
NEGRO	37	35	1						1								
OTHER NONWHITE	53	36	1	3	1			1	1	4	3	1	1				1
PENNSYLVANIA																	
WHITE: ONE STATE	30549	28099	336	291	229	211	212	252	224	218	203	116	89	38	15	12	4
OTHER U S	5005	4631	58	44	31	38	36	27	33	30	31	19	14	10	2	1	
FOREIGN	540	425	5	5	9	13	12	21	14	12	11	6	4		2	1	
NEGRO	1537	1253	20	28	25	14	14	34	31	40	24	20	13	12	4	3	2
OTHER NONWHITE	32	29										2				1	
RHODE ISLAND																	
WHITE: ONE STATE	1839	1724	17	15	12	12	13	6	7	11	11	5	1	2	2		1
OTHER U S	542	507	2	5	4	6	2	1	4	1	4	2	1	2		1	
FOREIGN	79	72	1	1				2		2							
NEGRO	29	24	1							1			2		1		
OTHER NONWHITE	8	7								1							
SOUTH CAROLINA																	
WHITE: ONE STATE	4063	3639	73	103	88	48	34	17	21	8	22	6	1	2		1	
OTHER U S	1400	1276	30	24	17	11	11	9	7	8	4	1	1	1			
FOREIGN	206	183	5	4	7	2		1	2	1				1			
NEGRO	565	432	7	27	19	16	21	12	8	9	7	3	3	1			
OTHER NONWHITE	5	4						1									
SOUTH DAKOTA																	
WHITE: ONE STATE	1935	1848	16	16	6	2	12	11	6	5	6	2	3			1	1
OTHER U S	1105	1041	11	16	6	6	1	6	5	3	4	3	1			2	
FOREIGN	69	66		1								1				1	
NEGRO	7	5										1	1				
OTHER NONWHITE	143	71			3		1	2	8	20	6	10	12	6	3		1

196

INDURATION TO PPD-S (IN GROUPS OF 2 MILLIMETERS)

	TOTAL	0	2	4	6	8	10	12	14	16	18	20	22	24	26	28	≥30
TENNESSEE																	
WHITE: ONE STATE	6020	5487	68	80	28	53	46	61	53	47	45	22	20	5	2	2	1
OTHER U S	2841	2561	42	37	17	21	24	33	32	18	26	12	11	6	1		
FOREIGN	212	186	5	10		1	3	2	1	1			1		1	1	
NEGRO	896	755	7	21	9	9	10	20	20	23	10		5	3	4		
OTHER NONWHITE	3	2										1					
TEXAS																	
WHITE: ONE STATE	19268	16873	358	458	323	238	231	215	155	135	110	84	37	28	14	7	2
OTHER U S	8965	8013	140	200	146	96	77	69	85	43	44	22	19	9	1	1	
FOREIGN	1347	1123	21	24	22	18	20	19	23	32	18	14	8	3	1	1	
NEGRO	2069	1627	31	72	69	51	56	35	38	26	18	14	14	13	2	2	1
OTHER NONWHITE	352	255	8	6	10	7	10	5	9	11	11	7	7	4	1	1	
UTAH																	
WHITE: ONE STATE	1818	1736	19	17	11	7	11	7	3		4	2	1				
OTHER U S	1192	1102	11	19	11	12	12	4	5	7	2	2	1	2		2	
FOREIGN	110	84	3	2	3	2	3	2	3	1	3	4					
NEGRO	6	6															
OTHER NONWHITE	33	30	1			1							1				
VERMONT																	
WHITE: ONE STATE	1307	1232	21	4	3	4	4	5	5	9	4	4	11				1
OTHER U S	554	528	4	4	3		3		1	2	3	5	1				
FOREIGN	70	65	1			1			1			2					
NEGRO	4	3										1					
VIRGINIA																	
WHITE: ONE STATE	4457	4081	53	63	35	32	37	48	30	30	22	16	6	4			
OTHER U S	2333	2109	38	35	22	24	26	22	18	14	11	11	1	2			
FOREIGN	396	348	5	4	1	5	6	6	7	6	3	4	1				
NEGRO	1087	920	16	16	12	17	16	10	26	9	17	12	7	4		2	
OTHER NONWHITE	7	5		1							1						
WASHINGTON																	
WHITE: ONE STATE	7140	6790	64	60	35	16	23	22	31	21	25	15	16	10	7	4	1
OTHER U S	5648	5304	66	59	26	18	24	28	26	32	21	23	9	9	3		
FOREIGN	855	760	9	9	8	12	8	16	9	9	5	1	5	1	1	1	1
NEGRO	82	70	2	2	1			1	1		3		1		1		
OTHER NONWHITE	112	85	1		3	2	3	3	2	2	3	2	1	2	2	1	
WEST VIRGINIA																	
WHITE: ONE STATE	5001	4525	79	43	24	46	26	62	48	54	38	31	15	3	5	2	
OTHER U S	1403	1261	19	11	13	11	17	13	15	16	9	8	8		1		1
FOREIGN	108	91	2	2	1	1	2	1	1	4	1	2					
NEGRO	156	135	1	2	3	1	4	2	4	1	1	1	1				
OTHER NONWHITE	1	1															
WISCONSIN																	
WHITE: ONE STATE	9187	8790	90	57	41	30	24	34	25	24	33	18	8	5	3	3	2
OTHER U S	2358	2225	33	18	22	3	9	8	9	13	6	7	2	1			2
FOREIGN	161	126	1	3	2		2	5	6	7			4	5			
NEGRO	94	79	1	3		1			1		1		3	4	1		
OTHER NONWHITE	68	62		1	1				1				1	1	1		
WYOMING																	
WHITE: ONE STATE	874	820	5	12	6	1	2	5	3	9	5	3	1	2			
OTHER U S	1077	1011	8	14	10	7	4	8	4	2	4	2	3				
FOREIGN	77	66	1	1	2	1		2	2			1		1			
OTHER NONWHITE	28	22				1		1				1	1		1	1	

197

Table C.6. Number of Negro Navy recruits tested, and percent with reactions of 10 or more mm to 0.0001 mg PPD-S, by type of residence, by state (ages 17–21, tested 1958–64)

	NUMBER TESTED			PERCENT REACTORS*		
	Total	Lifetime One-state	Not One-state	Total	Lifetime One-state	Not One-state
TOTAL	26,129	17,221	8,908	12.0	11.4	13.1
Alabama	705	540	165	11.6	10.4	15.8
Arizona	122	34	88	13.1	(3)	(13)
Arkansas	508	377	131	9.4	9.8	8.4
California	2,075	771	1,304	11.4	10.6	11.8
Colorado	88	22	66	(3)	(0)	(3)
Connecticut	112	48	64	13.4	(3)	(12)
Delaware	113	72	41	13.3	(9)	(6)
Dist. of Columbia	506	358	148	11.1	11.2	10.8
Florida	517	352	165	14.9	12.8	19.4
Georgia	951	774	177	10.4	10.1	11.9
Idaho	2	–	2	(0)	–	(0)
Illinois	2,329	1,363	966	16.9	17.5	16.1
Indiana	537	307	230	12.8	12.7	13.0
Iowa	80	48	32	(2)	(2)	(0)
Kansas	389	245	144	6.9	3.7	12.5
Kentucky	501	409	92	10.8	10.3	(12)
Louisiana	1,431	1,199	232	11.7	11.2	14.7
Maine	5	4	1	(0)	(0)	(0)
Maryland	540	422	118	18.7	18.7	18.6
Massachusetts	126	81	45	11.9	(9)	(6)
Michigan	1,078	576	502	12.3	10.6	14.3
Minnesota	89	40	49	(10)	(0)	(10)
Mississippi	403	287	116	9.7	8.7	12.1
Missouri	877	548	329	10.6	11.3	9.4
Montana	5	4	1	(0)	(0)	(0)
Nebraska	99	52	47	(16)	(8)	(8)
Nevada	50	7	43	(3)	(0)	(3)
New Hampshire	4	3	1	(0)	(0)	(0)
New Jersey	822	505	317	11.9	12.7	10.7
New Mexico	46	9	37	(4)	(2)	(2)
New York	1,119	629	490	15.2	13.2	17.8
North Carolina	988	744	244	10.1	9.0	13.5
North Dakota	–	–	–	–	–	–
Ohio	1,885	1,145	740	11.5	11.4	11.6
Oklahoma	458	345	113	11.8	10.7	15.0
Oregon	37	15	22	(1)	(1)	(0)
Pennsylvania	1,537	1,091	446	12.8	12.7	13.0
Rhode Island	29	15	14	(4)	(1)	(3)
South Carolina	565	445	120	11.3	10.8	13.3
South Dakota	7	4	3	(2)	(1)	(1)
Tennessee	896	647	249	10.6	10.7	10.4
Texas	2,069	1,703	366	10.6	9.9	13.7
Utah	6	2	4	(0)	(0)	(0)
Vermont	4	3	1	(1)	(1)	(0)
Virginia	1,087	815	272	9.5	8.7	11.8
Washington	82	18	64	(7)	(1)	(6)
West Virginia	156	119	37	9.0	9.2	(3)
Wisconsin	94	24	70	(10)	(3)	(7)
Wyoming	–	–	–	–	–	–

* Where less than 100 tested, the number of reactors is given in parentheses.

198

Table C.7. Distributions by sizes of reactions to 0.0001 mg PPD-S for Navy recruits, tuberculosis contacts, and non-contacts, by state (tested 1960–64)

WHITE, AGES 17 TO 21 YEARS, LIFETIME U.S. RESIDENTS

	TOTAL	INDURATION TO PPD-S (IN GROUPS OF 2 MILLIMETERS)															
		0	2	4	6	8	10	12	14	16	18	20	22	24	26	28	≥30
ALABAMA																	
TB CONTACTS	137	87	3		1	6	8	4	8	6	10	1	3				
NON CONTACTS	4314	3904	61	75	60	58	37	36	24	22	19	10	3	1	1	1	2
ARIZONA																	
TB CONTACTS	197	123	3	2	3		11	10	9	12	7	7	4	4	1	1	
NON CONTACTS	3855	3480	54	69	38	32	32	33	34	26	26	14	11	1	2	1	2
ARKANSAS																	
TB CONTACTS	139	96	2	1	4	2	2	4	5	4	5	8	5		1		
NON CONTACTS	3596	3256	65	66	46	34	21	29	33	19	15	7	4		1		
CALIFORNIA																	
TB CONTACTS	1209	922	14	9	14	8	18	26	40	38	43	22	32	12	5	4	2
NON CONTACTS	33483	31263	342	377	280	170	197	172	182	152	116	101	64	36	19	9	3
COLORADO																	
TB CONTACTS	175	134	2	1		3		3	6	8	5	3	4	3	1		2
NON CONTACTS	5477	5112	54	62	48	35	28	25	27	23	25	16	13	7		1	1
CONNECTICUT																	
TB CONTACTS	134	90	2	2	1	2	3	2	6	9	7	5	3		1		1
NON CONTACTS	4850	4646	26	36	20	22	13	20	20	13	18	7	6	1	1	1	
DELAWARE																	
TB CONTACTS	25	17	2				1	1	1	1		2				
NON CONTACTS	841	804	2	3	11	3	5	3	3	2	4		1				
DIST. OF COL.																	
TB CONTACTS	22	14		·		1				2	5					
NON CONTACTS	630	576	5	2	6	9	4	7	10	2	3	4	1		1		
FLORIDA																	
TB CONTACTS	202	136	2	9	4	6	1	10	7	11	8	3	2	2	1		
NON CONTACTS	8790	7879	140	182	176	145	94	54	51	27	24	10	5	1	1	1	
GEORGIA																	
TB CONTACTS	157	114	3	2		5	4	7	9	2	8	1	1		1		
NON CONTACTS	6227	5613	88	129	114	78	59	39	34	28	21	11	11	2			
IDAHO																	
TB CONTACTS	62	51		1				2	3	2		2		1		
NON CONTACTS	2078	1989	20	24	9	9	6	7	5	2	2	3	1	1			
ILLINOIS																	
TB CONTACTS	431	321	2	3	5	4	14	11	12	21	12	13	7	2	1	1	2
NON CONTACTS	14882	14027	106	111	94	94	84	83	84	63	55	42	14	18	6		1
INDIANA																	
TB CONTACTS	271	211	1	3	3	1	2	7	5	11	10	9	4	3	1		
NON CONTACTS	8665	8179	70	49	54	33	38	51	54	38	41	29	15	8	2	3	1
IOWA																	
TB CONTACTS	166	125	4	1	1		2	4	8	4	5	6	5	1			
NON CONTACTS	7568	7207	53	70	45	41	42	31	22	16	19	6	10	4	1	1	
KANSAS																	
TB CONTACTS	166	134		3	1	2	3	3	3	5	4	5	2			1	
NON CONTACTS	6330	5966	59	87	44	38	29	32	27	20	11	8	7	2			
KENTUCKY																	
TB CONTACTS	197	130			2	1	4	8	10	13	15	7	1	4	1	1	
NON CONTACTS	4034	3669	28	27	27	26	37	58	54	39	32	18	10	9			
LOUISIANA																	
TB CONTACTS	143	94	4	8	4	7	2	6	4	4	3	3	4				
NON CONTACTS	5678	4826	139	190	140	135	93	63	37	19	16	13	3	2	1		1

	TOTAL	INDURATION TO PPD-S (IN GROUPS OF 2 MILLIMETERS)															
		0	2	4	6	8	10	12	14	16	18	20	22	24	26	28	≥30
MAINE																	
TB CONTACTS	75	53					2			4	4	4	1	5	2			
NON CONTACTS	2414	2332	5	9	15	7	13	4	5	9	4	4	5	2			
MARYLAND																	
TB CONTACTS	130	80	3		2	4	9	7	4	9	7	2	1	1		1	
NON CONTACTS	4627	4055	39	55	73	85	76	67	63	51	30	14	13	5	1		
MASSACHUSETTS																	
TB CONTACTS	248	171	1	2	4	1	5	7	10	14	17	5	4	6		1	
NON CONTACTS	9910	9509	41	49	44	40	38	34	30	37	36	19	18	9	3		3
MICHIGAN																	
TB CONTACTS	416	326	2	1	4	2	6	7	12	11	16	15	6	7			1
NON CONTACTS	15203	14618	82	68	52	41	51	57	59	42	50	41	22	11	4	2	3
MINNESOTA																	
TB CONTACTS	274	225	3		3		2	6	3	4	10	9	5	3	1		
NON CONTACTS	10616	10260	65	59	32	48	37	25	21	10	20	16	10	6	5	1	1
MISSISSIPPI																	
TB CONTACTS	59	43	1	1	1	1	3	1	2	2	2	2					
NON CONTACTS	2243	1995	31	59	49	28	28	17	11	12	6	3	3	1			
MISSOURI																	
TB CONTACTS	342	251	4	4	4	7	6	3	14	11	14	10	10	3	1		
NON CONTACTS	9541	8949	76	92	71	58	51	62	60	44	31	20	14	5	5	2	1
MONTANA																	
TB CONTACTS	64	61						1				1					1	
NON CONTACTS	2301	2178	21	25	17	11	9	9	7	11	7		5	1			
NEBRASKA																	
TB CONTACTS	83	63	1	1		1	4	3	3		1	2	2		1	1	
NON CONTACTS	4111	3878	44	64	28	19	16	14	9	13	10	8	2	1	2	1	2
NEVADA																	
TB CONTACTS	33	25	2		1		1	1		1	1				1		
NON CONTACTS	923	867	11	8	8	4	4	8	2	7	1	2	1				
NEW HAMPSHIRE																	
TB CONTACTS	44	34				1	2				2	1	1	1			1	1
NON CONTACTS	1798	1751	7	4	7	5	2	5	6	2	4	3	2				
NEW JERSEY																	
TB CONTACTS	241	162	2	3	2	4	6	7	8	14	11	10	7	2	3		
NON CONTACTS	11186	10507	73	90	97	63	65	63	57	44	50	28	27	15	5	1	1
NEW MEXICO																	
TB CONTACTS	90	66		1	1	2	4	1	2	4	4	2	1	1	1		
NON CONTACTS	2611	2402	30	27	27	18	10	19	18	21	14	12	8	4	1		
NEW YORK																	
TB CONTACTS	550	370	2	5	8	7	22	14	26	31	21	28	10	3	3		
NON CONTACTS	24640	23333	153	148	129	99	119	172	129	124	93	65	49	16	6	2	3
NORTH CAROLINA																	
TB CONTACTS	151	110		2	1	2	2	5	8	7	7	6	1				
NON CONTACTS	5921	5485	69	97	82	53	34	30	25	18	18	5	5				
NORTH DAKOTA																	
TB CONTACTS	46	36				1				2	2	2		2		1	
NON CONTACTS	1767	1704	8	7	7	10	4	5	7	5	5	1	1	1	2		
OHIO																	
TB CONTACTS	565	421	4	2	5	9	12	14	25	18	20	17	7	8	2		1
NON CONTACTS	19818	18767	114	134	94	94	110	99	118	96	83	57	29	13	3	2	5

	TOTAL	INDURATION TO PPD-S (IN GROUPS OF 2 MILLIMETERS)															
		0	2	4	6	8	10	12	14	16	18	20	22	24	26	28	≈30
OKLAHOMA																	
TB CONTACTS	166	124	1	1	3	2	3	1	7	11	5	2	3	2	1		
NON CONTACTS	5202	4781	68	76	68	41	34	36	29	27	19	12	5	3	2	1	
OREGON																	
TB CONTACTS	272	217	1	1	2	1	1	3	7	5	12	10	4	5	2	1	
NON CONTACTS	6115	5852	51	46	33	17	21	17	14	20	17	16	6	3			2
PENNSYLVANIA																	
TB CONTACTS	460	296	2	3	7	4	12	17	29	26	23	21	12	4	2	1	1
NON CONTACTS	22765	21345	157	166	139	141	146	154	143	131	110	57	40	20	8	6	2
RHODE ISLAND																	
TB CONTACTS	52	34			1	2	1	3	3	2	4	1		1			
NON CONTACTS	1637	1563	8	10	12	8	7	2	5	8	7	4	1	2			
SOUTH CAROLINA																	
TB CONTACTS	58	39	1	1	1	2	1	1	3	3	5	1					
NON CONTACTS	3434	3123	53	71	67	35	30	18	13	4	13	4	1	1		1	
SOUTH DAKOTA																	
TB CONTACTS	38	33		1					3			1					
NON CONTACTS	2005	1925	10	19	9	8	7	10	5	2	4	1	2			2	1
TENNESSEE																	
TB CONTACTS	236	169			3		2	6	14	8	9	9	7	5	3	1	
NON CONTACTS	5492	5077	49	55	32	31	40	53	52	36	37	14	11	3	1	1	
TEXAS																	
TB CONTACTS	538	366	8	10	11	17	11	19	26	16	18	11	14	9	2		
NON CONTACTS	18475	16373	308	414	339	221	200	186	132	107	75	63	20	19	9	7	2
UTAH																	
TB CONTACTS	25	18			1	1	1		2		1			1			
NON CONTACTS	1833	1727	20	26	16	9	14	6	5	3	3	1	1	1		1	
VERMONT																	
TB CONTACTS	23	19									1	1	1				1
NON CONTACTS	1173	1127	5	6	5	1	3	5	3	7	3	3	5				
VIRGINIA																	
TB CONTACTS	127	87			4	1	1	3	3	11	3	4	8	2			
NON CONTACTS	4245	3955	35	53	30	24	38	41	16	21	17	10	3	2			
WASHINGTON																	
TB CONTACTS	280	228	2	2			2	4	3	10	6	7	6	7	2	1	
NON CONTACTS	7748	7416	59	50	35	23	30	20	29	19	22	22	9	7	6	1	
WEST VIRGINIA																	
TB CONTACTS	104	66	2	1			4	7	9	4	7	4					
NON CONTACTS	3672	3414	31	23	21	29	20	37	21	26	19	16	9	3	3		
WISCONSIN																	
TB CONTACTS	167	138	1		4			3	3	6	1	4	4	2			1
NON CONTACTS	7058	6832	32	26	33	19	25	21	15	18	18	14	3			1	1
WYOMING																	
TB CONTACTS	30	24						1	1	1	2	1					
NON CONTACTS	1274	1196	12	17	12	5	3	8	4	6	5	2	2	2			

NEGRO, AGES 17 TO 21 YEARS, LIFETIME U.S. RESIDENTS

	TOTAL	0	2	4	6	8	10	12	14	16	18	20	22	24	26	28	≈30
TB CONTACTS	537	317	2	12	7	8	15	22	24	37	24	32	13	11	7	5	1
NON CONTACTS	16847	13902	197	373	349	279	297	298	288	244	244	167	114	64	12	11	8

Table C.8. Distributions by sizes of reactions to 0.0001 mg PPD-S for school, university, and community programs, by age and race (tested 1956–64)

	TOTAL	INDURATION TO PPD-S (IN GROUPS OF 2 MILLIMETERS)															
		0	2	4	6	8	10	12	14	16	18	20	22	24	26	28	≥30
SCHOOL PROGRAMS																	
GEORGIA:																	
Augusta — White	762	704	8	6	9	3	5	3	4	3	7	7	2	1			
Augusta — Negro	331	262	4	9	9	16	3	5	2	6	4	7	2	1	1		
Columbus Area — White	3631	3307	181	51	21	16	10	8	11	12	6	5	3				
Columbus Area — Negro	3845	3421	116	72	55	38	32	16	20	23	20	17	10	4	1		
Jones-Twiggs Counties — White	1608	1450	85	31	10	11	6	5	3	2	2	3					
Jones-Twiggs Counties — Negro	2060	1752	122	36	21	38	23	20	6	8	6	9	12	1	3	2	1
Stewart County — White	436	236	158	28	7		2		2		2		1				
Stewart County — Negro	1444	706	447	147	48	41	19	12	7	6	5	3	2		1		
Whitfield-Murray Counties — White	8006	4858	2317	489	71	36	20	23	41	45	32	32	23	9	6	3	1
Whitfield-Murray Counties — Negro	272	133	99	13	2	1		2	3	2		3	4	8	2		
MARYLAND:																	
Montgomery County — White	2785	1881	614	165	29	17	16	14	13	13	11	8	3				1
Montgomery County — Negro	407	232	105	29	3	3	2		6	3	7	6	3	2	2	4	
Washington County — White	7637	7317	45	55	47	42	26	17	26	30	17	12	2	1			
Washington County — Negro	138	127			5			1	1	1	1	2					
MASSACHUSETTS:																	
Holyoke — White	1144	1046	31	11	8	6	10	6	2	4	7	6	4	2	1		
MINNESOTA:																	
Robbinsdale — White	12862	12523	117	60	47	31	35	21	8	7	9	2	2				
NORTH DAKOTA:																	
Williston — White	1045	991	11	12	10	8	7			2	2	1	1				
UNIVERSITY PROGRAMS																	
Univ. of Alabama — White	1592	1359	16	45	53	38	30	23	14	6	4	2	1	1			
Univ. of Kentucky — White	1889	1777	20	12	16	11	8	13	9	7	8	5	3				
Univ. of N. Dakota — White	799	739	25	6	1	2	4	1	4	4	5	3	5				
Univ. of Wisconsin — White	2085	1825	113	67	19	14	8	10	6	4	9	5	5				
Utah Universities — White	4755	4203	144	111	109	56	47	29	15	12	8	6	6	3	3	1	2
Georgia Colleges — White	3595	3129	137	85	50	36	45	30	34	16	19	8	4	1		1	
Georgia Colleges — Negro	264	189	9	6	4	8	15	11	2	10	3	3	4				
COMMUNITY PROGRAMS																	
MASSACHUSETTS:																	
Plainville (White) Ages 0–19	1636	1493	100	22	1	7	3			1	4	1	2			1	1
Plainville (White) 20–39	543	329	40	19	8	10	9	24	19	20	22	10	25	6	2		
Plainville (White) 40–59	419	109	9	14	10	15	15	28	36	51	57	22	32	9	8	3	1
Plainville (White) 60+	99	26	2	6	4	4	4	6	13	8	10	7	2	5	2		
MINNESOTA:																	
Austin (White) Ages 0–19	76	72		3		1											
Austin (White) 20–39	2096	1596	19	63	36	68	98	81	62	34	27	9	2		1		
Austin (White) 40–59	1670	738	14	42	65	112	181	205	149	80	61	17	4	2			
Austin (White) 60+	257	84	2	9	17	28	30	37	19	16	11	3	1				
Polk County (White) Ages 0–19	5002	4712	140	45	22	25	16	12	2	4	5	7	8	1	2	1	
Polk County (White) 20–39	2012	1633	40	36	19	19	24	29	31	40	47	23	34	15	16	4	2
Polk County (White) 40–59	2162	1350	34	27	15	17	43	49	80	117	112	95	108	50	41	9	15
Polk County (White) 60+	1006	446	5	19	16	22	31	51	71	74	75	50	64	40	22	2	18
NORTH CAROLINA:																	
Pamlico Co. (White) Ages 0–19	1882	1566	104	90	47	28	19	13	7	7		1					
Pamlico Co. (White) 20–39	793	470	57	66	29	28	30	34	31	22	10	7	5	1	2	1	
Pamlico Co. (White) 40–59	838	410	49	55	32	41	50	59	48	48	15	15	7	5	2	1	1
Pamlico Co. (White) 60+	398	172	31	20	19	19	29	32	21	22	21	8	3	1			
Pamlico Co. (Negro) Ages 0–19	1473	1069	122	78	53	33	30	22	23	21	12	7	1		1	1	
Pamlico Co. (Negro) 20–39	552	225	38	28	32	22	22	36	46	37	31	15	12	3	2	2	1
Pamlico Co. (Negro) 40–59	397	87	17	12	18	16	24	41	46	50	44	17	13	7	3	2	
Pamlico Co. (Negro) 60+	171	35	5	6	8	3	14	14	21	26	12	15	5	4	3		

References / I

CHAPTER 1

1. Winslow, C.-E. A., Smillie, W. G., Doull, J. A., and Gordon, J. E., *The History of American Epidemiology* (St. Louis: C. V. Mosby Co., 1952).

Gordon, M. B., *Aesculapius Comes to the Colonies: The Story of the Early Days of Medicine in the Thirteen Original Colonies* (Ventnor, N.J.: Ventnor Publishers, 1949).

Smith, S., *The City That Was* (New York: F. Allaben, 1911).

Cummins, S. L., *Tuberculosis in History, from the 17th century to Our Own Times* (London: Baillière, Tindall & Cox, 1949).

2. Morse, D., Brothwell, D. R., and Ucko, P. J., "Tuberculosis in Ancient Egypt," *Am. Rev. Resp. Dis.*, 90:524–541 (1964).

3. Pott, P., *Remarks on That Kind of Palsy of the Lower Limbs, Which Is Frequently Found to Accompany a Curvature of the Spine* (London: J. Johnson, 1779).

4. Castiglioni, A., *History of Tuberculosis* (New York: Medical Life Press, 1933).

Webb, G. B., "Tuberculosis," *Clio Medica*, vol. 16 (New York: Paul B. Hoeber, 1936).

5. Walsh, J., "Galen's treatment of pulmonary tuberculosis," *Am. Rev. Tuberc.*, 24:1–14 (1931).

6. Burke, R. M., *An Historical Chronology of Tuberculosis*, 2nd ed. (Springfield: Charles C Thomas, 1955).

7. Laënnec, R. T. H., *De l'Auscultation médiate* (Paris: J. A. Brosson & J. S. Chande, 1819).

8. Villemin, J. A., "Cause et nature de la tuberculose: Son inoculation de l'homme au lapin," *Compt. Rend. Acad. Sci.*, 61:1012–1015 (1865); *Etudes sur la tuberculose, preuves rationelles et expérimentales de sa spécificité et de son inoculabilité* (Paris: J. B. Ballière, 1868).

9. Koch, R., "Die Aetiologie der Tuberkulose," *Berliner Klinische Wochenschrift*, 19:221–230 (1882).

10. Osler, Sir William, *The Evolution of Modern Medicine* (New Haven: Yale University Press, 1923).

11. Holyoke, E. A., "A bill of mortality for the town of Salem, for the year 1782," *Mem. Am. Acad. Arts and Sciences*, 1:546 (1783).

Shattuck, L., "On the vital statistics of Boston," *Am. J. Med. Sci.*, 1:369 (1841).

12. Shattuck, L., *Report of the Sanitary Commission of Massachusetts, 1850*, reprinted (Cambridge, Mass.: Harvard University Press, 1948).

13. U.S. Department of Health, Education, and Welfare, *The Future of Tuberculosis Control: A Report to the Surgeon General of the Public Health Service by a Task Force on Tuberculosis Control*, Public Health Service Publication No. 1119 (Washington, D.C., December, 1963).

14. Winslow, C.-E. A., *The Life of Hermann M. Biggs* (Philadelphia: Lea & Febiger, 1929).

15. Philip, Sir R. W., *Public Aspects of the Prevention of Consumption* (Edinburgh: Morrison and Gibb, 1908).

Philip, Sir R. W., *Collected Papers on Tuberculosis* (London: Oxford University Press, 1937).

16. Drolet, G. J., and Lowell, A. M., *A Half Century's Progress against Tu-*

berculosis in New York City, 1900–1950 (New York Tuberculosis and Health Association, 1952).

17. Tocqueville, Alexis de, *Democracy in America,* vol. 2, trans. Henry Reeve, Esq., ed. Francis Bowen (Cambridge: Sever and Francis, 1862).

18. Jacobs, P. P., *The Control of Tuberculosis in the United States,* rev. ed. (New York: National Tuberculosis Association, 1940).

Knopf, S. A., *A History of the National Tuberculosis Association: The Antituberculosis Movement in the United States* (New York: National Tuberculosis Association, 1922).

Gunn, S. M., and Platt, P. S., *Voluntary Health Agencies* (New York: The Ronald Press, 1945).

19. Flick, L. F., *Development of Our Knowledge of Tuberculosis* (Philadelphia: privately printed, 1925).

20. Biggs, H. M., *The Administrative Control of Tuberculosis, in Henry Phipps Institute,* First Annual Report (Philadelphia: Henry Phipps Institute, 1905).

Craig, F. A., *Early Days at Phipps* (Philadelphia: Henry Phipps Institute, 1952).

21. Trudeau, E. L., *An Autobiography* (New York: National Tuberculosis Association, 1928).

22. Knopf, S. A., *Tuberculosis, A Disease of the Masses and How to Combat It,* first Am. ed. (New York, M. Firestack, 1901).

Charity Organization Society, *A Handbook on the Prevention of Tuberculosis,* First Annual Report of the Committee on the Prevention of Tuberculosis (New York: The Charity Organization Society, 1903).

23. Devine, E. T., *When Social Work Was Young* (New York: The Macmillan Co., 1939).

24. Brandt, L., *A Directory of Institutions and Societies Dealing with Tuberculosis in the United States and Canada* (New York: Charity Organization Society, 1904).

Paterson, R. G., "The evolution of official tuberculosis control in the United States," *Pub. Health Rep.,* 62:336–341 (1947).

25. Shryock, R. H., *National Tuberculosis Association, 1904–1954: A Study of the Voluntary Health Movement in the United States* (New York: National Tuberculosis Association, 1957).

26. *Transactions of the International Congress on Tuberculosis,* Washington, D.C., 1908 (Philadelphia: William F. Fell Co., 1908).

27. U.S. Public Health Service, "Public Health Service Act," *Pub. Health Rep.,* 59:916–919 (1944).

28. Blomquist, E. T., "The Tuberculosis Program of the U.S. Public Health Service," *NTA Bull.,* 47:9–11 (1961).

Blomquist, E. T., "Prospect of tuberculosis eradication," Tuberculosis Program, Communicable Disease Center, Public Health Service, *Pub. Health Rep.,* 78:507–509 (1963).

29. Drolet, G. J., "Epidemiology of tuberculosis," chap. 1 in *Clinical Tuberculosis,* vol. 1, ed. Benjamin Goldberg (Philadelphia: F. A. Davis Co., 1944).

30. Downing, T. K., Table of semicentennial mortality of the City of New York, compiled from the records of the City Inspectors Department, comprising the full period from Jan. 1, 1804, to Dec. 31, 1853, New York Public Library.

Hoffman, F. L., "The decline in the tuberculosis death rate, 1871–1912," *Transactions of the National Association for the Study and Prevention of Tuberculosis* (Philadelphia: William F. Fell Co., 1913).

Gray, C. E., "Tuberculosis mortality in the original death-registration states: A statistical study of the death rates from 1900 to 1924 and of the influence of certain factors upon them," *Am. Rev. Tuberc.*, 18:687–719 (1928).

Pearson, K., *The Fight against Tuberculosis and the Death Rate from Phthisis* (London: Dulan & Co., 1911).

31. Dubos, R., and Dubos, J., *The White Plague* (Boston: Little, Brown and Co., 1952).

Grigg, E. R. N., "The arcana of tuberculosis," *Am. Rev. Tuberc. Resp. Dis.*, 78:151–172, 426–453, 583–603 (1958).

Sigerist, H. E., *A History of Medicine*, vol. 1 (New York: Oxford University Press, 1951).

32. Edwards, P. Q., and Edwards, L. B., "Story of the tuberculin test—from an epidemiological viewpoint," *Am. Rev. Resp. Dis.*, 81:1–47 (1960).

Mantoux, C., *L'Intradermo-réaction à la tuberculine et son interprétation clinique* (Presse méd., 1910).

Seibert, F., "History of the development of purified protein derivative tuberculin," *Am. Rev. Tuberc.*, 44:1–8 (1941).

Whitney, J. S., and McCaffrey, I., "Summary of the results of group tuberculin testing with PPD in the United States," *Am. Rev. Tuberc.*, 35:597–608 (1937); "A statistical study: The results of group tuberculin-testing with M.A.-100," *Am. Rev. Tuberc.*, 33:78–90 (1936).

33. Frost, W. H., "Risk of persons in familial contact with pulmonary tuberculosis," *Am. J. Pub. Health*, 23:426–432 (1933).

Frost, W. H., "The age selection of mortality from tuberculosis in successive decades," *Am. J. Hyg.*, 30:91–96 (1939).

34. Myers, J. A., *Man's Greatest Victory over Tuberculosis* (Springfield: Charles C Thomas, 1940).

Myers, J. A., "Eighty years after the first glimpse of the tubercle bacillus," *Dis. Chest*, 51:500–521 (1967).

35. Smith, T., "Two varieties of the tubercle bacillus from mammals," *Tr. A. Am. Physicians*, 11:75 (1896); "A comparative study of bovine tubercle bacilli and of human bacilli from sputum," *J. Exper. Med.*, 3:451–511 (1898).

CHAPTER 2

1. Perkins, J. E., "Airborne infection and tuberculosis," *Arch. Environ. Health*, 16:738–743 (1968).

Riley, R. L., "The J. Burns Amberson Lecture: Aerial dissemination of pulmonary tuberculosis," *Am. Rev. Tuberc.*, 76:931–941 (1957).

"Conference on airborne infection," reprinted from *Bacteriological Reviews*, 25:173–377 (1961).

2. Rich, A., *Pathogenesis of Tuberculosis*, 2nd ed. (Springfield: Charles C Thomas, 1951).

Pinner, M., *Pulmonary Tuberculosis in the Adult* (Springfield: Charles C Thomas, 1945).

Amberson, J. B., "Evaluation of the present-day treatment of pulmonary tuberculosis," *An. Int. Med.*, 43:1209–1217 (1955).

Amberson, J. B., "A retrospect of tuberculosis," *Am. Rev. Resp. Dis.*, 93: 343–351 (1966).

Brown, L., *Story of Clinical Pulmonary Tuberculosis* (Baltimore: Williams and Wilkins Co., 1941).

Wallgren, A., "The time-table of tuberculosis," *Tubercle*, 29:245–251 (1948).

Cameron, V., and Long, E. R., *Tuberculosis medical research: National Tuberculosis Association, 1904–1955* (New York, 1959).

3. National Tuberculosis Association, *Diagnostic Standards and Classification of Tuberculosis* (New York, 1961); new edition, National Tuberculosis and Respiratory Disease Association (New York, 1969).

4. Wilson, J. L., "Curing and learning: 100 years of sanatoriums," the 1964 Baker Lecture, Michigan Tuberculosis and Respiratory Disease Association, 1964; Editorial, "Rise and decline of the tuberculosis sanatorium," *Am. Rev. Resp. Dis.,* 98:515–516 (1968).

U.S. Department of Health, Education, and Welfare, *Areawide Planning of Facilities for Tuberculosis Services,* Public Health Service Publication No. 930-B-4 (1963).

5. Alexander, J., *The Surgery of Pulmonary Tuberculosis* (Philadelphia and New York: Lea and Febiger, 1925).

Francis, R. S., and Curwen, M. P., "Major surgery for pulmonary tuberculosis: Final report," *Tubercle,* 35suppl.:1–69 (1964).

Medlar, E. M., "The behavior of pulmonary tuberculosis lesions: A pathological study," *Am. Rev. Tuberc.,* 71pt. 2:1–244 (1955).

6. Carson, J., *Essays, Physiological and Practical* (Liverpool: F. B. Wright, 1822).

7. Forlanini, C., "A contribuzione della terapia chirurgica della tisi ablazione del pulmone? Pneumotorace artificiale?" *Gazz. d. Osp. Clin.,* Agosto, Settembre–Ottobre–Novembre, 1882.

8. Murphy, J. B., "Surgery of the lung," *J. Am. Med. Assn.,* 31:151–165, 208–216, 281–297, 341–356 (1898).

9. Des Prez, R. M., and Muschenheim, C., "The chemoprophylaxis of tuberculosis," *J. Chr. Dis.,* 15:599–610 (1962).

10. U.S. Department of Health, Education, and Welfare, Public Health Service, *Laboratory Methods for Clinical and Public Health Mycobacteriology,* National Communicable Disease Center, Atlanta, Georgia, Public Health Service Publication No. 1547 (April 1967).

Middlebrook, G., and Cohn, M. L., "Bacteriology of tuberculosis: Laboratory methods," *Am. J. Pub. Health,* 48:844–853 (1958).

Russell, W. F., and Middlebrook, G., *Chemotherapy of Tuberculosis* (Springfield: Charles C Thomas, 1961).

Long, E. R., *The Chemistry and Chemotherapy of Tuberculosis,* 3rd ed. (Baltimore: Williams and Wilkins Co., 1958); see also "Tuberculosis," *Encyclopaedia Britannica,* 22:298–302 (1967 edition).

11. McDermott, W., "Chemotherapy of microbial diseases," in R. J. Dubos, ed. *Bacterial and Mycotic Infections of Man,* 3rd ed. (Philadelphia: J. B. Lippincott Co., 1958), pp. 694–726.

Hart, P. d'Arcy, "Chemotherapy of tuberculosis: Research during the past 100 years," *Brit. Med. J.,* 2:805, 849–855 (1946).

12. Waksman, S. A., *The Literature on Streptomycin, 1944–1952* (New Brunswick: Rutgers University Press, 1952).

Waksman, S. A., *The Conquest of Tuberculosis* (Berkeley and Los Angeles: University of California Press, 1964).

13. Hinshaw, H. C., and Feldman, W. H., "Streptomycin in treatment of clinical tuberculosis: A preliminary report," *Proc. Mayo Clin.,* 20 (1945).

14. Robitzek, E. H., Selikoff, I. J., and Ornstein, G. G., "Chemotherapy of human tuberculosis with hydrazine derivatives of isonicotinic acid" (preliminary report of representative cases), *Quart. Bull. Sea View Hospital,* 13:27–51 (1952).

Domagk, G., Behnisch, R., Mietzsch, F., and Schmidt, H., "On a new class of compounds effective in vitro against tubercle bacilli," *Die Naturwissenschaften,* 33:315 (1946), trans. Shenley Laboratories in *Am. Rev. Tuberc.,* 61:8–18 (1950).

15. Chaves, A. D., Dangler, G., Abeles, H., Robins, A. B., and Widelock, D., "The prevalence of drug-resistant strains of mycobacterium tuberculosis isolated from untreated patients in New York City during 1960," *Am. Rev. Resp. Dis.,* 84:647–656 (1961).

16. Anderson, R. J., Sauer, H. I., Smith, V., and Roberts, D. E., "The nonhospitalized tuberculosis patient: Program implications," *Pub. Health Rep.,* 71:888–896 (1956).

Blomquist, E. T., "The nonhospitalized tuberculosis patient," *Am. J. Pub. Health,* 46:149–155 (1956).

17. U.S. Department of Health, Education, and Welfare, *The Arden House Conference on Tuberculosis,* Tuberculosis Program, Communicable Disease Center, Public Health Service Publication No. 784 (reprinted 1961).

Blomquist, E. T., "Chemotherapy: A public health measure against tuberculosis," Tuberculosis Program, Communicable Disease Center, Public Health Service, *Pub. Health Rep.,* 75:1069–1076 (1960).

18. U.S. Department of Health, Education, and Welfare, Public Health Service, Tuberculosis Program, *Report of First Annual National Tuberculosis Conference,* National Communicable Disease Center, Atlanta, Georgia (1967).

19. U.S. Department of Health, Education, and Welfare, *Identification and Treatment of Tuberculous Infection: A Statement of the U.S. Public Health Service,* National Communicable Disease Center, Atlanta, Georgia (June 13, 1967).

U.S. Department of Health, Education, and Welfare, United States Public Health Service, Tuberculosis Program:

"Prophylactic effects of isoniazid on primary tuberculosis in children," by Ferebee, S. H., Mount, F. W., and Anastasiades, A. A., *Am. Rev. Resp. Dis.,* 76:942–963 (1957);

"Tuberculosis morbidity in a controlled trial of the prophylactic use of isoniazid among household contacts" by Ferebee, S. H., and Mount, F. W., *Am. Rev. Resp. Dis.,* 85:490–521 (1962);

"The effect of isoniazid prophylaxis in tuberculosis morbidity among household contacts of previously known cases of tuberculosis by Mount, F. W., and Ferebee, S. H., *Am. Rev. Resp. Dis.,* 85:821–827 (1962);

"A controlled trial of isoniazid prophylaxis in mental institutions" by Ferebee, S. H., Mount, F. W., Murray, F. J., and Livesay, V. T., *Am. Rev. Resp. Dis.,* 88:161–175 (1963);

"A controlled trial of community-wide isoniazid prophylaxis in Alaska" by Comstock, G. W., Ferebee, S. H., Hammes, L. M., *Am. Rev. Resp. Dis.,* 95:935–943 (1967).

20. U.S. Department of Health, Education, and Welfare, Public Health Service, *Public Health Service Recommendations on the Use of BCG Vaccination in the United States,* National Communicable Disease Center, Morbidity and Mortality Report, vol. 15 (Oct. 15, 1966).

21. Calmette, L. C. A., *Tubercle Bacillus Infection and Tuberculosis in Man and Animals* (Baltimore: Williams and Wilkins, 1933).

22. Aronson, J. D., and Aronson, C. F., "Appraisal of protective value of BCG vaccine," *J. Am. Med. Assn.,* 149:334–335 (1952).

23. Rosenthal, S. R., *BCG Vaccination against Tuberculosis* (Boston: Little, Brown and Co., 1957).

24. International Tuberculosis Campaign, Final Report, *Mass BCG Vaccination Campaigns* (Copenhagen, 1954).

25. Hilleboe, H. E., and Morgan, R. H., *Mass Radiography of the Chest* (Chicago, Ill.: The Year Book Publishers, Inc., 1945).

Blakeslee, A. L., *And the Spark Became a Flame: The Beginnings of Mass Chest X-rays* (New York: National Tuberculosis Association, 1954).

Edwards, H. R., "Tuberculosis case-finding: Studies in mass surveys," *Am. Rev. Tuberc.*, 41suppl.:1–159 (1940).

Blomquist, E. T., "Tuberculosis case-finding, 1961," Tuberculosis Program, Communicable Disease Center, Public Health Service, *Pub. Health Rep.*, 76:871–876 (1961).

26. U.S. Department of Health, Education, and Welfare, *Community-wide Chest X-ray Survey Data,* Public Health Service (April 1953); *Community-wide Chest X-ray Survey,* Public Health Service Publication No. 222 (Washington, D.C., 1952).

27. U.S. Department of Health, Education, and Welfare, Public Health Service, *Special Tuberculosis Projects, June 1967,* National Communicable Disease Center, Tuberculosis Program, Atlanta, Georgia (February 1968); *Tuberculosis —Program Reports, December 1967,* National Communicable Disease Center, Tuberculosis Program, Atlanta, Georgia (October 1968).

28. "Hospitals," Guide Issue, pt. 2, *Jour. Am. Hosp. Assn.* (Aug. 1, 1968).

29. U.S. Department of Health, Education, and Welfare, *Tuberculosis Beds in Hospitals and Sanatoria, June 30, 1967,* Tuberculosis Program, National Communicable Disease Center, Public Health Service Publication No. 801 (1968 edition, also earlier editions with data as of: Jan. 1, 1946, Jan. 1, 1947, Jan. 1, 1950, Jan. 1, 1951, Jan. 1, 1952, April 1, 1953, April 1, 1954, April 1, 1955, May 1, 1957, April 1, 1959, June 1, 1961, June 30, 1963, June 30, 1965).

Drolet, G. J., "Tuberculosis hospitalization," *Am. Rev. Tuberc.*, 14:1–25 (1926).

Whitney, J. S., *Tuberculosis Hospitalization in the United States* (New York: National Tuberculosis Association, 1933).

30. U.S. Department of Health, Education, and Welfare, Public Health Service, "Program analysis," Tuberculosis control programs, National Communicable Disease Center, Tuberculosis Program, Atlanta, Georgia (unpub. ms., May 1967).

CHAPTER 3

1. Russell Sage Foundation, *The Campaign against Tuberculosis in the United States,* Charities Publication Committee, compiled under the direction of the National Association for the Study and Prevention of Tuberculosis by Philip P. Jacobs (New York, 1908).

U.S. Department of Health, Education, and Welfare, *Manual of Procedures for National Morbidity Reporting and Surveillance of Communicable Disease, Effective January 1968,* National Communicable Disease Center, Public Health Service (March 1968).

2. U.S. Department of Health, Education, and Welfare, Public Health Service, *Tuberculin Testing in Special Tuberculosis Projects, Summary Tables, 1966–1967,* National Communicable Disease Center, Tuberculosis Program, Atlanta, Georgia (March 1968); *Tuberculosis—Program Reports, Tuberculin Testing during 1966–1967 School Year,* National Communicable Disease Center, Tuberculosis Program, Atlanta, Georgia (December 1968).

3. U.S. Department of Health, Education, and Welfare, *Public Health Service*

Recommendations on the Reporting of Tuberculosis—1961, Tuberculosis Program, Communicable Disease Center, Public Health Service (Washington, D.C. 1962).

4. U.S. Department of Health, Education, and Welfare, *Reported Tuberculosis Data—1967*, Tuberculosis Program, National Communicable Disease Center, Public Health Service Publication No. 638 (1969, also earlier editions with data for years 1952, 1953, 1954, 1955, 1956, 1957–58, 1959–60, 1961–62, 1963, 1964, 1965, 1966).

U.S. Department of Health, Education, and Welfare, *Tuberculosis Chart Series*, Tuberculosis Program, Communicable Disease Center, Public Health Service (1961, also earlier editions 1956, 1957, 1958, 1959, 1960, and new series, *A Graphic Presentation: Tuberculosis in the United States*, 1967 and 1968 editions).

5. Simpson, D. G., and Lowell, A. M., "Tuberculosis first registered at death," *Am. Rev. Resp. Dis.*, 89:165–174 (1964).

Simpson, D. G., "Tuberculosis first registered at death," *Am. Rev. Resp. Dis.*, 92:863–869 (1965).

6. Horwitz, O., *New Trends in Tuberculosis Research*, the Danish National Association for the Fight against Tuberculosis, Supplement to the Annual Report for the year 1965–66.

Groth-Petersen, E., Knudsen, J., and Wilbek, E., "Epidemiological basis of tuberculosis eradication in an advanced country," *Bull. WHO*, 21:5–49 (1959).

Horwitz, O., and Palmer, C. E., "Epidemiological basis of tuberculosis eradication: II, Dynamics of tuberculosis morbidity and mortality," *Bull. W H O*, 30:609–621 (1964).

CHAPTER 4

1. Spiegelman, M., *Significant Mortality and Morbidity Trends in the United States since 1900* (Bryn Mawr: American College of Life Underwriters, 1964).

Edwards, H. R., and Drolet, G. J., "The implications of changing morbidity and mortality rates from tuberculosis," *Am. Rev. Tuberc.*, 61:39–50 (1950).

Dublin, L. I., *A 40 Year Campaign against Tuberculosis* (New York: Metropolitan Life Insurance Co., 1952).

2. U.S. Department of Health, Education, and Welfare, *Vital Statistics of the United States*, 1955, Supplement: Mortality Data, Multiple Causes of Death, Public Health Service, National Center for Health Statistics (1965).

3. U.S. Department of Health, Education, and Welfare, *Death Rates by Age, Race, and Sex, United States, 1900–1953, Tuberculosis All Forms, Vital Statistics*—Special Reports, National Office of Vital Statistics, Public Health Service, 43 (April 4, 1956).

U.S. Department of Health, Education, and Welfare, Public Health Service, *Tuberculosis in the United States: Graphic Presentation*, vol. 1, *Mortality Statistics for State and Geographic Divisions by Age, Sex, and Race* (1943); vol. 2, *Proportionate Mortality Statistics for States and Geographic Divisions by Age, Sex, and Race* (1944); vol. 3, *Mortality Statistics for Large Cities by Age, Sex, and Race* (1945); vol. 4, *Mortality Statistics for Counties* (1946) (New York: Medical Research Committee, National Tuberculosis Association, 1943–1946).

U.S. Department of Health, Education, and Welfare, Vital Statistics Division, National Center for Health Statistics, related reports prepared by the National Office of Vital Statistics and the Bureau of the Census: *Mortality Statistics, Annual, 1900–1966; Vital Statistics of the United States, 1937–1962; Vital Statistics Rates in the United States, 1900–1940; Mortality Summaries,* Vital Statistics, Special Reports, vol. 16 (1944); *Age-Adjusted Death Rates in the United States, 1900–1940,* Vital Statistics, Special Reports, vol. 23, no. 1 (1945); *Mortality Summaries for the United States, 1941–1945,* Vital Statistics, Special Reports, vol. 27, nos. 14 to 51 (1948); *The Effect of the Sixth Revision of the International Lists of Diseases and Causes of Death upon Comparability of Mortality Trends,* Vital Statistics, Special Reports, vol. 36, no. 10 (1951).

U.S. Department of Health, Education, and Welfare, *Tuberculosis in 1963: An Overview,* Tuberculosis Branch, Communicable Disease Center, Public Health Service (1963).

U.S. Department of Health, Education, and Welfare, *Tuberculosis in the United States: Status of the Disease in the Early Sixties,* Tuberculosis Program, Communicable Disease Center, Public Health Service Publication No. 1036 (1963).

4. Drolet, G. J., and Lowell, A. M., "Tuberculosis mortality among children —The last stage," *Dis. Chest,* 42:364–371 (1962).

Lincoln, E. M., and Sewell, E. M., *Tuberculosis in Children* (New York: McGraw-Hill, Inc., 1962).

5. U.S. Department of Health, Education, and Welfare, *Final Table Specifications for Monographs on Vital and Health Statistics, 1959–1961,* Public Health Service, National Center for Health Statistics (April 1965).

American Public Health Association, Tabulations for Monographs on Vital and Health Statistics, 1959–1961, monograph no. 11, *Tuberculosis Mortality Tabulations, White and Nonwhite by Sex and Age.*

Table M.S. 1—Cause list, 038, 038.1, 038.2, 038.3, (Intl. list nos., 001–019, 001–008, 010–019, 011–018), U.S. totals, regions, and states.

Table M.S. 2—Cause list, 038, 038.1, 038.2, 038.3, (Intl. list nos., 001–019, 001–008, 010–019, 011–018), U.S. totals, regions, total metropolitan and non-metropolitan counties, total metropolitan counties, metropolitan with central city, metropolitan without central city, non-metropolitan counties.

Table M.S. 3—Cause list 038 (Intl. list nos. 001–019), U.S. totals, regions, all marital status, single, married, widowed, divorced, not stated.

Table M.S. 4—Cause list 038 (Intl. list nos. 001–019), U.S. totals, regions, white total, native, foreign born, not stated, and non-white.

Table 1, Part 1—Cause list 038 (Intl. list nos. 001–019), Economic subregions (121), U.S. totals, total metropolitan and non-metropolitan counties, total metropolitan counties, metropolitan counties with central city, metropolitan counties without central city, non-metropolitan counties.

Table 1, Part 2—Cause list 038 (Intl. list nos. 001, 019), Standard metropolitan statistical areas (201).

Table 5—Cause list 38.4 (Intl. list separately nos. 001 to 018), U.S. totals, divisions, consolidated age groups.

Spiegelman, M., *Introduction to Demography,* rev. ed. (Cambridge, Mass.: Harvard University Press, 1968).

6. Dublin, L. I., Lotka, A. J., and Spiegelman, M., *Length of Life, A Study of the Life Table* (New York: Ronald Press Co., 1949).

Dublin, L. I., and Lotka, A. J., *Twenty-five Years of Health Progress* (New York: Metropolitan Life Insurance Company, 1937).

Dublin, L. I., *Health Progress, 1936–1945* (New York: Metropolitan Life Insurance Company, 1948).

CHAPTER 5

1. Veiller, L., *Housing and Tuberculosis,* Transactions of the National Association for the Study and Prevention of Tuberculosis (1915).

Kraus, A. K., "Environmental factors in tuberculosis," *Am. Rev. Tuberc.,* 4:713–727 (1920).

Collins, S. D., *Economic Status and Health,* Public Health Bulletin 165, U.S. Public Health Service (Washington, D.C., 1926).

Green, H. W., *Tuberculosis and Economic Strata, Cleveland's Five-city Area, 1928–1931* (Cleveland: Anti-Tuberculosis League of Cleveland, 1932).

National Health Survey, 1935–1936, Preliminary Reports, Sickness and Medical Care Series, Bulletin 9, National Institutes of Health, Public Health Service (Washington, D.C., 1938).

Britten, R. H., "Illness and accidents among persons living under different housing conditions," *Pub. Health Rep.,* 56:609–640 (1941).

Allen, F. P., *People of the Shadows: Studies of Mortality in Cincinnati* (Cincinnati: Public Health Federation, 1954).

Pond, M. A., "Interrelationship of poverty and disease," *Pub. Health Rep.,* 76:967–974 (1961).

2. Dubos, R. J., "Biological and social aspects of tuberculosis," The Hermann M. Biggs lecture, *Bull. N.Y. Acad. Med.,* 27:351–369 (1951).

Wolff, G., "Tuberculosis mortality and industrialization: With special reference to the United States," *Am. Rev. Tuberc.,* 42:1–27, 214–242 (1940).

Selye, H., "Stress and disease," *Science,* 122:625–631 (1955); also *Annual Report on Stress* (Montreal, Canada: Aacta, Inc., 1951).

Guralnick, L., *Socio-economic Differences in Mortality by Cause of Death: United States, 1950, and England and Wales, 1949–53,* prepared for National Vital Statistics Division, Public Health Service (Washington, D.C., 1963).

3. Stockwell, E. G., "A critical examination of the relationship between socio-economic status and mortality," *Am. J. Pub. Health,* 53:956–964 (1963).

Anderson, R. J., Enterline, P. E., and Turner, O. D., "Undetected tuberculosis in various economic groups," *Am. Rev. Tuberc.,* 70:593–600 (1954).

Terris, M., and Monk, M. A., "The validity of socio-economic differentials in tuberculosis mortality," *Am. Rev. Resp. Dis.,* 81:513–517 (1960).

Terris, M., "Relation of economic status to tuberculosis mortality by age and sex," *Am. J. Pub. Health,* 38:1061–1070 (1960).

Yerushalmy, J., and Silverman, C., "Tuberculosis mortality in communities of different size," *Am. Rev. Tuberc.,* 51:413–431 (1945).

Guerrin, R. F., and Borgatta, E. F., "Socio-economic and demographic correlates of tuberculosis incidence," *Milbank Memorial Fund Quarterly,* 43:269–290 (1965).

4. Lowell, A. M., *Socio-economic conditions and tuberculosis prevalence, New York City* (New York: New York Tuberculosis and Health Association, 1956).

5. Morton, L. T., *Garrison and Morton's Medical Bibliography: An Annotated Check-list of Texts Illustrating the History of Medicine,* 2nd ed. (New York: Argosy, 1954).

Thackrah, C. T., *The Effect of the Principal Arts, Trades, and Professions, and of Civic States and Habits or Living on Health and Longevity* (London: Longman, Rees, Orme, Brown, Green, and Longman, 1832).

7. Robinson, D. E., and Wilson, J. G., *Tuberculosis among Industrial Work-*

ers, Public Health Bulletin No. 73, U.S. Public Health Service (Washington, D.C., 1916).

Warren, B. S., and Sydenstricker, E., "Health of garment workers," *Pub. Health Rep.*, 31:1298–1305 (1916).

Hoffman, F. L., *Mortality from Respiratory Diseases in Dusty Trades,* Bulletin U.S. Bureau of Labor Statistics, no. 231 (Washington, D.C., 1918).

Sydenstricker, E., *Health and Environment* (New York: McGraw-Hill, Inc., 1933).

8. Neil, C. P., and Perry, A. R., *Report on Conditions of Women and Child Wage-earners, in the United States,* U.S. Senate Document No. 645, 61st Congress, 2nd sess. (Washington, D.C., 1912).

9. Gardner, L. U., *Tuberculosis in Industry* (New York: National Tuberculosis Association, 1942).

Gardner, L. U., *Industry, Tuberculosis, Silicosis, and Compensation: A Symposium* (New York: National Tuberculosis Association, 1945).

Lanza, A. J., and Vane, R. J., "The prevalence of silicosis in the general population and its effects upon the incidence of tuberculosis," *Am. Rev. Tuberc.*, 29:8–16 (1934).

Moriyama, I. M., and Guralnick, L., *Occupational and Social Class Differences in Mortality,* Milbank Memorial Fund (New York, 1955).

10. Lincoln, E. M., "Epidemics of tuberculosis," *Advances in Tuberculosis Research* (Karger: Basel, Switzerland), 14:157–201 (1965).

Bryant, W. F., Hutcheson, R. H., and Dillon, A., "An epidemiologic investigation of tuberculosis in a Tennessee high school following discovery of a student case," *J. Tennessee Med. Assn.*, 57:41–44 (1964).

11. Dublin, L. I., and Vane, R. J., *Causes of Death by Occupation,* Bulletin U.S. Bureau of Labor Statistics, No. 507 (1930).

Dublin, L. I., *Causes of Death by Occupation,* Bulletin U.S. Bureau of Labor, No. 207 (1917).

12. Whitney, J. S., *Death Rates by Occupation* (New York: National Tuberculosis Association, 1934).

13. U.S. Department of Health, Education, and Welfare, *Mortality in 1950 by Occupation and Industry,* no. 1, *The Comparability of Reports on Occupation from Vital Records and the 1950 Census;* no. 2, *Mortality by Occupation and Industry among Men 20 to 64 Years of Age, United States, 1950;* no. 3, *Mortality by Occupation and Cause of Death among Men 20 to 64 Years of Age, United States, 1950;* no. 4, *Mortality by Industry and Cause of Death among Men 20 to 64 Years of Age, United States, 1950;* no. 5, *Mortality by Occupation Level and Cause of Death among Men 20 to 64 Years of Age, United States, 1950,* Vital Statistics, Special Reports, vol. 53, nos. 1–5, Vital Statistics Division, National Center for Health Statistics, Public Health Service.

14. Dominion Bureau of Statistics, *Special Report on Occupational Mortality in Canada, 1931–32.*

15. Kitagawa, E. M., and Hauser, P. M., "Educational differentials in mortality by cause of death, United States, 1960," *Demography,* vol. 5 (1968).

CHAPTER 6

1. [Argentina] *Epidemiologia de la tuberculosis en la Republica Argentina,* Poder Ejectivo Nacional, Ministerio de Asistencia Social y Salud Publica (Buenos Aires, 1961).

Baldo, J. I., "El problema de la tuberculosis en las Américas," *Boletín de la Oficina Sanitaria Panamericana,* pp. 37–65 (January 1965).

Blanco-Rodriguez, F., "Changes in the control of tuberculosis as a result of modern therapy," *Bull. Internat. Union against Tuberc.* (July–October 1954).

Bogen, E., "Tuberculosis in Australia," *Am. Rev. Tuberc.*, 57:155–161 (1948).

Boardman, D. W., "Tuberculosis among persons of Japanese ancestry in the United States," *Am. Rev. Tuberc.*, 54:227–238 (1946).

Btesh, S., "Tuberculosis in Israel," *Israel Medical Journal*, 17:245–252 (1958).

Buraczewski, O., and Juchniewicz, M., *Tuberculosis Control in Poland*, Ministry of Health and Social Welfare, Tuberculosis Institute (Warsaw: Polish State Medical Publishers, 1961).

Dominion Bureau of Statistics, *Tuberculosis Statistics*, vol. 1, *Tuberculosis Morbidity and Mortality, 1962* (Ottawa, Canada, 1965).

Drolet, G. J., and Lowell, A. M., "Whither tuberculosis? A statistical review of reports from selected American and European communities," *Dis. Chest*, 21:3–37 (1952).

Drolet, G. J., and Lowell, A. M., "Whereto tuberculosis? The first seven years of the antimicrobial era, 1947–1953," *Am. Rev. Tuberc.*, 72:419–452 (1955); "Qué pasa con la tuberculosis?" *Revista Española de Tuberculosis*, 25:73–88, 119–144 (Madrid, 1956).

Dunn, H. L., *Summary of International Vital Statistics, 1937–1944*, Vital Statistics Division, National Center for Health Statistics, Public Health Service (Washington, D.C., 1947).

[Finland] "Tuberculosis mortality in Finland," WHO Tuberculosis Research Office, *Bull. WHO* 12:211–246 (1955).

Härö, A. S., *TB-Statistics in Finland*, Eripainos Suomen Lääkärilehdestä–Finlands Läkartidning, 18 (1963).

Holm, J., *Final Report of the International Tuberculosis Campaign* (Copenhagen, Denmark, 1951).

[Korea] "Summary report on a national tuberculosis prevalence survey in Korea, June–November 1965," *WHO, TB, Techn. Information*, 67.57.

Kreuser, F., *Tuberkulose—Jahrbuch, 1963*, Deutsches Zentralkomitee zur Bekampfung der Tuberkulose (1965).

[Kuwait, State of] The Planning Board, Central Statistical Office, *Statistical Abstract*, p. 38, (1964).

Large, S. E., "Tuberculosis in the Gurkhas of Nepal," *Tubercle*, 45:321–336 (1964).

League of Nations, *Mortality from Tuberculosis*, Monthly Epidemiological Report, 147 and 148 (February–March 1931).

L'Eltore, G., "La mortalità tubercolare in Italia nel tempo," *Revista della tuberculosi e delle malattie dell'apparato respiratorio*, 13:338–392 (1965).

Lindhardt, M., *Tuberculosis Statistics: The Fight against Tuberculosis in Denmark*, Nat. Assn. against Tuberc. (Copenhagen, 1950).

Lotte, A., "Remarques à propos de l'épidémiologie de la tuberculose en France comparativement aux autres pays européens," *Gazette Médicale de France*, no. 10 (1963); "Mortalité par tuberculose en France," Situation actuelle: 1965 et 1966, et évolution depuis 1950 (et chiffres provisoires pour 1967 et partiels pour 1968, *Bulletin de l'Institut National de la Santé et de la Recherche Médicale*, 23 (1968).

Lowell, A. M., "A view of tuberculosis morbidity and mortality fifteen years after the advent of the chemotherapeutic era, 1947–1962," *Advances in Tuberculosis Research* (Karger: Basel, Switzerland), 15:55–124 (1966).

Lowell, A. M., *Tuberculosis in New York City, 1956: A City's Problem in a World-wide Epidemic*, New York Tuberculosis and Health Association (1957), pp. 92–106.

Lugosi, L., Nyárády, I., Csordás, I., Tusnádi, G., *Analyse statistique comparative de l'efficacité de la vaccination par le BCG en Hongrie entre 1959 et 1966*, Laboratoire du BCG, Institut d'Hygiène Publique, Services de Statistique, Institut National de Tuberculose "Korányi," (Budapest, 1967).

Machuca, R. V., "Factores que influyen en la epidemiologia de la tuberculosis en el Perú," *Revista Peruana de tuberculosis y enfermedades respiratorias* (January–December 1963); "Consideraciones epidemiológicas sobre el estado actual de la tuberculosis, mortalidad y morbilidad tuberculosa en el Perú, 1941–1952," *Revista Peruana de tuberculosis*, 14:3–79 (1954).

McDougall, J. B., *Tuberculosis: A Global Study in Social Pathology*, (Baltimore: The Williams & Wilkins Co., 1949).

Metzger, N. J., *Tuberculosis in Israel, 1962* (State of Israel, Ministry of Health, 1964).

Ministry of Health and Welfare, Japanese Government, *A Brief Report on Public Health Administration in Japan* (Tokyo, 1964).

Narain, D., *Tuberculosis Control in India* National Tuberculosis Institute (Bangalore, April 1965).

[Norway] *Official Publications of Statistisk Sentralbyra*, Oslo.

Okada, H., *et. al., Global Epidemiology of Tuberculosis*, Department of Preventive Medicine, Nagoya University School of Medicine (Nagoya, April 1967).

Pastor, J. R., and Janer, J. L., "Tuberculosis in the Island of Puerto Rico," *Am. Rev. Tuberc.*, 67:132–153 (1953); Pastor, J. R., "Problems in pulmonary tuberculosis," *Dis. Chest*, 51:422–426 (1967).

Payne, H. M., "The problem of tuberculosis control among American Negroes," *Am. Rev. Tuberc.*, 60:332–342 (1949).

Prasad, B. G., "Pulmonary tuberculosis in India," *Brit. J. Dis. Chest*, 55:169–184 (1961).

[Puerto Rico, Department of Health] *Annual Vital Statistics Report* (San Juan, 1964).

Puffer, R. R., and Griffith, G. W., *Patterns of Urban Mortality*, Scientific Publication no. 151, Pan American Health Organization, World Health Organization (Washington, D.C., September 1967).

Rakower, J., "Tuberculosis among Jews," *Am. Rev. Tuberc.*, 67:85–93 (1953).

Shimao, T., *Analysis on the Factors Contributed to the Reduction of Tuberculosis in Japan in the Recent Years* (Japan Anti-Tuberculosis Association, Tokyo, 1966).

Sigurdsson, S., and Edwards, P. Q., "Tuberculosis morbidity and mortality in Iceland," *Bull. WHO*, no. 7, 1952.

[Sweden] *Official publications of Statistiska Centralbyran*, Stockholm.

[Taiwan Provincial Health Administration] *Annual Report 1961*, Taiwan Tuberculosis Control Program (Taipei, Taiwan).

Townsend, J. G., Aronson, J. D., Saylor, R., and Parr, I., "Tuberculosis control among the North American Indians," *Am. Rev. Tuberc.*, 45:41–52 (1942).

[Vietnam, Health Data Publications] *The Republic of Viet-Nam, South Viet-Nam*, no. 5, revised (January 1966), p. 30; *Democratic Republic of Viet-Nam, North Viet-Nam*, no. 25, revised (October 1966), p. 20, Walter Reed Army Institute of Research. Walter Reed Army Medical Center (Washington, D.C., 1966).

Wolff, G., "Tuberculosis and civilization," *Human Biology*, 10:106–123, 251–284 (1938).

World Health Organization, *Reported Cases of Notifiable Diseases*, Scientific Publication no. 58 (1959–1960), no. 86 (1961), no. 102 (1962), no. 114 (1963), no. 135 (1964), no. 149 (1965), Pan Amer. San. Bureau (Washington, D.C.).

World Health Organization Tuberculosis Research Office, "Tuberculosis mortality in Finland," *Bull. WHO*, 12:211–246 (1955). (See also official publications of Statistiska Centralbyran, Helsinki, Finland.)

World Health Organization, official publications of WHO, *Annual Epidemiological and Vital Statistics*, Epidemiological and Vital Statistics Report (monthly since 1948).

Yelton, S. E., "Tuberculosis throughout the world: The pre-war distribution of tuberculosis throughout the world," *Pub. Health Rep.*, 61:1144–1160 (1946).

Zaki, M. H., "On the epidemiology of tuberculosis in some selected countries: Highlights and prospects for control and eradication," pt. 1, *Am. J. Pub. Health*, 58:1692–1712 (1968).

CHAPTER 7

1. Department of Health, Education, and Welfare, Public Health Service, *Report of the Ad Hoc Advisory Committee on Surveillance Reporting of Tuberculosis*, Second Annual National Tuberculosis Conference, April 3–4, 1968, National Communicable Disease Center (Atlanta, Georgia, 1968).

Additional References / I

Amberson, J. B., "Symposium on Tuberculosis," *Am. J. Med.*, 9:571–677 (1950).

Armstrong, D. B., Framingham Monograph no. 10, *Final summary report, 1917–1923*, National Tuberculosis Association (Framingham, Mass., 1924).

Aronson, J. D., and Palmer, C. E., "Experience with BCG vaccine in the control of tuberculosis among North American Indians," *Pub. Health Rep.*, 61:802–820 (1946).

Billings, J. S., *Vital Statistics of New York City and Brooklyn, Six years ending May 31, 1890*, Census Office, Department of the Interior (Washington, D.C., 1894).

Bowditch, H. I., "Consumption in America," *Atlantic Monthly*, 23:51–61, 177–187, 315–323 (1869).

Brailey, M. E., "A study of tuberculosis infection and mortality in the children of tuberculous households," *Am. J. Hyg.*, 31:1–43 (1940).

Brownlee, J., *An Investigation into the Epidemiology of Phthisis in Great Britain and Ireland*, Medical Research Committee (London, 1918).

Bushnell, G. E., *Epidemiology of Tuberculosis* (New York: William Wood and Co., 1922).

Chadwick, H. D., and Pope, A. S., *The Modern Attack on Tuberculosis*, The Commonwealth Fund (New York, 1946).

Chaillé, S. E., "The American Mountain Sanitarium for Consumption, at Asheville, N.C.," *New Orleans, Med. and Surg., J.* (April 1878).

City of New York, *Cost Analysis*, Department of Hospitals, Bureau of Business Administration, Division of Audits and Accounts, Year Ended December 31, 1967.

Comstock, G. W., and Sartwell, P. E., "Tuberculosis studies in Muscogee County, Georgia," *Am. J. Hyg.*, 61:261–285 (1955).

Comstock, G. W., "Untreated inactive pulmonary tuberculosis, risk of reactivation," *Pub. Health Rep.*, 77:461–470 (1962).

Comstock, G. W., "Community research in tuberculosis, Muscogee County, Georgia," *Pub. Health Rep.*, 79:1045–1056 (1964).

Comstock, G. W., and Palmer, C. E., "Long-term results of BCG vaccination in the southern United States," *Am. Rev. Resp. Dis.*, 93:171–183 (1966).

Corper, H. J., "Founders of our knowledge of tuberculosis," *Hygeia, The Health Magazine* (October–November 1929).

De Abreu, M., and De Paula, A., *Roentgenfotografia* (Rio de Janeiro: Livraria Ateneu, 1940).

Dressler, S. H., "The changing focus in tuberculosis control," *Med. Times* (July 1965).

Excerpta Medica: Section 15, *Tuberculosis*, vols. 1–8; *Chest Diseases*, vols. 8–17; Section 17, *Public Health, Social Medicine and Hygiene*, vols. 1–10 (Amsterdam: Medica Foundation).

Ferebee, S. H., "An epidemiological model of tuberculosis in the United States," *NTA Bull.*, 53:4–7 (1967).

Grigg, E. R. N., "Historical and bibliographical review of tuberculosis in the mentally ill," *J. Hist. Med. and Allied Sci.*, 10:58–108 (1955).

Hill, A. B., *Statistical Methods in Clinical and Preventive Medicine,* chaps. 12 and 13 (Edinburgh and London: E. & S. Livingstone, Ltd., 1962).

Holguin, A. H., "The vast potential for prevention of tuberculosis," *NTA Bull.,* 52:4–6 (1966).

Holguin, A. H., "The child-centered program to prevent tuberculosis," *NTA Bull.,* 50:4–7 (1966).

Lawson, L. M., *Practical Treatise on Phthisis Pulmonalis* (Cincinnati, 1861).

Lumsden, L. L., and Dearing, W. P., "Epidemiological studies of tuberculosis," *Am. J. Pub. Health,* 30:219–228 (1940).

Lurie, M. B., "Heredity, constitution and tuberculosis: An experimental study," *Am. Rev. Tuberc.,* 44 suppl.: 1–125 (1941).

Magnus, K., *Epidemiological Studies of Bovine Tuberculous Infection in Man,* from the Danish Tuberculosis Index, Universitetsforlaget (Oslo, 1968).

Massachusetts Tuberculosis and Health League, *A Century of Tuberculosis Control in Massachusetts* (Boston, 1951).

Moorman, L. J., *Tuberculosis and Genius* (Chicago: University of Chicago Press, 1940).

Moorman, L. J., *American Sanatorium Association: A Brief Historical Sketch,* National Tuberculosis Association (1947).

Morton, S. G., *Illustrations of Pulmonary Consumption* (Philadelphia: Key and Biddle, 1834).

Pearson, K., *Heredity and environment* (London: Cambridge University Press, 1912).

Public Health Service, "Tuberculosis Control Issues," nos. 1–70, extracts from *Pub. Health Rep.,* 61–66 (1946–1951).

Puffer, R. R., *Familial Susceptibility to Tuberculosis* (Cambridge, Mass.: Harvard University Press, 1944).

Ramazzini, Bernardino, *De morbis artificum diatriba.* (Mutinae, A. Capponi, 1700, first systematic treatise on occupational diseases, translated into English in 1705, and new translations with notes by Wilmer Cave Wright, University of Chicago Press, 1940).

Röntgen, W. C., *Üeber eine neue Art von Strahlen, Sitzungsberichte der physikalisch-medicinische gesellschaft* (Wurzburg, 1895); See also Glasser, O., *Dr. W. C. Röntgen,* (Springfield: Charles C Thomas, 1945).

Rosen, G., *History of Miner's Diseases: A Medical and Social Interpretation* (New York: Shuman, 1943).

Shryock, R., *The Development of Modern Medicine* (New York: Knopf, 1947).

Society of Actuaries, "Mortality trends and projections," *Transactions of the Society of Actuaries,* 19:D428–D493 (1967).

Soper, F. L., "Problems to be solved if eradication of tuberculosis is to be realized," *Am. J. Pub. Health,* 52:734–748 (1962).

Spiegelman, M., "Segmented Generation Mortality," Population Association of America, Annual Meeting, mimeo., Boston, April 18–20, 1968.

U.S. Department of Health, Education, and Welfare, *List of Available Tuberculosis Literature,* Tuberculosis Program, National Communicable Disease Center, Public Health Service (Atlanta, Georgia, 1968).

U.S. Department of Health, Education, and Welfare, *Illness among Indians: Reported Incidence of Notifiable Diseases among Indians and Alaska Natives, 1962,* Public Health Service, Division of Indian Health, 1963.

U.S. Department of the Navy, "Tuberculosis control in the United States Navy: 1875–1966," *Arch. Environ. Health,* 16:4–50 (1968).

Venezian, E. C., *Quantitative Planning Tools for Tuberculosis Control and Eradication,* interim report to Seton Hall College of Medicine and Dentistry (Cambridge, Mass.: Arthur D. Little, Inc., April 1964).

Waring, J. J., The history of artificial pneumothorax in America," *J. Outdoor Life,* September, October, November, December, 1933, January 1934.

Webb, G. B., *René Théophile Hyacinth Laënnec* (New York: P. B. Hoeber, 1928).

World Health Organization, Tuberculosis Program, Public Health Service, U.S.A., "Experimental studies of vaccination, allergy, and immunity in tuberculosis," *Bull WHO,* 12:13–62 (1955).

Zeidberg, L. D., Gass, R. S., Dillon, A., and Hutcheson, R. H., "The Williamson County Tuberculosis Study, A Twenty-four Year Epidemiological Study," *Am. Rev. Resp. Dis.,* 87 pt. 2:1–88 (1963).

References / II

PREFACE
1. Palmer, C. E., Ferebee, S. H., and Peterson, O. S., "Studies of pulmonary findings and antigen sensitivity among student nurses. VI Geographic differences in sensitivity to tuberculin as evidence of nonspecific allergy," *Pub. Health Rep.,* 65:1111–1131 (1950).

Edwards, L. B., and Palmer, C. E., "Georgraphic variations in naturally acquired tuberculin sensitivity," *The Lancet,* 1:53–57 (1953).

Edwards, L. B., Edwards, P. Q., and Palmer, C. E., "Sources of tuberculin sensitivity in human populations. A summing up of recent epidemiologic research," *Act. Tuberc. Scand.,* 47 (suppl.):77–97 (1959).

CHAPTER 1
1. Seibert, F. B., and Glenn, J. T., "Tuberculin purified protein derivative: Preparation and analysis of a large quantity for standard," *Am. Rev. Tuberc.,* 44:9–25 (1941).

2. *WHO Expert Committee on Biologic Standardization,* Fifth Report. World Health Organ., Technical Report Series, 56:6–7 (1952).

3. Shaw, L. W., Howell, A., Jr., and Weiss, E. S., "Biological assay of lots of histoplasmin and the selection of a new working lot," *Pub. Health Rep.* 65:583–609 (1950).

4. Affronti, L. F., "Purified protein derivatives (PPD) and other antigens prepared from atypical acid-fast bacilli and *Nocardia asteroides,*" *Am. Rev. Tuberc. Pulm. Dis.,* 79:284–295 (1959).

5. Seibert, F. B., and DuFour, E. H., "Comparison between the international standard tuberculins, PPD-S and old tuberculin," *Am. Rev. Tuberc.,* 69:585–594 (1954).

6. Edwards, L. B., Cross, F. W., and Hopwood, L., "Effect of duration of storage on the potency of dilutions of PPD antigens," *Tubercle,* 44:153–161 (1963).

CHAPTER 2
1. Palmer, C. E., Krohn, E. F., Manos, N. E., and Edwards, L. B., "Tuberculin sensitivity of young adults in the United States," *Pub. Health Rep.,* 71:633–645 (1956).

2. U.S. Bureau of the Census, *U.S. Census of Population: 1960. Selected Area Reports. State Economic Areas, Final Report PC (3)-1A,* Washington, D.C.: U.S. Government Printing Office (1963).

3. Mollohan, C. S., and Romer, M. S., "Public health significance of swimming pool granuloma," *Am. J. Pub. Health,* 51:883–891 (1961).

Schaefer, W. B., and Davis, C. L., "A bacteriologic and histopathologic study of skin granuloma due to *Mycobacterium balnei,*" *Am. Rev. Resp. Dis.,* 84:837–844 (1961).

Palmer, C. E., and Edwards, L. B., "Geographic variations in the prevalence of sensitivity to tuberculin (PPD-S) and to the battey antigen (PPD-B) throughout the United States," *Bull. Int. Union against Tuberc.,* 32:373–383 (1962).

4. U.S. Bureau of the Census, *U.S. Census of Population: 1960. Number of Inhabitants, United States Summary, Final Report PC (1)-1A,* Washington, D.C.: U.S. Government Printing Office (1961).

5. Comstock, G. W., and Palmer, C. E., "Long-term results of BCG vaccination in the southern United States," *Am. Rev. Resp. Dis.,* 93:171–183 (1966).

6. Edwards, L. B., "Current status of the tuberculin test," *Ann. N.Y. Acad. Sci.,* 106:32–42 (1963).

7. Palmer, C. E., "Tuberculin sensitivity and contact with tuberculosis: Further evidence of nonspecific sensitivity," *Am. Rev. Tuberc.,* 68: 678–694 (1953).

8. WHO/UNICEF BCG Vaccination Programme, *Quarterly Summary Report, Third Quarter, 1965,* Geneva: World Health Organization (1966).

CHAPTER 3

1. Edwards, L. B., and Smith, D. T., "Community-wide tuberculin testing study in Pamlico County, North Carolina," *Am. Rev. Resp. Dis.,* 92:43–54 (1965).

2. Magnus, K., "Epidemiological basis of tuberculosis eradication: Risk of pulmonary tuberculosis after human and bovine infection," *Bull. WHO,* 35:483–508 (1966).

3. U.S. Bureau of the Census, *U.S. Census of Population: 1960, vol. 1, Characteristics of the Population,* pts. 23, 25, 35, Washington, D.C.: U.S. Government Printing Office (1963).

4. Groth-Peterson, E., Knudson, J., and Wilbek, E., "Epidemiological basis of tuberculosis eradication in an advanced country," *Bull. WHO,* 21:5–49 (1959).

Palmer, C. E., Shaw, L. W., and Comstock, G. W., "Community trials of BCG vaccination," *Am. Rev. Tuberc. Pulm. Dis.,* 77:877–907 (1958).

Frimodt-Moller, J., Thomas, J., and Parthasarathy, R., "Observations on the protective effect of BCG vaccination on a South India rural population," *Bull. WHO,* 30:545–574 (1964).

5. Comstock, G. W., "Isoniazid prophylaxis in an undeveloped area," *Am. Rev. Resp. Dis.,* 86:810–822 (1962).

Ferebee, S. H., and Mount, F. W., "Tuberculosis morbidity in a controlled trial of the prophylactic use of isoniazid among household contacts," *Am. Rev. Resp. Dis.,* 85:490–521 (1962).

Index

Abeles, Hans, 209

Adirondack Cottage Sanitarium (Sanatorium; *1884*), 11, 12, 32

Administrative control, development of tuberculosis programs: governmental, 13; pioneer, 9; voluntary, 12

Admissions to tuberculosis hospitals, 34. *See also* Hospitals

Adults: tested in community surveys, 168-175, 179

Africa, cases, deaths, and rates, 98

Age: of recruits, 126; of student nurses *1943–1949*, 162; and tuberculin sensitivity, 167-175

Agricola, Georgius, 87

Airborne transmission, 22

Alcoholism among patients, 25, 26

Alexander, John, 208

Allen, Floyd P., 213

Amberson, J. Burns, 207, 218

American Thoracic Society, 22

Anastasiades, A. A., 209

Ancient evidence of disease, 5; Egyptian and Nubian remains, 5

Anderson, Robert J., 209, 213

Antigens: dosage, 130, 131; histoplasmin, 131; PPD-B, 130, 131, 132; PPD-S tuberculin, 130, 131; preparation, 130, 131; protein content, 130, 131

Antigua: cases and case rates, 95; deaths and death rate, 96

Anti-tuberculosis drugs, *see* Chemotherapy; Chemoprophylaxis; Treatment

Arden House Conference (*1959*), 26

Argentina, cases and case rates, 95

Armstrong, Donald B., 218

Aronson, Charlotte F., 209

Aronson, Joseph D., 28, 209, 216, 218

Asia, cases, deaths, and rates, 98

Athens, Greece, death rate (*1935*), 9

Atypical microorganisms, 16

Auenbrugger, Leopold, 5

Australia: cases and case rates, 98; deaths and death rates, 98

Austria, deaths and death rates, 100

Average daily census in tuberculosis hospitals, 34

Bacillus Calmette Guérin (BCG), 28

Bahama Islands: cases and case rates, 95; deaths and death rate, 96

Bailey, Mary V., 36

Baldo, Jose Ignacio, 214

Baltimore, Md., death rate (*1821–1830*), 7

Bantu, cases and case rates, 98

Barbados: cases and case rates, 95; deaths and death rate, 96

Battey antigen (PPD-B), 130, 131, 132

BCG vaccination, 28, 163-166; trials in Georgia, 146; U.S. Public Health Service recommendations, 28

BCG vaccine, 28

Bedrest, 23

Beds, hospital, 31. *See also* Hospitals

Behnisch, Robert, 209

Belgium: cases and case rates, 99; deaths and death rates, 100

Berlin Phthisiological Society, 6

Bermuda: cases and case rates, 95; deaths and death rate, 96

Biggs, Hermann M., 9, 10, 12, 206

Billings, John S., 9, 218

Biological attrition, 18

Bissell, Emily P., 12

Blake, James, 32

Blakeslee, Alton L., 210

Blanco-Rodriguez, F., 215

Blomquist, Edward T., 206, 209, 210

Boardman, Donnell W., 215

Bogen, Emil, 215

Bolivia, cases and case rates, 95

Borgatta, Edgar F., 213

Boston, Mass., death rates (*1810–1820*), 7

Bovine tuberculin testing, U.S., 20, 21; in accredited areas, 20

Bovine tuberculosis, 171; economic loss, 20; eradication in cattle, 20; eradication in other mammals, 21

Bowditch, Henry I., 218

Bowditch, Vincent Y., 32

Brailey, Miriam E., 218

Brandt, Lilian, 206

Brazil, cases and case rates, 95

British Guiana: cases and case rates, 95; deaths and death rate, 96

British Honduras: cases and case rates, 95; deaths and death rate, 96

Britten, Rollo H., 213

Brooklyn Home for Consumptives (*1881*), 32

Brothwell, Don R., 205

Brown, Lawrason, 207

Brownlee, John, 218

Bryant, Joseph D., 10

Bryant, William F., 214

Btesh, S., 215

Budapest, Hungary, death rate (*1919*), 9

Bulgaria, deaths and death rates, 100

Bunyan, John, 6

Buraczewski, O., 215

Burke, Richard M., 205

Bushnell, George E., 218

Calmette, Leon Charles Albert, 28, 209